Vital Notes for Nurses:
Health Assessment

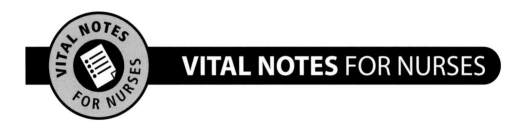

VITAL NOTES FOR NURSES

Health Assessment

Edited By

Anna T Crouch

RGN, RMN, SCM, TCPC, ADM, CertEd,
BA (Midwifery Studies),
Ed Couns Skills Cert, MA (Ed) Open, ILM Cert
Senior Lecturer
The University Of Northampton

Clency Meurier

RGN, RMN, DipN, CertEd, FETC Cert, BEd (Hons), MSc, PhD,
Research Degree Supervision Cert
Senior Lecturer
The University Of Northampton

Blackwell
Publishing

© 2005 by Blackwell Publishing Ltd

Editorial offices:
Blackwell Publishing Ltd, 9600 Garsington Road, Oxford OX4 2DQ, UK
    Tel: +44 (0)1865 776868
Blackwell Publishing Inc., 350 Main Street, Malden, MA 02148-5020, USA
    Tel: +1 781 388 8250
Blackwell Publishing Asia Pty Ltd, 550 Swanston Street, Carlton, Victoria
3053, Australia
    Tel: +61 (0)3 8359 1011

First published 2005 by Blackwell Publishing Ltd

ISBN-10: 1-4051-1458-4
ISBN-13: 978-1-4051-1458-5

Library of Congress Catalogining-in-Publication Data

Vital notes for nurses : health assessment / edited by Anna T. Crouch,
Clency Meurier.
    p. ; cm.
  Includes bibliographical references and index.
  ISBN-13: 978-1-4051-1458-5 (alk. paper)
  ISBN-10: 1-4051-1458-4 (alk. paper)
  1. Nursing assessment.   2. Holistic nursing.
  [DNLM: 1. Nursing Assessment.   2. Holistic Nursing. WY 100.4 V836
2005]   I. Title: Health assessment.   II. Crouch, Anna T.   III. Meurier,
Clency.
RT48.V58   2005
616.07′5–dc22

                                                                        2005013099

A catalogue record for this title is available from the British Library

Set in 10/12 pt Palatino
by SNP Best-set Typesetter Ltd., Hong Kong
Printed and bound in Great Britain
by TJ International Ltd, Padstow, Cornwall

For further information on Blackwell Publishing, visit our website:
www.blackwellnursing.com

Contents

Preface

The healthcare climate has been undergoing rapid changes, with renewed emphasis on holistic assessment and evidence-based care of clients and patients. There is also the broadening of the scope of practice for nurses, professional academic awards and professional standing for nurses. Nurses are also accountable for their practice and must be able to apply theory to practise safely and effectively. Hence, the knowledge and skills underpinning holistic health assessment to practise effectively to ensure protection of the public are of vital importance. Crucial to this will be the nurse's ability to assess patients and clients holistically in a variety of settings, to identify their needs, plan and deliver evidence-based and holistic healthcare. Programmes for the education and preparation of nurses should therefore foster an enquiring approach to care. They should also encourage progressive development and the use of appropriate analytical, critical and problem-solving skills. It is important to provide opportunities for nursing students to gain the theoretical knowledge which informs the assessment of patients and clients, enabling them to become competent nurses, able to work safely, confidently and flexibly within a multidisciplinary team setting.

Most current books on health assessment in nursing tend to focus on detailed physical assessment of the client with little or no emphasis on a holistic approach. They are also based on American rather than on generic models of assessment. Moreover, there is little focus on the fundamental knowledge informing health assessment. The intention of this book is to fill such gaps.

This book will therefore be of particular relevance for undergraduate nursing students in foundation programmes both nationally and internationally. It will also be useful to return-to-nursing students and already qualified staff would find it a helpful teaching tool.

Anna Crouch and Clency Meurier

Acknowledgements

Special thanks to Blackwell Publishing for permission to use figures from Bray *et al.* (1999), Mallet and Dougherty (2000), Ellis (2002) and Cox (2004), as acknowledged within the text. Thanks also to Heinemann Professional Publishing for permission to use Figure 9.1 from Burnard (1990). Thanks to RCN Publishing Company Ltd and the World Health Organisation for giving us permission to adapt and use some of their material and information. Special thanks also to Beth Knight, Lisa Whittington and Amy Brown for their guidance and support.

We also wish to express thanks to Doreen Addicott HND Computing, Cert Ed, BTEC, for all the advice and help she gave in relation to the management of large documents to Gehric Barreau (IT Services), and to Ann Turner T.Dip COT, NA, FCOT (Principal Lecturer OT) for her advice and encouragement.

Special thanks to Sue Allen (Dean, School of Health) for her encouragement and support and to the following students, working colleagues and clinical staff for their comments and suggestions: Claire Barton (Student Nurse), Celina Mfukuo (Student Nurse), Evelyn Osei-Twum (Student Nurse, London South Bank University), Roberta Blankson (BSc Hons Nursing, Postregistration Student Nurse), A Salat (Student Nurse), Angela Hicks (RN, Dip HE, Clinician), Gloria Price (SRN SCM, Clinician), Julie Quilter (SRN, RM, ADM, CertEd, BSc, MA, Senior Lecturer), C Ager (SRN, SCM, DN, MTD, BSc Hons, MA, Principal Lecturer), David Bird (RGN, Adv Cert (HE), Burns & Plastic Nursing (ENB), BSc Hons (Human Biology), MSc, Senior Lecturer), Linda Lilley (RGN, RNT, DMS, FETC, BEd, Senior Lecturer), Penny Paradine (support staff).

Thanks also to A Crouch for the following line drawings: Figures 1.1, 1.3a, 1.4, 1.15b, 1.16a, 2.1, 3.1, 3.2, 5.1, 5.2, 6.13, 6.14, 6.15, 6.16, 6.17, 6.18, 6.19, 6.20, 8.1, 8.2. Thanks also to J Aldridge for Figure 8.3.

Last but not least, thanks to Ian and Peter for their patience and support when needed, and to our Lord Jesus who made the writing of this book possible.

Anna Crouch and Clency Meurier

Dedication

I would like to dedicate this book to the Lord Jesus.

Anna Crouch

I would like to dedicate the book to Marnie,
Christopher and Annabel

Clency Meurier

List of contributors

John Aldridge RMN, RMNH, CertEd, MA
Senior Lecturer, The University Of Northampton

Sue Allen SRN, SCM, DipNurs, DipNursEd, RNT, MSc
Dean, School of Health, The University Of Northampton

Janis Brown RGN, Clin Teaching Cert, CertEd, BSc (Hons) Open, MSc (Science) Open
Senior Lecturer, The University Of Northampton

Anna T Crouch RGN, RMN, SCM, TCPC, ADM, CertEd, BA (Midwifery Studies), Ed Couns Skills Cert, MA (Ed) Open, ILM Cert
Senior Lecturer, The University Of Northampton

Adelaide Eshun RGN, Cert HSM, BSc (Hons) (Health Sc)
Lecturer, The University Of Northampton

Moira Ingham RGN, RNT, MA (Hons) (English & History), MSc (Nursing)
Associate Dean, The University Of Northampton

Clency Meurier RGN, RMN, DipNurs, CertEd, FETC Cert, BEd (Hons), MSc, PhD, Research Degree Supervision Cert
Senior Lecturer, The University Of Northampton

Stephen O'Brien RGN, RMN, RCNT, BEd (Hons), MSc
Principal Lecturer, The University Of Northampton

James O'Reilly BSc, MSc, PhD
Senior Lecturer in Human Nutrition, University College of Chester

Jackie H Parkes RMN, BA (Hons), MMedSci, PGDip
Principal Lecturer, The University Of Northampton

Graham Rumbold RGN, RNT, CHNT, NDN, BA, MSc
Senior Lecturer, The University Of Northampton

Michelle Thompson SRN, RNT, CertEd, FETC, BSc, MSc
Principal Lecturer, The University Of Northampton

Wendy Turner RN (LD), RNDip HE Child, ENB 998, PG CertEd, BA
(Hons) Evidence Based Practice
Senior Lecturer, The University Of Northampton

The human body

C Meurier

Learning objectives

- Use appropriate anatomical terminologies to describe the location of the different organs of the body.
- Discuss the relationship between cells, tissues, organs and systems in relation to the whole organism.
- List the components of each body system and explain how they contribute to the function of the system.
- Discuss how the different parts and systems of the body work together to maintain homeostasis.

Section 1: Introduction

Whether a health assessment is being performed to identify a health problem or to evaluate risk factors for health education purposes, a good understanding of biological knowledge is important (Carroll, 2004). Familiarisation with the common terminologies used for the different structures of the body, for example, enables effective communication of assessment findings to colleagues and other health professionals. Disease states and their impact can only be fully appreciated against the background of normal body structure and functions. In this chapter, the body will be looked at in a systematic way, starting from an examination of its basic organisation and the maintenance of internal stability to looking at individual organ systems.

1

Anatomical terms

To begin with, it is useful to provide an orientation of the body – looking at body regions, directional terms to describe one body part relative to another, and spaces and cavities that contain the different internal organs. This will facilitate precise and concise reporting of the assessment of the body. By using the exact anatomical term to describe the area of complaint of a particular symptom, attention can be focused more quickly to that specific area (Thibodeau & Patton, 2004).

Body regions

The body is conventionally divided into two major regions:

- *Axial.* This consists of the head, face, neck and trunk or torso.
- *Appendicular.* This consists of the shoulder girdles, the upper limbs, pelvic girdles and lower limbs.

Directional terms

Directional terms are used to locate body structures. They are usually grouped in opposite pairs, e.g. superior/inferior, anterior/posterior. Directional terms only make sense when they are used to describe one structure relative to another. We refer, for example, to the elbow being superior to the wrist although they are both located in the superior aspect of the body. Directional terms are shown in Table 1.1.

Body cavities

The internal organs are located within spaces in the body called cavities. There are two main cavities: dorsal and ventral. The *dorsal cavity*, situated near the dorsal surface of the body, contains the brain in the cranial cavity and the spinal cord in the vertebral canal. The *ventral cavity*, located near the anterior part of the body, can be further divided into three cavities, namely thoracic, abdominal and pelvic. The diaphragm separates the thoracic cavity from the abdominal cavity. The largest organs in the thoracic cavity are the lungs. The heart is embedded in the mediastinum, i.e. the space between the two lungs. There is no physical separation between the abdominal and pelvic cavities and they are often referred to as the *abdominopelvic cavity*. The cavities contain internal organs that are collectively called viscera. To enable the precise location of organs, the abdominopelvic cavity is divided into nine smaller compartments as shown in Figure 1.1.

Table 1.1 Directional terms.

Directional term	Definition	Examples
• Superior	• Towards the top. Upper part of a structure. Towards the head (cephalic or cranial)	• The head is superior to the lower limbs and the knee is superior to the ankle
• Inferior	• Towards the bottom. The lower part of a structure. Away from the head	• The diaphragm lies inferiorly to the lungs
• Anterior or ventral	• Towards the front	• The sternum is anterior to the heart
• Posterior or dorsal	• Towards the back	• The thoracic vertebrae are posterior to the heart
• Medial	• Towards the midline	• The heart is medial to the lungs
• Lateral	• Further away from the midline. Towards the sides	• The lungs are lateral to the heart
• Proximal	• Refers to a structure that is closer to any point of reference	• The proximal part of the nerve running along the arm is the part closest to the spinal cord
• Distal	• Further away from a point of reference	• In the hand, the phalanges are distal to the carpals
• Superficial	• Towards or on the surface of the skin	• The skin is superficial to the muscles
• Deep	• Away from the surface of the body	• The intestines are deep to the surface of the skin of the abdomen

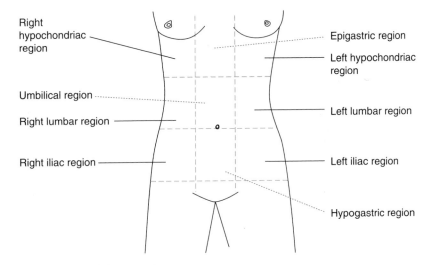

Figure 1.1 Abdomino-pelvic regions

Levels of organisation of the body

The human body and its many parts are categorised into six levels of organisation, which influence body structure and functions. Ranging from the smallest to largest, these differing levels are as follows.

Chemical level

The body is made up of atoms and molecules. Atoms (e.g. carbon, oxygen, hydrogen) are the smallest units of matter. When two or more atoms joined together, they become molecules (e.g. water). Molecules in turn combine with other atoms and molecules to form macromolecules in the cytoplasm of the cells, which enables normal cellular functions. If this is not maintained, disease or death may result.

Cellular level

Cells are the basic structural and functional units of an organism. They consist of atoms and molecules. Each human organism begins life as a single cell, when the sperm fertilises the ovum. The fertilised ovum, now called a zygote, then divides into two cells, four cells, eight cells and so on. During development, these cells undergo differentiation, i.e. the transformation of unspecialised cells into specialised cells.

Tissue level

Tissues are aggregates of cells that work together to perform a particular function. The cells of the body are organised into four primary tissues: epithelial, connective, muscle and nervous. *Epithelial tissue* covers body surfaces and, lines cavities, hollow organs and ducts. *Connective tissue* is mainly a support tissue, connecting, anchoring and supporting the structures of the body. Connective tissue is characterised by large amount of extracellular material, called matrix, in the spaces between the connective tissue cells. *Muscle tissue* is responsible for movement. *Nervous tissue* consists of neurons and neuroglia. Neurons generate and transmit messages whereas neuroglia provide neurons with anatomical and functional support.

Organ level

Two or more different types of tissues join together to form an organ. For example, the heart is an organ and is composed of three different types of tissues: epithelial (endothelial), muscle and connective. Organs have specific functions. The specific function of the heart is to pump blood.

System level

A system is a group of organs that work together to perform a common function. The heart and blood vessels work together to transport blood around the body and is referred to as the cardiovascular system. The other systems of the body are integumentary, skeletal, muscular, nervous, respiratory, lymphatic and immune, gastrointestinal, urinary, endocrine and reproductive.

Organism level

All structures and systems in the body combine to make the human organism.

Hierarchy of functions

The levels of organisation show something of a hierarchy but each level in the hierarchy is as important as the other. Disturbance at one level may affect the activity of the other levels. This can go up or down the hierarchy as shown in Figure 1.2. For example, the chemicals within the cells influence their function, which in turn affects the activity at the next level and so on. Events at the level of the organism (and ultimately in the environment) can also affect activities of the lower levels. For instance, the availability or choice of diet can affect the functions of the cells.

The basic structure of cells

The human body is composed of billions of cells and the functions of these cells ultimately determine the function of the human organism.

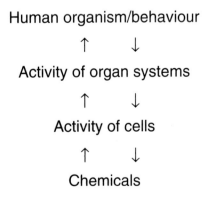

Figure 1.2 Hierarchy of phenomena in organisation of the human body

Cells are the basic unit of structure and function of the body. Cells become specialised for different tasks but their basic structure remains essentially the same. A cell has three parts (Figure 1.3):

- an outer membrane or plasma membrane
- cytoplasm
- nucleus (some cells, e.g. erythrocytes do not have a nucleus).

The plasma membrane

The plasma membrane is a phospholipid bilayer, into which a variety of proteins are immersed, that forms the boundary between the intracellular and extracellular environments of the cell. It controls the selective passage of substances into and out of the cell. The proteins within the cell membrane have a variety of functions. Some proteins form channels for substances to pass through. Others act as receptors, cell recognition molecules, adhesion molecules and enzymes.

The cytoplasm

The cytoplasm consists of all the contents, including the intracellular fluid (cytosol) and organelles, between the nucleus and the cell membrane. The organelles (listed in Table 1.2) are necessary for the biological processes of cellular life.

The nucleus

The nucleus is the most prominent intracellular structure and is found in most cells. Cells like the skeletal cells have multiple nuclei, while erythrocytes or red blood cells have none (Widmaier *et al.*, 2004). The nucleus contains the genetic material, deoxyribonucleic acid (DNA). The DNA molecules are organised into genes, which carry the information that passes from one generation to the next and also contain the code for protein synthesis. Genes are arranged into single files of DNA called chromosomes. Chromosomes also contain a special class of proteins called histone proteins or histones. In humans, there are 46 chromosomes.

Although the DNA contains the code for specifying the amino acid sequences in proteins, it does not itself participate directly in the synthesis of proteins in the ribosomes (Widmaier *et al.*, 2004). Information is transferred to the ribosomes for the assembly of proteins by the ribonucleic acid (RNA). The process of making a copy of the code, whereby information is transferred from the DNA to RNA, is called *transcription*. The RNA, also known as messenger RNA, then leaves the nucleus to travel to the ribosomes where the coded information in the RNA is used to assemble the protein – a process known as *translation*. An alteration in the sequence of the DNA is known as a *mutation*. The

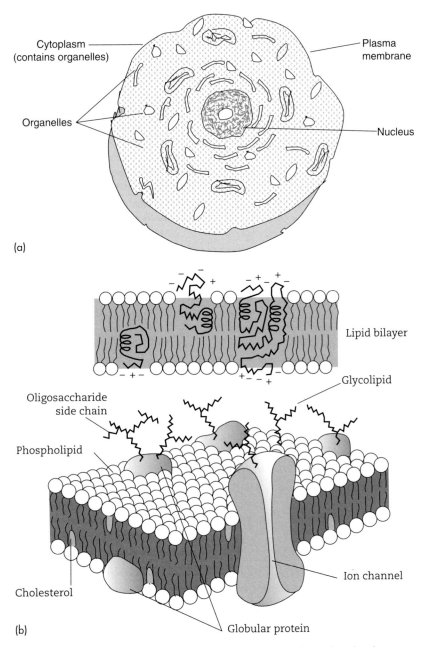

Figure 1.3 (a) A typical cell. (b) The plasma membrane (reproduced with permission from Bray *et al.*, 1999)

Table 1.2 Organelles and their functions.

Organelles	Functions
• Mitochondria	• Scattered throughout the cells, they are the sites of energy (ATP) production
• Ribosomes	• Sites of protein synthesis
• Rough endoplasmic reticulum (rough ER)	• A network of folded membranes. Rough ER is studded with ribosomes
• Smooth endoplasmic reticulum (smooth ER)	• Smooth ER has no ribosomes attached to its surface. Fatty acids, steroids and cholesterol are synthesised in smooth ER
• Golgi complex	• Flat membrane-like sacs. Newly synthesised proteins are modified in the Golgi complex and packed into vesicles that are then transported to where they are needed in the cell or exported out of the cell by a process called exocytosis
• Lysosomes	• Vesicles which contain digestive enzymes for the breakdown of molecules
• Centrosome	• Consists of two centrioles and is important in cell division
• Cytoskeleton	• A network of microfilaments in the cytoplasm contributing to the cell's strength and shape. Also helps to generate movements

resulting faulty code can lead to the synthesis of an abnormal protein, e.g. faulty haemoglobin in sickle cell disease.

The environment of the cells

Cells have a fluid environment. There is fluid within the cells, around the cells and in the blood vessels. The fluid inside the cells is called intracellular fluid and that outside the cells extracellular or interstitial fluid. The fluid contains various salts or electrolytes as well as many dissolved substances, such as nutrients and oxygen. The composition of the intracellular fluid differs from that of extracellular fluid. Body fluids are located within two main compartments:

- intracellular fluid (28 L in a 70 kg person) and
- extracellular fluid (14 L in a 70 kg person, of which 11 L is interstitial fluid and 3 L plasma).

Homeostasis

For the body to function normally, the internal environment of the cells has to stay relatively constant. Variables such as the chemical composition of the fluid that surrounds the cells, its temperature, acid level (pH) and glucose level have to remain stable for the cells to function optimally. Homeostasis is defined as a state of relative constancy of the internal environment (Fox, 2004). This is achieved by the balancing of inputs and outputs (Widmaier *et al.*, 2004). All organ systems contribute to homeostasis but the nervous and endocrine systems in particular play a vital role.

Feedback systems

The stability of the internal environment is maintained by feedback systems or feedback loops (Figure 1.4), which is a concept derived from engineering. A feedback system is a cycle of events whereby the status of a controlled condition is continually monitored and adjusted as required. It has three basic components:

- *Receptor.* The receptor monitors changes in the controlled condition and sends the input to the control centre.
- *Control or integrating centre.* The control centre evaluates the input and sends an output to the effector.
- *Effector.* The effector receives the output from the control centre and produces a response to the changes in the controlled condition.

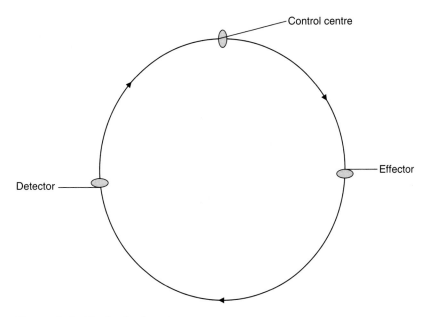

Figure 1.4 The feedback system

Table 1.3 Major organ systems.

System	Organs and tissues	Functions
• Integumentary	• Skin, appendages	• Protection against injury and dehydration. Defence against micro-organisms. Temperature regulation
• Musculoskeletal	• Bones, cartilage, ligaments, tendons, joints, skeletal muscle	• Support. Protection. Movement. Red bone marrow produces blood cells
• Nervous	• Brain, spinal cord, peripheral nerves, cranial nerves, special sense organs	• States of consciousness. Regulation and co-ordination of many body functions. Detection of changes in internal and external environment
• Endocrine	• Glands producing hormones – pituitary, thyroid, parathyroid, adrenal, pancreas, testes, ovaries	• Regulation and co-ordination of activities such as growth, metabolism, reproduction, blood pressure, water and electrolytes balance
• Respiratory	• Nose, pharynx, larynx, trachea, bronchi, lungs	• Exchange of carbon dioxide and oxygen. Regulation of blood pH
• Cardiovascular	• Heart, blood vessels (arteries, veins, capillaries), blood, lymphatic vessels and lymph	• Transport of blood and other materials
• Lymphatic and immune	• Lymph vessels and nodes, spleen, thymus, white blood cells	• Return of lymph to the blood. Defence against foreign invaders
• Digestive	• Mouth, pharynx, oesophagus, stomach, intestines and accessory organs such as salivary glands, pancreas, liver and gall bladder	• Digestion and absorption of nutrients, water and salts
• Urinary	• Kidneys, ureters, bladder, urethra	• Regulation and composition of body fluids through control secretions of salts, water and wastes
• Reproductive	• Male: testes, penis and associated ducts and glands • Female: ovaries, fallopian tubes, vagina, mammary glands	• Production of sperm, transfer of sperm to females • Production of eggs, provision of a conducive environment for the developing embryo and foetus, nutrition of the infant

Negative and positive feedback systems

There are two types of feedback system: negative and positive. The negative feedback system reverses or opposes changes in a controlled condition. For example, if the blood glucose is rising or falling, it returns it to normal through a series of actions. A negative system is important for the maintenance of health. A positive feedback system reinforces changes in a controlled condition and is on the whole detrimental to health, e.g. if the body temperature starts to rise, the positive feedback system will amplify the rise.

Homeostasis and disease

Homeostasis promotes normal cellular activity (Tortora & Grabowski, 2004). Homeostatic functions operate with maximum efficiency and effectiveness during childhood and young adulthood but become less and less efficient in late adulthood and old age (Thibodeau & Patton, 2004). A disorder or disease may occur if the normal balance of the body's processes is disturbed. If the homeostatic imbalance is severe, death may result. Tortora & Grabowski (2004) define a *disorder* as any disturbance of structure and/or function, and a *disease* as an illness characterised by a recognisable set of symptoms (subjective changes of body functions) and signs (observable changes).

Organ systems

Most of the cells of the body are isolated from the external environment. Consequently, they rely on the organ systems for their 'servicing', i.e. obtaining materials that are needed for their functions and removing the waste products of metabolism. As discussed, through the homeostatic regulatory mechanisms, the organ systems also ensure that the internal environment of the cells stays relatively stable. Widmaier *et al.* (2004) identify ten major organ systems. These are listed in Table 1.3.

Section 2: The integumentary system

The integumentary system includes the skin and its appendages, i.e. hair, nails and specialised sweat- and oil-producing glands. The skin covers the external surface and is the largest organ of the body, accounting for about 16% of the total body weight. Knowledge of anatomy and physiology of the skin and its major roles in thermoregulation, protection, sensation and vitamin D metabolism can assist nurses in assessment of skin conditions and general physiological disturbances (Casey, 2002). In fact, the skin acts as a window for many systemic disorders. For example, signs of cardiovascular, respiratory, renal, hepatic and digestive disorders may be observed in the skin. Because of its exposed location, the skin is also vulnerable to damage from trauma and pressure, burns, ultraviolet light, micro-organisms, parasites, fungi, pollutants and allergens. Inspection of skin is a fundamental part of health assessment.

Structure of the skin

The skin consists of two main parts:

- epidermis
- dermis.

Subcutaneous (adipose) tissue connects the skin to underlying structures but is not part of the skin. It stores fat and also contains large blood vessels and pressure receptors.

Epidermis

The epidermis is the outer epithelial layer of the skin. It is composed of four or five distinct layers or strata. The deepest layer is the stratum basale, which continually undergoes mitotic activity or cell division to produce new skin cells. These are slowly pushed to the surface. The stratum basale also contains melanocytes, which produce melanin. Melanin provides protection from ultraviolet radiation. Ultraviolet radiation, as well as systemic hormones such as adrenocorticotrophic hormone (ACTH), stimulates production of melanin. Excess ACTH production by the pituitary gland, as in adrenal insufficiency or Addison's disease, results in the skin becoming very tanned (Porth, 1998). If the stratum basale is destroyed, the skin cannot regenerate itself and scar tissue is formed. The outermost layer of the skin consists of dead keratinised cells that act as a strong protective barrier. Protection against mechanical abrasion is linked to the ability of the skin to desquamate (Tortora & Grabowski, 2004).

Dermis

The dermis is the inner layer of the skin and is connected to the epidermis by papillae. It is made of connective tissue containing collagen and elastic fibres, which give the skin its strength and elasticity. The dermis contains blood vessels and various sensory receptors as well as hair follicles and sweat glands. The deep veins in the dermis act as a reservoir for approximately 1.5 litres of blood (Bray *et al.*, 1999). This blood is pushed back into the general circulation during haemorrhage or shock through the action of the sympathetic nervous system. This diversion of blood makes the skin look pale, cool and mottled in appearance (Porth, 2005).

The hypodermis or subcutaneous tissue

This is not strictly speaking part of the skin. The hypodermis contains a layer of subcutaneous fat cells (or adipose tissue), which forms the link between the skin and the rest of the body. The hypodermis provides a cushioning layer and some thermal insulation (Tortora & Grabowski, 2004).

The appendages or accessory structures of the skin

The hair

The human skin is covered with millions of hairs, most visible in the scalp, eyelids and eyebrows while the lips, palms of the hands and soles of the feet are hairless (Thibodeau & Patton, 2004). In response to hormone secretion at puberty, coarse hair develops in the pubic area and axilla.

Hair consists of a shaft and root. The root penetrates deep into the dermis and surrounding it is the hair follicle. Hair growth begins from a cluster of cells called the hair papilla located at the base of the hair follicle. The papilla is nourished by a dermal blood vessel. Sebaceous glands and arrector pili muscles are associated with the hair follicle.

The nails

The nails are plates of hard keratinised cells, consisting of a nail body, free edge and nail root. Under the nail is a layer of epithelium called the nail bed. The nail bed has a pink tinge as a result of the rich blood supply underneath and low oxygen levels in the blood cause the nail bed to turn blue or cyanosed (Thibodeau & Patton, 2004).

Skin glands

These are of two types: *sudoriferous* or sweat glands and *sebaceous* glands. The sweat glands are grouped into eccrine and apocrine glands. The eccrine glands are numerous and they produce a watery substance called perspiration or sweat, the main function of which is to assist in the reduction of body temperature. Indeed, evaporation of sweat from the skin surface is responsible for about 15% of heat loss at room temperature (Bray *et al.*, 1999). The apocrine glands are found primarily in the skin of the armpit and around the genitals and produce a thick fluid. The odour associated with this secretion is due to contamination and decomposition of skin bacteria (Thibodeau & Patton, 2004).

The sebaceous glands secrete an oily substance known as sebum in the hair and skin. This lubricates the skin and hair. The increase in dryness and cracking of the skin in late adulthood and old age is due to a reduction of sebum secretion (Thibodeau & Patton, 2004).

Thermoregulation and the skin

By regulating sweat secretion and the flow of blood close to the surface of the body, the skin plays a key role in the regulation of body temperature (Thibodeau & Patton, 2004). This is achieved by a negative feedback system in which an 'increase or decrease in the variable being regulated brings about responses that tend to move the variable in the direction opposite the direction of the original change' (Widmaier *et al.*, 2004: p9). Any changes in body temperature are detected by thermoreceptors in the skin and deeper organs. The information is fed back to the control centre (i.e. hypothalamus), which in turn will send impulses to the effector organs to adjust the body temperature. If the body temperature is high, there is vasodilation of the blood vessels in the skin, allowing warm blood to flow close to the skin surface, hence causing heat loss to the environment. Conversely, when the body temperature drops, vasoconstriction of the skin blood vessels takes blood away from the surface to effect a reduction in heat loss.

Section 3: The musculoskeletal system

The musculoskeletal system consists of the bones, skeletal muscles and joints. The overall function of the musculoskeletal system is to provide a rigid framework and support structure for the body as well as allowing movement in conjunction with the nervous system. Familiarity with the names, shapes and positions of individual bones enables one to locate other organs, e.g. the radial artery, where the pulse is usually taken, is named for its closeness to the radius (Tortora & Grabowski, 2004).

The human skeleton

The skeleton has two principal divisions: axial and appendicular. The axial skeleton includes the bones of the skull, face, ossicles, hyoid bone, ribs, sternum and vertebrae. The appendicular skeleton consists of the bones of the upper and lower limbs as well as the girdles (shoulder and pelvic), which connect the limbs to the axial skeleton. There are 206 bones in the adult (although there may be some biological variations): 80 in the axial skeleton and 126 in the appendicular skeleton (Tortora & Grabowski, 2004).

Bone

Bone is a connective tissue, consisting of a hard matrix that surrounds widely separated cells. The matrix also contains collagen fibres and calcium phosphate, providing flexibility and hardness. There are two types of bone: compact and cancellous. Compact bone is hard and dense and forms the external layer of all bones and the bulk of the diaphyses or shafts of long bones. Cancellous or spongy bone tissue makes up the ends (epiphyses) and centres of the bones.

Functions of skeleton and bone tissue

Bones perform the following functions:

- support for the body and soft tissues
- protection of internal organs
- movement, in conjunction with the skeletal muscles and motor neurons
- production of blood cells in the red bone marrow
- storage of calcium and phosphate.

Joints

The joint is the point of contact between bones, between cartilage or between teeth and bones (Tortora, 2005). There are three types of joints: synovial, cartilaginous and fibrous:

- *Synovial joints* have space between the articulating bones, allowing them to be freely movable. Figure 1.5 shows the special characteristics of synovial joints.
- *Cartilaginous joints* are held together by cartilage and only allow slight movement. There is no cavity between the bones.
- *Fibrous joints* are joined together by fibrous connective tissue. They permit no movement, e.g. cranial joints.

Types of movements at synovial joints

The shapes of the articulating surfaces in synovial joints dictate the types of movements that are possible. The principal movements are shown in Table 1.4.

Table 1.4 Movements at synovial joints.

Movements	Description
<ul><li>Flexion</li><li>Extension</li><li>Abduction</li><li>Adduction</li><li>Circumduction</li></ul>	<ul><li>Bending</li><li>Stretching out</li><li>Movement away from the midline</li><li>Movement toward the midline</li><li>Movement of the distal part of the body in a circle. The ball and socket joints (e.g. shoulder and hip joints) permit circumduction</li></ul>

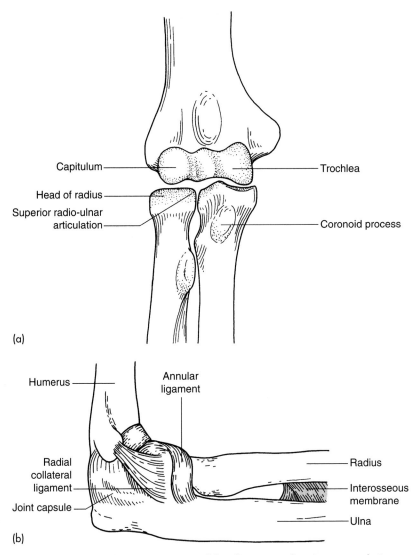

Figure 1.5 (a) The bony components of the elbow joint. (b) A joint capsule (reproduced with permission from Ellis, 2002)

Muscular tissue

There are three types of muscular tissue: skeletal, smooth and cardiac.

Skeletal muscles are attached to bones by tendons and move the skeleton. A few skeletal muscles (e.g. facial muscles) are attached to structures other than bone. When skeletal muscle tissues are examined under the microscope, alternating light and dark bands are visible;

hence they are called striated muscles. As skeletal muscles can be consciously controlled, they are also referred to as voluntary muscles (Tortora, 2005) and are supplied by the voluntary nervous system. Skeletal muscles also assist with posture and produce body heat when contracting.

Smooth muscles are located in the walls of hollow organs (e.g. blood vessels, digestive tract, bronchi). They appear non-striated under the microscope, hence the term smooth. Smooth muscles control internal processes such as peristalsis and blood pressure. They are termed involuntary muscle because they are not under our conscious control but are regulated by the autonomic division of the nervous system.

Cardiac muscle is the middle layer (myocardium) of the heart. Contraction of the heart muscle enables blood to be pumped round the body. The action is involuntary, i.e. cannot be consciously controlled. The heart muscle has the property of autorhythmicity, i.e. it has a built-in rhythm whereby each cardiac contraction is initiated by its own pacemaker or sinoatrial node, although its rate is adjusted by the autonomic nervous system (Tortora, 2005).

Section 4: The nervous system

Along with the endocrine system (see page 28), the nervous system is responsible for co-ordinating and regulating body functions, thus playing a crucial part in the maintenance of homeostasis. The nervous system has a rapid mode of action whereas the endocrine system acts more slowly.

Structure and function of the nervous system

The functional units of the nervous system are the neurons. Neurons are specialised to respond to physical and chemical stimuli and conduction of nerve impulses (Fox, 2004). They are supported by neuroglia. Unlike mature neurons, neuroglia are able to multiply and divide. In fact, brain tumours are derived from neuroglia and not neurons (Fox, 2004).

A neuron (Figure 1.6) is divided into three parts: a cell body, dendrites and an axon. The cell body and dendrites receive the input or stimulus to the cell; the outputs are sent down by the axon in the form of impulses (action potentials). The points of contacts between neurons are called synapses. When an impulse reaches the end of an axon terminal, it triggers the release of neurotransmitters from vesicles, enabling the impulse to cross the synapse and depolarise the next neuron. Figure 1.6 shows the structure of a motor neuron.

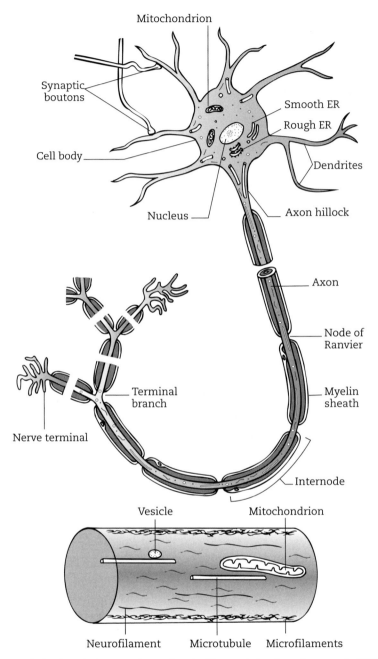

Figure 1.6 A typical neuron (reproduced with permission from Bray *et al.*, 1999)

The nervous system consists of two structural divisions: the central nervous system (CNS) and the autonomic nervous system (ANS).

The central nervous system (CNS)

The CNS is composed of the brain and spinal cord. These are very delicate structures and, besides being encased in bones, are protected by three connective tissues layers: the dura mater, arachnoid mater and pia mater. There is a space called the subarachnoid space between the dura and arachnoid mater, into which cerebrospinal fluid (CSF) circulates. The CSF acts as a shock absorber as well as providing nourishment for the nervous tissue. Inflammation of the meninges is called meningitis and is usually caused by bacterial or viral infection.

The brain

The brain is located within the cranial cavity. It can be subdivided into four major divisions: the cerebrum, diencephalon (thalamus and hypothalamus), the brainstem (midbrain, pons and medulla) and cerebellum. Figure 1.7 shows the brain.

The cerebrum

The cerebrum is the most prominent part of the human brain, accounting for about 80% of its mass, and is divided into the right and left cerebral hemispheres (Fox, 2004). The corpus callosum, a bundle of nerve fibres, connects the two hemispheres across the midline; it enables transfer of information between the two hemispheres. The outer layer of the cerebrum, called the cerebral cortex, consists of grey matter or cell bodies, which are responsible for higher functions such as motor and sensory functions, speech, memory and other intellectual faculties. The inner layer of the cerebrum, or white matter, consists mostly of myelinated nerve fibres, enabling communication to various regions of the brain as well as the spinal cord.

Each cerebral hemisphere can be anatomically divided into four major lobes: frontal, temporal, parietal and occipital lobes. Each lobe is responsible for a specific function. For instance, the primary motor cortex, located in the frontal lobe, initiates voluntary motor movement to the opposite sides of the body and Broca's area is responsible for motor speech (Tortora & Grabowski, 2004). The primary somatosensory area is located in the parietal lobe and receives sensory information from the body via the thalamus. The cerebral cortex has projection fibres that connect the cortex to the spinal cord. These projection fibres, also called the pyramidal tract, cross over at the medulla oblongata so that fibres from the left hemisphere supply the right side

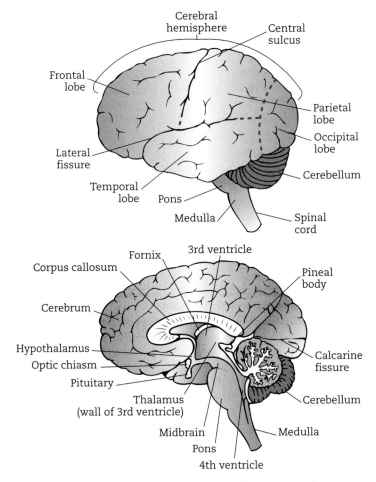

Figure 1.7 The brain (reproduced with permission from Bray *et al.*, 1999)

of the body and vice versa. Afferent or sensory fibres also cross over in the CNS so that sensory information from the right side of the body is taken to the sensory cortex in the left hemisphere and that of the left side of the body to the right hemisphere. Thus, damage to the left hemisphere, as in a stroke, will cause paralysis and loss of sensation to the right side of the body. Wernicke's area is located in the temporal lobe and parietal lobes and is responsible for interpreting the meaning of speech by recognising the spoken word (Tortora & Grabowski, 2004).

The basal ganglia or basal nuclei are located deep within the white matter of the cerebrum and are essential for producing automatic movements and postures (Thibodeau & Patton, 2004).

The diencephalon

This is located beneath the cerebral hemispheres and contains the thalamus and hypothalamus. The thalamus is a sensory relay centre and conveys sensory information from the periphery to the sensory cortex and from one brain area to another. It also processes incoming sensory signals, determining whether sensory information will reach the cerebral cortex. The thalamus is part of the system that promotes alertness and causes arousal from sleep (Fox, 2004). The hypothalamus, located below the thalamus, is concerned with maintaining the internal environment of the body. It links the nervous system to the endocrine system through its connection to the pituitary gland.

The brainstem

The brainstem is formed by the midbrain, pons varolii and medulla oblongata. Located between the cerebral cortex and the spinal cord, it is concerned with the basic activities necessary for life. Vital centres such as the cardiac, respiratory and vasomotor centres are located in the medulla. The brainstem also consists of clusters of nuclei known as the reticular formation that modulate the activity of neurons in other brain regions and in the spinal cord (Fox, 2004). The ascending part of the reticular formation, called the reticular activating system (RAS), regulates the sleep–wake cycle. A state of wakefulness or consciousness is maintained when the RAS stimulates the cerebral cortex. Loss of consciousness results from damage to the RAS and/or cerebral cortex.

The cerebellum

The cerebellum lies behind the brainstem and under the cerebrum. It is concerned with co-ordinating body movements, maintaining posture and learning motor skills. Lesions in the cerebellum affect muscle co-ordination, causing a condition of ataxia.

The spinal cord

The spinal cord is a long, thin cylinder of nervous tissue located in the vertebral canal. It extends from the medulla oblongata to the first lumbar vertebra. The spinal cord consists of two regions: an H-shaped inner region of grey matter and an outer region of white matter. The grey matter consists of two dorsal horns and two ventral horns. Sensory or afferent nerves enter the spinal cord at the dorsal horns and motor or efferent nerves exit at the ventral horns. Each sensory nerve brings sensory information from very specific areas of the skin called dermatomes. Each motor neuron, on the other hand, innervates a small number of muscle fibres, controlling their contraction. The spinal cord has 31 segments (a thoracic segment is shown in Figure 1.8), giving rise to 31 pairs of spinal nerves (also called *peripheral nerves*) as follows:

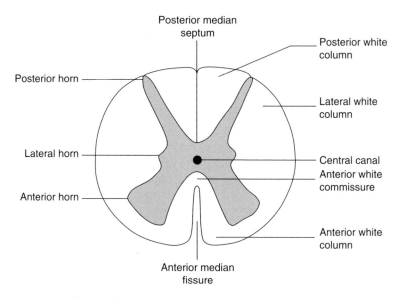

Figure 1.8 The spinal cord – transverse section through thoracic segment (reproduced with permission from Ellis, 2002)

- *Cervical nerves* (C1 to C8): supplying the neck, arms and hands.
- *Thoracic nerves* (T1 to T12): supplying the chest or thorax, the upper abdomen and back.
- *Lumbar nerves* (L1 to L5): supplying lower abdomen, the back and front of legs.
- *Sacral nerves* (C1 to C5): supplying the genitals, regions surrounding the anus and back of the leg.
- *Coccygeal nerve* (co1).

Besides the 31 pairs of spinal nerves, the peripheral nervous system also consists of 12 pairs of cranial nerves, so called because they evolve from the brain or brainstem. Thus the brainstem controls motor output and receives sensory information from areas above the neck via the cranial nerves.

The autonomic nervous system (ANS)

The ANS regulates the internal organs of the body such as cardiac muscle, smooth muscle and glands. It is responsible for maintaining an optimal environment or homeostasis for the cells to function. It consists of two divisions: sympathetic and parasympathetic. The sympathetic and parasympathetic nervous systems have opposing actions. For instance, mass activation of the sympathetic system helps us to respond to physical activity in emergencies and prepares the body for 'fight' or 'flight' (Fox, 2004). In sympathetic stimulation, the heart rate increases, blood glucose rises and blood is diverted from visceral organs and skin to the skeletal muscles. The parasympathetic nervous system is responsible for maintaining our body in a resting state. Its activation results in slowing of the heart rate, dilation of visceral blood vessels and increased activity of the digestive tract. Normally the actions of the two divisions must be balanced to maintain homeostasis.

Sensations

The sensory cortex receives and processes sensory information such as hearing, vision, smell, taste, touch, temperature, pain and posture. This enables conscious or subconscious awareness of external or internal conditions of the body. Sensations can be divided into general senses and special senses (Thibodeau & Patton, 2004). General senses include somatic senses (from the skin and joints) and visceral senses (from internal organs). Special senses are smell, taste, vision, hearing and balance.

Somatic senses

There are a number of receptors in the skin, mucous membranes, muscles, tendons and joints that will respond to physical stimuli and produce specific sensations. Mechanoreceptors respond to deformation of the skin and provide information on texture. Thermoreceptors are activated by changes in temperature while nociceptors respond to tissue damage and produce pain sensation. Proprioceptors in joints and muscles give information on the position and movement of body parts.

Pain

The nociceptors are the sensory receptors for pain. These free nerve endings are widespread in the body and respond to intense mechanical deformation, excessive heat and various types of chemicals such as bradykinin, histamines, cytokines and prostaglandins normally released by damaged tissue. Stimulation of the nociceptors by these noxious stimuli generates impulses that travel to the cortex to be interpreted as pain. The sensory cortex recognises the type, location and intensity of pain. However, in visceral pain, the sensation is not always projected back to the point of stimulation and is felt instead in another area, a phenomenon called referred pain (Widmaier *et al.*, 2004). For instance, cardiac pain is typically felt on the skin over the heart, the jaw, throat and the left arm. This is because both visceral and somatic afferents converge on the same neurons in the spinal cord and as excitation of somatic afferents is the most common source of afferent discharge, the sensation is incorrectly perceived to have come from these somatic areas (Widmaier *et al.*, 2004).

The perception of pain is modulated by past experiences, emotions (anxiety) and suggestion as well as simultaneous stimulation of other sensory modalities. Thus the level of pain experienced is not solely the result of the stimulus (Widmaier *et al.*, 2004).

Section 5: The special senses

The receptors for special senses are located in specialised sensory organs such as the eyes, ears, olfactory epithelium in the superior aspect of nasal cavity, and taste buds in the tongue and mouth.

The eye

The eye (Figure 1.9) is the organ of vision. The photoreceptors located deep in the eye pick up light stimuli and transmit the visual impulses

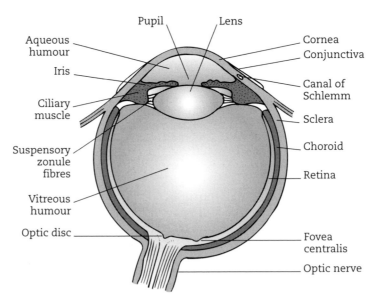

Figure 1.9   Eye in horizontal section (reproduced with permission from Bray *et al.*, 1999)

to the brain (mostly the occipital cortex) for interpretation. The eyeball is located in the eye orbit.

The accessory structures of the eye

The accessory structures of the eyes are as follows:

- Upper and lower *eyelids*, which protect the eyes from foreign objects and excessive light. The meibomian glands secrete an oily substance that lubricates the eyes.
- The *eyebrows* and *eyelashes*, which protect the eyes from foreign objects and perspiration.
- The *lacrimal apparatus*, which is a group of glands, ducts, canals and sacs that produce and drain tears.
- The *six eye muscles* that move the eyeball right, left, down, up and diagonally.
- The *conjunctiva*, a thin membrane lining the inside of the eyelids and covering most of the anterior eye.

The eyeball is divided into three layers: outer fibrous layer, middle vascular layer and an innermost layer (retina).

The outer layer consists of an anterior cornea and a posterior sclera. The cornea is a transparent and curved coat which helps to focus the light rays onto the retina. The sclera or the 'white' of the eye covers the eyeball, except the cornea.

The middle layer consists of the choroid, ciliary body and iris. This very vascular tissue provides nourishment to the retina. The ciliary body consists of ciliary muscles that alter the shape of the lens. The iris is a circular disc of muscle that contains the pigments responsible for eye colour. The hole in the centre of the iris is called the pupil. The smooth muscles of the iris control the size of the pupil. The lens is a transparent structure that focuses the light rays onto the retina. It also divides the eyeball into cavities: the anterior cavity filled with aqueous humour and the vitreous chamber that contains a jelly-like substance. The aqueous humour is continuously secreted by blood capillaries of the ciliary's processes into the anterior chamber, which is then drained into the canal of Schlemm, an opening where the sclera and cornea meet (Tortora & Grabowski, 2004). The intraocular pressure (normally 12–20 mmHg) is produced mainly by the aqueous humour and is maintained by a balance between production and drainage of the fluid (McBean, 2003). If the pressure is raised, a pathological condition called *glaucoma* occurs which can cause irreparable damage to the retina and optic nerve.

The retina is the inner coat of the eye, lining the posterior three-quarters of the eyeball. It consists of layers of nerve cells, including the rods and cones which are photoreceptors. The rods function in dim light whereas the cones respond to bright lights. The optic disc is round

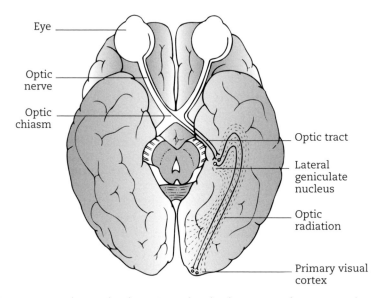

Eye

Optic
nerve

Optic
chiasm

Optic tract

Lateral
geniculate
nucleus

Optic
radiation

Primary visual
cortex

Figure 1.10   The visual pathway (reproduced with permission from Bray *et al.*, 1999)

or oval in shape and is located towards the medial or nasal side of the
eye. It is here that the optic nerve (cranial nerve II) exits the eyeball.
There are no rods and cones in this area and it is referred to as the blind
spot.

The visual pathway

When light rays enter the eyes, they stimulate the rods and cones, triggering electrical impulses which are conducted to the brain via the
optic nerve and interpreted as sight. At the optic chiasm, the nerve
fibres from the nasal quadrant of each retina cross over to the opposite
side. After the optic chiasm, the neurons then become the optic tract
and they terminate in the thalamus where they synapse with neurons
whose axons project to the visual areas in the occipital lobes. Figure
1.10 shows the visual pathway.

The ear

The ear is the sense organ for hearing and balance. It is divided into
three parts as shown in Figure 1.11: external ear, middle ear and inner
ear. The tympanic membrane or eardrum separates the external ear
from the middle ear. Descriptions and functions of the three structures
are given in Table 1.5.

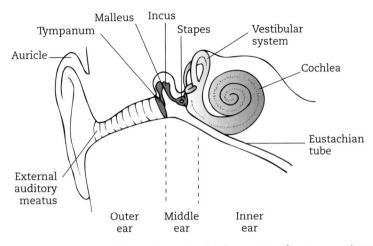

Figure 1.11   Structure of the ear (reproduced with permission from Bray *et al.*, 1999)

Table 1.5 The three main parts of the ear and their functions.

Parts	Description	Functions
• External ear	• Composed of the auricle (pinna) and external auditory canal. Eardrum separates it from middle ear	• Collects sound waves and passes them inward towards the eardrum
• Middle ear	• Air-filled cavity between eardrum and inner ear. Auditory tube (Eustachian) connects middle ear to the nasopharynx. There are three ossicles between the eardrum and the oval window	• The ossicles receive the vibrations from the eardrum and transmit them to the oval window
• Inner ear	• There are three areas: vestibule and semicircular canals (concerned with equilibrium) and cochlea (concerned with hearing). Has an outer bony labyrinth and inner membranous labyrinth, both containing fluid	• Movement of the oval window causes pressure waves in the fluid of the cochlea, stimulating the hair cells. This produces an impulse, which travels along the auditory nerve • The inner ear is also responsible for maintaining static and dynamic equilibrium or balance. Changes in position cause movement of fluid in the semicircular canals, generating an impulse which is conducted by the vestibular branch of the vestibulocochlear nerve

Section 6: The endocrine system

The endocrine system consists of a number of organs scattered throughout the body. The glands produce hormones, which circulate in the blood and act on target cells and organs. Like the nervous system, the endocrine system is a control system, co-ordinating the functioning of body parts and maintaining homeostasis. These two control systems often work together but the endocrine system is slower to act than the nervous system (Tortora, 2005).

Hormones

Hormones are produced by the endocrine glands and are transported by the blood. There are two basic types of hormones: peptides and steroids. Peptide hormones act on cell receptors on the plasma membrane, triggering a 'second messenger' within the cell that carries out various cellular activities. In contrast, steroid hormones enter the cell and act directly on receptors within the cytoplasm. Hormones help maintain homeostasis on a daily basis (Tortora, 2005).

Negative and positive feedback mechanisms

The hormone levels in the blood are regulated by homeostatic negative feedback mechanisms, often involving the hypothalamus and pituitary glands (Thibodeau & Patton, 2004). For example, the level of thyroxine (T_4) and tri-iodothyronine (T_3) in the blood is monitored by the hypothalamus. If the level drops, the hypothalamus produces a releasing hormone, which triggers the anterior pituitary gland to produce thyroid-stimulating hormone (TSH). This stimulates the thyroid gland to produce more T_4 and T_3. The reverse happens if the levels of T_4 and T_3 become raised. Positive feedback mechanisms amplify changes rather than reversing them, hence usually threatening homeostasis (Thibodeau & Patton, 2004). However, in labour, positive feedback helps the body to maintain stability by making uterine contractions become stronger and stronger by means of a mechanism that regulates the secretion of the hormone oxytocin (Thibodeau & Patton, 2004). A full list of endocrine glands and their functions is given in Table 1.6.

Section 7: The respiratory system

The two major functions of the respiratory system are to supply oxygen to all the cells of the body for the production of energy and remove carbon dioxide as a waste product of energy production and cellular metabolism.

Table 1.6 Endocrine glands, their hormones and their functions.

Gland	Location	Hormones	Functions
• Hypothalamus	• Brain (diencephalon). Connected to the pituitary gland. Forms part of nervous system	• Releasing hormones	• Stimulates anterior pituitary gland • Influences functions of posterior pituitary
• Anterior pituitary	• Brain. Inferior to hypothalamus	• Thyroid-stimulating hormone (TSH) • Adrenocorticotrophic (ACTH) hormone • Gonadotrophic hormone • Follicle-stimulating hormone (FSH) • Luteinising hormone (LH) • Growth hormone • Prolactin	• Stimulates thyroid • Stimulates adrenal cortex • Stimulates gonads • Regulates egg and sperm production • Regulates production of sex hormones • Promotes growth • Stimulates milk production
• Posterior pituitary	• Inferior to hypothalamus	• Antidiuretic hormone (ADH) • Oxytocin	• Promotes reabsorption of water in the kidneys • Causes uterine contraction and milk secretion
• Thymus	• Midthoracic cavity	• Thymosin	• Regulates development and function of T-cells
• Thyroid	• Just below the larynx in the neck	• Thyroxine • Calcitonin	• Increases metabolic rate • Decreases plasma level of calcium
• Parathyroid	• Four small glands embedded in posterior surface of thyroid	• Parathormone	• Increases plasma level of calcium
• Adrenal cortex	• Upper pole of kidneys	• Glucocorticoids (cortisol) • Mineralocorticoids (aldosterone)	• Causes gluconeogenesis • Causes sodium retention and potassium excretion by kidneys
• Adrenal medulla	• Innermost layer of adrenal glands	• Adrenaline • Noradrenaline	• Promote 'fight or fight' response
• Pancreas (islets of Langerhans)	• Curve of duodenum in abdominal cavity	• Insulin • Glucagon	• Lowers blood glucose • Increases blood glucose
• Testes	• Scrotum	• Testosterone	• Promotes secondary sexual characteristics
• Ovaries	• Pelvic cavity	• Oestrogen	• Promotes secondary female characteristics

The oxygen has to be taken from the atmosphere into the lungs and then diffuses into the blood to be transported to all parts of the body. Carbon dioxide is transported from the body by the blood to the lungs to be expelled into the atmosphere. The structures necessary for the exchange of gases between the atmosphere and the lungs are the:

- *upper respiratory system*, which includes the nose, pharynx and associated structures
- *lower respiratory system*, which consists of the larynx, trachea, bronchi, bronchioles, alveoli and lungs
- *respiratory pump*, which consists of the ribcage, respiratory muscles, pleura and respiratory control centre in the brainstem.

Figure 1.12 shows the structure of the upper and lower respiratory system.

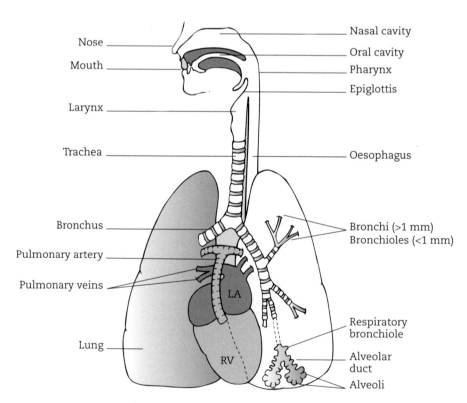

Figure 1.12 The upper and lower respiratory system (reproduced with permission from Bray *et al.*, 1999)

The mechanism of breathing

The mechanism of breathing consists of inspiration and expiration. In *inspiration*, the contraction of the diaphragm and external intercostal muscles causes an increase in the volume within the lungs and a reduction in pressure. This pressure gradient results in airflow from the atmosphere to the lungs.

Expiration occurs when the diaphragm and external intercostal muscles relax and there is elastic recoil of the chest wall and lungs, reducing the lung volume and increasing the pressure. The resulting pressure gradient enables air to flow outwards.

The pulmonary volumes and capacities

Spirometry is the measurement of lung volumes as follows:

* *Tidal volume.* The volume of one breath, normally 0.5 litre at rest.
* *Inspiratory reserve volume.* The additional inhaled air following deep inspiration, normally 3.1 litres.
* *Expiratory reserve volume.* The volume that can be exhaled in forced expiration, normally 1.2 litres.
* *Vital capacity.* The maximum amount of air that can be exhaled after maximal inspiration, normally 4.8 litres.

Exchange of oxygen and carbon dioxide in the lungs in adults at sea level (external respiration)

Gases diffuse from areas of high pressure to areas of low pressure. The pressure of a specific gas in a mixture is called partial pressure; pO_2 stands for partial pressure of oxygen and pCO_2 for partial pressure of carbon dioxide. Since pO_2 is higher in alveolar air than in pulmonary capillaries, O_2 diffuses from alveolar sacs into pulmonary capillaries. The reverse occurs with CO_2, the pCO_2 being higher in the blood than in the alveolar sacs.

Calculation of partial pressure

Atmospheric or barometric pressure is about 760 mmHg at sea level. This air contains 21% of oxygen. When we inhale atmospheric air, it becomes humidified and warmed. The water vapour so formed contributes about 47 mmHg of the inhaled air as it enters the lungs (Bray *et al.*, 1999). This alters the partial pressure of inhaled oxygen, which becomes 21% of 713 mmHg (i.e. 760 mmHg minus 47 mmHg) or 150 mmHg, and by the time the oxygen reaches the alveoli, the partial pressure will have fallen to 100 mmHg because the inhaled air has mixed with 'dead space' air (air in the trachea and bronchi) and residual air (Casey, 2001). Giving a person a higher percentage of oxygen can increase the partial pressure of inspired oxygen. For instance, by giving 40% of oxygen, the pO_2 becomes 285 mmHg (40% of 713 mmHg).

Rate of diffusion of oxygen from the alveoli into the blood

The rate of diffusion from the alveoli into the blood of the pulmonary capillaries is determined by three main factors: concentration gradient, surface area available for diffusion, and thickness of the alveolar–capillary membrane (Casey, 2001).

Concentration gradient

The blood coming into the lungs from the pulmonary arteries has a pO_2 of 40 mmHg whereas pO_2 in the alveoli is 100 mmHg. This creates a steep concentration gradient, enabling oxygen to diffuse from the alveoli into the blood until equilibrium is reached (Bray *et al.*, 1999).

Surface area available for diffusion

This is determined by the number of alveoli that are receiving both air and blood flow, estimated at between 50 and 90 square metres (Bray *et al.*, 1999). This can be affected by normal physiological factors (e.g. posture) as well as pathological conditions.

Thickness of the alveolar–capillary membrane

The alveolar–capillary membrane lies between the alveoli and pulmonary capillaries. It is normally very thin and allows rapid diffusion of oxygen into the blood. Any conditions that cause an increase in the thickness of the membrane or the distance between the air and the blood will slow down diffusion (Casey, 2001).

The transport of oxygen

About 98.5% of the oxygen that has diffused from the alveolar air into the blood is bound to haemoglobin in the red blood cells and transported as oxyhaemoglobin. The remaining 1.5% is dissolved in blood plasma. At the tissue level, the haemoglobin unloads its oxygen, which diffuses out of the blood capillaries into the interstitial fluid and cells along a pressure gradient. Because the tissue cells are constantly using up oxygen to produce adenosine triphosphate (ATP), the pO_2 in the blood capillaries is higher (100 mmHg) than that of the tissue cells (40 mmHg). This creates a pressure gradient enabling oxygen to diffuse from the capillaries into the interstitial fluid and cells.

The transport of carbon dioxide

Carbon dioxide diffuses out of the cells into the blood along a pressure gradient. The tissue cells are constantly producing carbon dioxide, a by-product of ATP production, making the pCO_2 in the tissue cells (45 mmHg) higher than that in the blood capillaries (40 mmHg) (Tortora, 2005). This causes carbon dioxide to diffuse from the tissue cells via the interstitial fluid into the blood capillaries along a concentration gradient. In the blood, the carbon dioxide is transported in three forms:

- 10% is dissolved in plasma, producing the pCO_2
- 30% is bound with haemoglobin
- 60% is converted to bicarbonate (HO_3) and transported in the plasma.

The carbon dioxide is returned to the right side of the heart by the veins to be pumped to the lungs for another cycle of external respiration (Tortora, 2005).

Section 8: The cardiovascular system

The cardiovascular system consists of the blood, the heart and a closed system of blood vessels. It is responsible for transporting materials (e.g. oxygen, nutrients, waste products), through the medium of blood, to and from the cells. Apart from its transportation functions, the cardiovascular system contributes to hormonal and temperature regulation and protects the body against blood loss from injury and against micro-organisms (Fox, 2004).

The blood

In an average-sized adult, the total volume of blood is 5 litres or 8% of body weight (Fox, 2004). The blood leaving the heart is called arterial blood, and that returning the heart venous blood. Blood consists of the following components:

- *Form elements.* These are the blood cells – erythrocytes, leucocytes and thrombocytes. *Erythrocytes* (red blood cells) lack nuclei and mitochondria and have a lifespan of approximately 120 days. They contain haemoglobin molecules, which are responsible for the transport of oxygen. *Leucocytes* or white blood cells are responsible for protecting the body against micro-organisms. *Thrombocytes* are fragments of cells which play an important role in blood clotting.

- *Plasma.* This is a straw-coloured liquid consisting of water and dissolved solutes such as sodium, various other salts, hormones, enzymes and antibodies. Plasma proteins (e.g. albumin, globulin, fibrinogen and prothrombin) constitute 7–9% of the plasma. Albumin provides the osmotic pressure required to draw fluid from the surrounding tissues back into the capillaries (Fox, 2004).

The heart

The heart is located in the mediastinum, an area in the thoracic cavity between the two lungs. It is about the size of the closed fist. It extends vertically from the second to the fifth intercostal space. The sternum lies anterior to the heart and the thoracic vertebrae lie posterior. The heart can be thought of as an inverted cone, with the tip or apex facing downward towards the fifth intercostal space and the base at the top near the second intercostal space. The major blood vessels (e.g. aorta, pulmonary artery, inferior and superior vena cava, pulmonary veins) enter and exit at the base.

The heart is a four-chambered organ. The two upper chambers are the atria and the two lower chambers are the ventricles. The heart has four valves located in the fibrous septum separating the upper from lower chambers. They open and close in response to pressure changes as the heart contracts and relaxes, and allow blood to flow in one direction only. The tricuspid valve lies between the right atrium and right ventricle, the bicuspid valve is between the left atrium and left ventricle, the pulmonary valve lies in the opening where the pulmonary trunk leaves the right ventricle and the aortic valve is located at the opening between the left ventricle and aorta. Figure 1.13 shows the structure of the heart and direction of flow of blood.

The heart wall

The heart has three layers: an outer layer of pericardium, a middle layer of cardiac muscle (myocardium) and an inner layer of endothelium. The pericardium has two layers: The outer, fibrous pericardium is a loose-fitting sac which surrounds and protects the heart. The serous pericardium forms a double layer around the heart: the parietal and visceral layers. The parietal layer lines the fibrous pericardium whereas the inner visceral layer adheres firmly to the surface of the heart. There is a thin film of fluid (pericardial fluid) between the parietal and visceral pericardium, which reduces friction when the heart contracts. The myocardium is a specialised muscle tissue responsible for the pumping action of the heart. The endocardium is a layer of squamous epithelium that lines the inside of the heart and blood vessels, providing a smooth surface for the flow of blood.

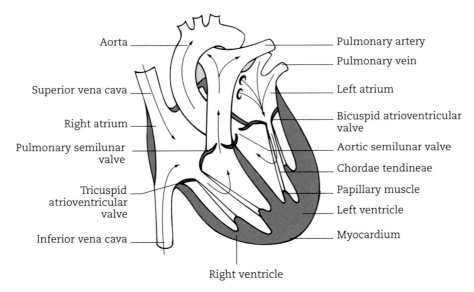

Aorta

Superior vena cava

Right atrium

Pulmonary semilunar
valve

Tricuspid
atrioventricular
valve

Inferior vena cava

Right ventricle

Pulmonary artery

Pulmonary vein

Left atrium

Bicuspid atrioventricular
valve

Aortic semilunar valve

Chordae tendineae

Papillary muscle

Left ventricle

Myocardium

Figure 1.13   The heart (reproduced with permission from Bray *et al.*, 1999)

Blood supply to the heart

The heart receives its circulation from the right and left coronary arteries, which are the first branches of the aorta. The coronary arteries and their branches deliver oxygen and nutrients to the myocardium. Deoxygenated blood is collected by the coronary sinus, which empties into the right atrium.

The conduction system of the heart

The conduction system of the heart (Figure 1.14a) ensures that the atria and ventricles contract in a co-ordinated manner (Tortora, 2005). The sinoatrial (SA) node, or pacemaker, is where the cardiac impulse begins, which then spreads throughout the atria, causing atrial contraction. The impulse then passes to the atrioventricular (AV) node. Here the impulse is delayed slightly, allowing the atria to contract first and emptying the blood into the ventricles. From the AV node, the impulse travels down the bundle of His and Purkinje fibres, which conduct the action potential to the ventricles, causing ventricular contraction. The cardiac control centre in the brain controls the activity of the heart through the autonomic nervous system (ANS). The parasympathetic nerve slows down the rate of firing of the SA node whereas sympathetic activity enhances contractility.

The electrocardiogram (ECG) is a record of the electrical activity that passes through the heart (Tortora, 2005). The P wave represents atrial

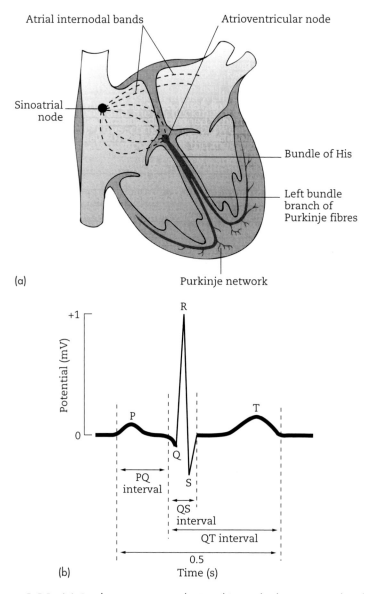

(a)

(b)

Figure 1.14   (a) Conduction system and ECG. (b) Standard ECG (reproduced with permission from Bray et al., 1999)

depolarisation. The PR interval represents the time delay that occurs at the AV node to allow the atria to contract before the ventricles. The QRS complex represents ventricular depolarisation. The T wave is the repolarisation of the ventricles. The TP interval represents the relaxation or diastole of the whole heart. The ECG is shown in Figure 1.14b.

The cardiac cycle

The cardiac cycle or heart beat consists of two phases: systole and diastole (Tortora, 2005). *Systole* refers to the phase of contraction and *diastole* is the period of relaxation. At rest, each cardiac cycle lasts approximately 0.8 seconds (systole lasts 0.3 seconds and diastole 0.5 seconds). Sympathetic and parasympathetic (vagus) nerve fibres to the heart are continuously active and modify the spontaneous depolarisation of the SA node (Fox, 2004). The rate of the cardiac cycle can be measured by palpating the pulse, which is the rhythmic expansion and recoil of the elastic arteries caused by the ejection of blood from the left ventricles (Jamieson *et al.*, 2002).

The heart sounds

The heart sounds are caused by the closure of the valves. When the pressure in the ventricles increases, the bicuspid and tricuspid valves shut and this is when we hear the first heart sound as *lubb*. The second heart sound or *dubb* occurs when the semilunar valves shut at the end of ventricular systole. Heart murmurs are abnormal heart sounds caused by defective valves.

Cardiac output

The volume of blood ejected by the left ventricle per minute is called the cardiac output (CO). It is the product of the heart rate (HR) multiplied by the stroke volume (SV). SV is the amount of blood pumped from each ventricle with each heart beat and is approximately 70 millilitres (ml) per heart beat (Bray *et al.*, 1999). Cardiac output is the volume of blood ejected by the heart per minute (Widmaier *et al.*, 2004). Cardiac output is roughly 5 litres per minute and is calculated as follows:

Cardiac output = HR × SV
$\qquad$ = 70 beats × 70 ml
$\qquad$ = 4900 ml/min

In clinical practice, cardiac output is estimated by measuring the patient's blood pressure and pulse (Casey, 2001).

Blood vessels: arteries, capillaries and veins

The heart pumps blood through a series of large distribution arteries, which subdivide into vessels that become progressively smaller until they finally become arterioles (Thibodeau & Patton, 2004). The arterioles control the flow of blood into microscopic vessels called capillaries where exchange of nutrients and gases takes place between the capillaries and the interstitial fluid. Blood is drained from the capillary beds into venules, which join together to become veins. The inferior and superior vena cavae are the two largest veins that return the blood to the heart.

Blood pressure

Blood pressure (BP) refers to the pressure of blood against the vessel walls (Kindlen, 2003). Systolic BP is the pressure at the peak of ventricular ejection and diastolic pressure is the pressure of blood in the vessels when the heart is not contracting (see also Chapter 6). In the blood vessels, there is a pressure gradient, with the mean pressure in the aorta being 100 mmHg and that in the vena cavae being 0 mmHg. It is this pressure gradient that enables the blood to flow (Thibodeau & Patton, 2004).

Section 9: The lymphatic and immune system

Components

The lymphatic and immune system has the following components (see Table 1.7):

- *Lymphatic vessels.*
- *Lymph.*
- *Lymphatic organs and tissues.* Lymph nodes, thymus, spleen, tonsils.
- *Immune system cells.* Phagocytes (neutrophils, monocytes, macrophages) and lymphocytes (T-lymphocytes and B-lymphocytes).

Functions

The lymphatic and immune system has three primary functions (Tortora, 2005):

- *Draining excess interstitial fluid.* Any excess fluid and protein molecules that cannot return through the blood capillary walls are returned to the blood as lymph.
- *Transporting dietary lipids.* Lymphatic vessels transport lipids that are absorbed through the lacteals of the small intestine.
- *Defence function.* Lymphatic tissue initiates specific responses against micro-organisms and abnormal cells. Two types of lymphocytes participate in specific immune responses and promote the development of immunity against infection: B-lymphocytes and T-lymphocytes. Phagocytes engulf bacteria.

Table 1.7 Components of lymphatic and immune system.

Components	Descriptions	Functions
• Lymph	• Fluid circulating in the lymphatic vessels	• Excess interstitial fluid that cannot be reabsorbed back into the blood capillaries is returned to the circulation as lymph
• Lymphatic vessels	• Begin as lymphatic capillaries located in the spaces between the cells. They join together to form larger vessels and eventually empty the lymph into the subclavian veins	• Vessels that collect excess interstitial fluid and return it to the blood circulation
• Lymph nodes	• Located along the lymphatic vessels. Scattered throughout the body but large concentrations are found near the mammary glands, in the axillae and groins	• Function as a type of filter, trapping and destroying foreign substances
• Thymus	• Located in the thoracic cavity. Grows during childhood but regresses in adulthood	• Transforms lymphocytes into T-cells
• Spleen	• Largest single mass of lymphatic tissue; located in the left hypochondriac region between the stomach and diaphragm	• Filters blood. Destroys bloodborne pathogens by phagocytosis
• Phagocytes	• Neutrophils, monocytes and macrophages	• Ingest and destroy bacteria, cellular debris, denatured proteins and toxins
• Complement proteins	• Immune proteins found in the plasma and other body fluids in inactive state, activated by attachments of antigens or antibodies	• Promote destruction of bacteria; enhance inflammatory response
• B-lymphocytes	• Produced by stem cells in the bone marrow	• When exposed to specific antigens, B-lymphocytes form specific antibodies against them
• T-lymphocytes	There are three types: • Killer or cytotoxic cells • Helper T-cells • Suppressor T-cells	• Effect cell-mediated destruction of specific victim cells • Both helper and suppressor T-cells regulate the responses of B-cells and killer T-cells

Section 10: The digestive system

Functions

The body requires nutrients for anabolism (i.e. building up of new tissues) and energy production. The digestive system consists of a number of organs whose functions are to get nutrients into the body by the following processes (Tortora, 2005):

- *Ingestion (or eating).* This involves taking food and liquids into the mouth.
- *Digestion.* The process of breaking down food into smaller components to enable absorption into the circulation. *Mechanical* digestion is the breaking down of food into smaller pieces. *Chemical* digestion is the breakdown of carbohydrate, fats and proteins by digestive enzymes into their individual components.
- *Absorption.* This is the passage of nutrients, fluids and ions through the epithelial lining of the digestive tract into the blood and lymph circulation.
- *Defaecation.* This is the process by which wastes, indigestible substances, bacteria and cells shed by the digestive tract leave the body through the anus.

Organs of the digestive system and their location

The digestive system (Figure 1.15a) consists of two groups of organs (Tortora, 2005):

- *The digestive tract.* This is a continuous tube that extends from the mouth to the anus and includes the mouth, pharynx, oesophagus, stomach, small intestine, large intestine, rectum and anus.
- *The accessory organs of digestion*, consisting of the teeth, tongue, salivary glands, liver, gall bladder and pancreas.

To describe the location of the abdominal organs precisely, the abdominal cavity can be divided into four quadrants (as shown in Figure 1.15b) by one horizontal and one vertical line crossing at the umbilicus. The quadrants are: right upper quadrant, left upper quadrant, right lower quadrant and left lower quadrant. The quadrants are commonly used in assessment to describe the site of abdominal pain, mass or other abnormality.

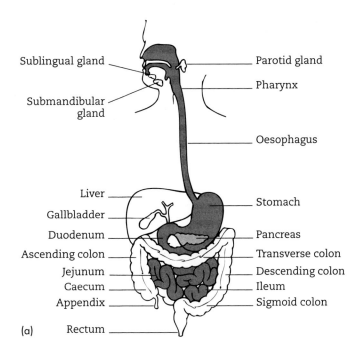

Sublingual gland

Submandibular gland

Parotid gland

Pharynx

Oesophagus

Liver

Gallbladder

Duodenum

Ascending colon

Jejunum

Caecum

Appendix

Rectum

Stomach

Pancreas

Transverse colon

Descending colon

Ileum

Sigmoid colon

(a)

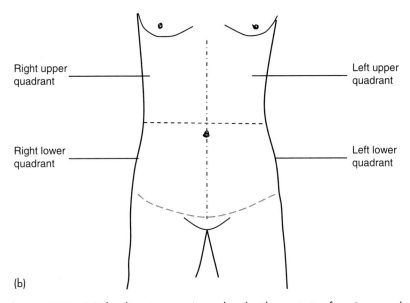

Right upper quadrant

Right lower quadrant

Left upper quadrant

Left lower quadrant

(b)

Figure 1.15 (a) The digestive tract (reproduced with permission from Bray *et al.*, 1999). (b) The abdominal quadrants

Table 1.8a Organs of the digestive system and their functions.

Organs	Special features	Functions
• Mouth (oral cavity)	• Teeth, tongue • Tongue • Salivary glands	• Mastication and chewing of food • Formation of bolus • Lubrication of food. Digestion of cooked starch
• Pharynx (oro and laryngo pharynx)	• Pharyngeal muscles • Soft palate • Epiglottis	• Swallowing • Common passage for food and air • Rises on swallowing to prevent entry of food into nasopharynx • Flap which prevent entry of food into larynx during swallowing
• Oesophagus	 • Cardiac sphincter	• Swallowing • Conveys food from pharynx to stomach by peristalsis • Prevents regurgitation of food from the stomach
• Stomach	• Three layers of smooth muscle • Pepsin • Pyloric sphincter	• Churning of food into a liquid called chyme • Digestion of proteins • Allows release of small amount of chyme at a time into the duodenum
• Small intestine (duodenum, jejunum and ileum) • Large intestine or colon	• Intestinal glands, villi	• Produce intestinal enzymes for digestion of food • Absorption of food • Absorption of water and electrolytes • Production of vitamin K by colonic bacteria • Storage of non-digestible remains
• Anus and rectum	• Internal and external sphincters	• Increase in rectal pressure by faecal content in rectum gives the urge to defaecate (Fox, 2004) • Defaecation

Table 1.8b Accessory organs of digestion.

Organs	Functions
• Liver	• Conversion and storage of glucose as glycogen • Destruction of worn-out red blood cells • Production of bile • Production of plasma proteins • Production of clotting factors • Production of urea from ammonia produced by deamination of amino acids • Storage of fat-soluble vitamins A, D, E and K • Chemical alteration of biologically active molecules such as hormones and drugs (Fox, 2004)
• Gall bladder	• Storage of bile, required for emulsification of dietary fats
• Pancreas	• Produces pancreatic juice, which contains digestive enzymes for carbohydrate, proteins and fats • Also an endocrine gland, producing primarily insulin and glucagon

Activity	
List the digestive organs located in the four abdominal quadrants.	

Quadrant	Organs
Right upper	
Left upper	
Right lower	
Left lower	

General plan of the digestive tract

From the oesophagus to the anus, the digestive tract has the same basic four-layered arrangement of tissues, although the layers are modified according to the special functions of each part of the digestive tract. The four layers, from the inside out, are as follows:

- The *mucosa* is the inner, epithelial lining of the tract.
- The *submucosa* is a connective tissue layer containing many blood and lymphatic vessels. It also contains the enteric nervous system, responsible for controlling gastrointestinal tract secretions and motility.
- The *smooth muscle* is arranged as an inner sheet of circular muscle and outer sheet of longitudinal muscle. Alternating contraction and relaxation of the smooth muscle (or peristalsis) allow mixing and movement of food along the digestive tract.
- The *serosa* is the outermost connective tissue layer of the digestive tract.

The peritoneum

The organs of the digestive system from below the diaphragm are covered by a double-layered serous membrane called the peritoneum. The visceral peritoneum covers the organs whereas the parietal peritoneum lines the abdominal cavity. The space between the two membranes is called the peritoneal cavity. *Peritonitis* is an acute inflammation of the peritoneum (Tortora, 2005).

The functions of the digestive and accessory organs are described in Tables 1.8a and 1.8b.

Section 11: The urinary system

The urinary system disposes of unwanted substances formed as a result of metabolic functions. It consists of the following organs (also see Figure 1.16a):

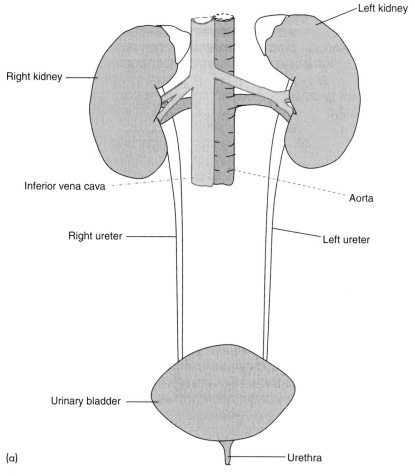

Figure 1.16(a) The urinary tract system

- kidneys (2)
- ureters (2)
- urinary bladder (1)
- urethra (1).

The kidney and its functions

The kidneys lie retroperitoneally on either side of the vertebral column. Internally, the kidneys have three regions: cortex, medulla and renal pelvis. Urine is produced by the nephrons (Figure 1.16b), the functional units of the kidneys, and is drained in the renal pelvis. The renal pelvis connects with the ureter, which conveys the urine to the bladder.

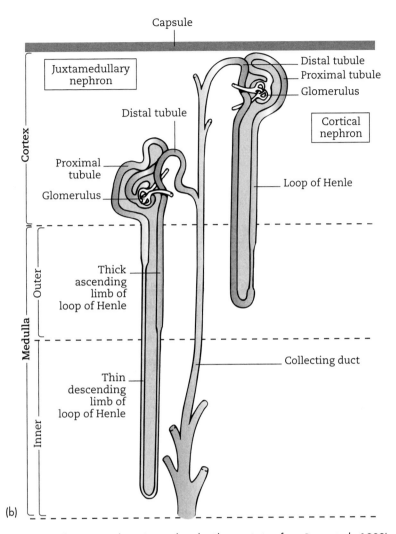

Figure 1.16(b)   A nephron (reproduced with permission from Bray *et al.*, 1999)

The blood supply to the kidneys is via the two renal arteries. The kidneys receive approximately 25% of cardiac output at rest per minute. The two renal veins drain blood from the kidneys. The overall functions of the kidneys are:

- regulation of electrolyte or ion levels in the body fluid
- regulation of blood volume
- regulation of blood pressure
- regulation of blood pH
- excretion of waste products (urea, uric acid, creatinine)
- production of hormones (e.g. erythropoietin, rennin and calcitriol).

Table 1.9 Processes in urine formation.

Processes	Functions
• Filtration	• Occurs in the glomeruli. Blood pressure (filtration pressure) forces water, nutrients, ions and waste products across the wall of the glomerular capillaries, forming the glomerular filtrate. Only molecules of certain molecular size can pass through the filtration membrane into the tubule. Large molecules such as blood cells and plasma proteins stay in the blood circulation. If they are found in the urine, they may indicate damage to the filtration membrane. In severe *hypotension*, filtration stops, leading to *acute renal failure*
• Reabsorption	• Occurs in the convoluted tubule. All nutrients and most ions as well as 99% of the water are reabsorbed back into the circulation. *Antidiuretic hormone (ADH)* regulates water absorption by negative feedback. *Aldosterone* regulates sodium reabsorption
• Secretion	• Transport of materials from the blood into the tubular fluid. These include hydrogen ions, potassium, ammonia, urea and creatinine

Processes in urine formation

Three basic processes are involved in the formation of urine by the nephrons: glomerular filtration, tubular reabsorption and tubular secretion. These are described in Table 1.9.

The passage of urine

Urine is produced by the kidneys at the rate of 1 ml per minute and is conveyed by peristaltic action by the ureters to the urinary bladder. Up to 600 ml of urine can be stored in the bladder. The bladder is a hollow muscular organ, lying in the pelvic cavity. A combination of voluntary and involuntary muscle contractions, involving both the autonomic and voluntary nervous systems, enables urine to be expelled by the bladder into the urethra. This process is termed *micturition, urination* or *voiding* (Tortora, 2005). *Incontinence* is an inability to control micturition.

Section 12: The reproductive system

The reproductive system produces sex cells or gametes (sperm cell in male and ovum in female) as well as sex hormones, which are necessary for the development of secondary sexual characteristics. The accessory reproductive organs (e.g. the penis and vagina) assist in the delivery and joining of the gametes necessary for fertilisation (Tortora, 2005).

Female reproductive system

The female reproductive system (Figure 1.17) consists of the:

- ovaries
- uterine (fallopian) tubes
- uterus
- vagina
- external organs (vulva)
- mammary glands or breasts (considered part of reproductive system).

The organs and functions of female reproductive system are given in Table 1.10.

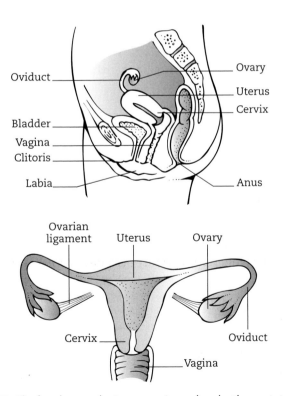

Figure 1.17   The female reproductive system (reproduced with permission from Bray *et al.*, 1999)

Table 1.10 Organs and functions of the female reproductive system.

Organs	Description	Functions
• Ovaries	• Paired organs, one on each side of upper pelvic cavity, containing sac-like structures called follicles in the cortex	• Produce ovum or egg and sex hormones, including oestrogen. Responsible for ovarian and uterine cycles (menstrual cycle)
• Two uterine tubes	• Extend from the uterus to the ovaries. Each tube measures 10–11.5 cm and is divided into 4 parts, namely the interstitial portion, the isthmus, ampulla and infundibulum (part with finger-like projections called fimbrae one of which is attached to the ovary)	• Transport ovum from ovaries to uterus. The sites where fertilisation occurs
• Uterus or womb	• Thick-walled, hollow, muscular, pear-shaped organ, lying above the urinary bladder. The uterine tubes join the uterus anteriorly. It has a fundus (top part), body of uterus and cervix (narrow portion that opens into the vagina). It has 3 layers: the endometrium (lining), myometrium (middle muscular coat) and perimetrium (outer layer of peritoneum)	• Site of implantation of fertilised ovum. Development of the embryo/foetus during pregnancy
• Vagina	• A tube that extends from the exterior of the body to the uterine cervix	• Receives penis during sexual intercourse and serves as birth canal
• Vulva (external genital organs)	• Consists of: *Mons pubis:* fat pad over the symphysis pubis; covered by pubic hair *Labia majora:* two folds of skin extending from the mons pubis to the perineum; contains adipose tissue, sebaceous and sweat glands; covered by pubic hair *Labia minora:* two folds of skin located inside the labia majora; contains numerous sebaceous glands *Clitoris:* located at the anterior end of labia minora *The vestibule:* the region between the labia minora containing the openings of the urethra and vagina to the exterior and mucus glands	• The vestibule contains the vaginal orifice inferiorly and external urethral orifice superiorly
• Mammary glands (breasts)	• Paired organs lying over the pectoralis major and serratus anterior muscles. Contain modified sudoriferous glands. Each mammary gland consists of 15–20 lobes. In each lobe are smaller lobules, which contain milk-secreting glands (alveoli). The nipple is the pigmented projection from each breast and has a series of openings or ducts where milk emerges	• Produce, secrete and eject milk for nourishment of newborn

The male reproductive organs

The male reproductive system (Figure 1.18) consists of:

- the testes
- a system of ducts (e.g. seminiferous tubules, vas deferens, ejaculatory duct and urethra)
- accessory sex glands (e.g. seminal vesicles, prostate and bulbourethral gland)
- supporting structures (e.g. scrotum and penis).

The organs and functions of male reproductive system are given in Table 1.11.

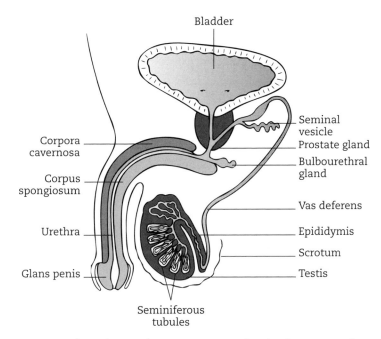

Figure 1.18 The male reproductive system (reproduced with permission from Bray *et al.*, 1999)

Table 1.11 Male reproductive organs.

Organs	Location	Function
• Testes (paired oval glands)	• Scrotum – a pouch outside the abdominal cavity	• Produce sperm and the male sex hormones (testoterone and androgen)
• Epididymis	• Testes (in scrotum)	• Stores sperm as they mature
• Vas deferens	• Scrotum, inguinal canal and pelvic cavity	• Transports and stores sperm
• Seminal vesicle	• Posterior to the base of urinary bladder	• Produces an alkaline secretion
• Prostate	• Lies inferior to the urinary bladder and surrounds the upper portion of urethra	• Secretes a milky, slightly acidic fluid that contains citric acid
• Bulbourethral (Cowper's) glands	• Inferior to the prostate on either side of the urethra	• Secrete an alkaline substance
• Ejaculatory ducts	• Formed by the union of the seminal vesicles and vas deferens	• Eject sperm into the urethra
• Urethra	• Passes through the prostate and penis	• Passageway of both semen and urine
• Penis	• Attached to the pubic arch by ligaments	• Contains urethra and is the passageway to the ejaculation of semen (mixture of sperm and secretions of Sertoli cells, seminal vesicles, prostate and Cowper's glands)

Summary

In this chapter, it was emphasised that a good understanding of body structure and function is important for effective health assessment. The contribution of each organ system in the maintenance of homeostasis was explained. It was pointed out that disease occurs as a result of breakdown in homeostasis. When performing a health assessment, it is important to identify not only what findings are abnormal but also what impact these may have on body functions. Monitoring and management of physiological problems are also dependent on sound biological knowledge. To enable a systematic method of health assessment, a body system approach is proposed whereby each organ system is assessed in order to identify the patient's problems. This approach will be further explained in Chapter 3 when discussing the taking of a health history and in Chapter 6 when covering physical assessment.

Activity

- Explain how changes in the normal structure of the body can affect body functions.
- Discuss the homeostatic functions of each organ system.
- The skin is often described as a window for many internal disorders. With reference to some specific internal disorders, discuss the changes that may occur in the skin.

References

Bray, J J, Cragg, P A, Macknight, A D C & Mills, R G (1999) *Lecture Notes on Human Physiology*, 4th edition. Blackwell Science, Oxford.

Carroll, L (2004) Clinical skills for nurses in medical assessment units. *Nursing Standard* 18 (42): 33–40.

Casey, G (2001) Oxygen transport and the use of pulse oximetry. *Nursing Standard* 15 (47): 46–55.

Casey, G (2002) Physiology of the skin. *Nursing Standard* 16 (34): 47–51.

Ellis, H (2002) *Clinical Anatomy: a revision of applied anatomy for clinical students*, 10th edition. Blackwell Publishing, Oxford.

Fox, S T (2004) *Human Physiology*, 8th edition. McGraw-Hill, Boston.

Jamieson, E M, McCall, J M & Whyte, L A (2002) *Clinical Nursing Practice*, 4th edition. Churchill Livingstone, Edinburgh.

Kindlen, S (2003) The cardiovascular circulatory system. In: Kindlen, S (ed.) *Physiology for Health Care and Nursing*, 2nd edition. Churchill Livingstone, Edinburgh.

McBean, D E (2003) Vision. In: Kindlen, S (ed.) *Physiology for Health Care and Nursing*, 2nd edition. Churchill Livingstone, Edinburgh.

Porth, C M (2005) Pathophysiology. In: *Concepts of Altered Health States*, 5th edition. Lippincott, Philadelphia.

Thibodeau, G A & Patton, K T (2004) *Structure and Function of the Body*, 12th edition. Mosby, St Louis.

Tortora, G J (2005) *Principles of Human Anatomy*, 10th edition. Wiley, New York.

Tortora, G J & Grabowski, S R (2004) *Introduction to the Human Body: the essentials of anatomy and physiology*, 6th edition. Wiley, New York.

Widmaier, E P, Raff, H & Strang, K T (2004) *Human Physiology: the mechanics of body function*, 9th edition. McGraw-Hill, Boston.

Nursing assessment and care planning

J. Aldridge, A. Eshun and C. Meurier

Learning objectives

- Describe the five stages of the nursing process.
- Identify subjective and objective data in an assessment.
- Discuss how you will use the subjective and objective data in the process of diagnosis and identifying the client's problems.
- Describe the four components of a nursing model.
- Explain how nursing frameworks/models can be used as a tool of assessment in various fields of nursing.
- Discuss the role of integrated care pathways in assessment and care delivery.
- Discuss the essential features of the Eshun–Smith model of nursing and its application for care of the older person.

Introduction

A health assessment is the collection and analysis of data in order to identify the client's problems. We perform assessments on our clients to make professional judgements about what care is required. Assessment takes place from the time we encounter the client and will be ongoing and continuous until discharge. Nurses use various tools to facilitate the process of assessment. For a holistic assessment, nurses commonly apply a nursing framework or model to organise the data obtained from a health assessment. The body systems approach is used to identify medical problems. This chapter will explore the concept of health assessment, with particular reference to the nursing process, the use of integrated care pathways and the application of frameworks or models in the collection and organisation of assessment data.

Nursing assessment and the nursing process

The nursing process is commonly described as a systematic problem-solving cycle, consisting of 4–5 interrelated steps or stages. For the purposes of this chapter we intend to adopt the five-stage model of nursing process (Hogston, 2002), with particular emphasis on the stages of assessment and diagnosis. The five stages are as follows:

- *Assessment.* Gathering data about the individual and their health, finding out about them and the influences on their health.
- *Nursing diagnosis.* Analysing the assessment data and deciding on the number and nature of problems.

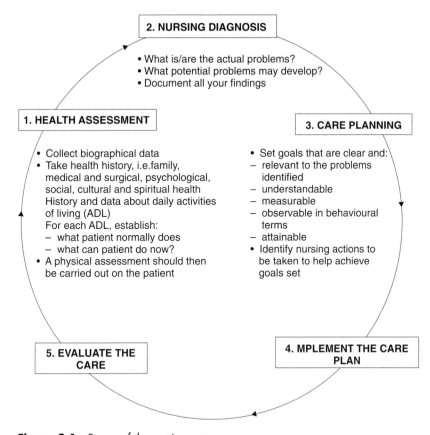

2. NURSING DIAGNOSIS
- What is/are the actual problems?
- What potential problems may develop?
- Document all your findings

1. HEALTH ASSESSMENT
- Collect biographical data
- Take health history, i.e.family, medical and surgical, psychological, social, cultural and spiritual health History and data about daily activities of living (ADL)
  For each ADL, establish:
  – what patient normally does
  – what can patient do now?
- A physical assessment should then be carried out on the patient

3. CARE PLANNING
- Set goals that are clear and:
  – relevant to the problems identified
  – understandable
  – measurable
  – observable in behavioural terms
  – attainable
- Identify nursing actions to be taken to help achieve goals set

5. EVALUATE THE CARE

4. MPLEMENT THE CARE PLAN

Figure 2.1 Stages of the nursing process

- *Care planning.* Deciding how to address the individual's health problems in order to achieve optimum health and well-being. Setting outcomes for nursing care.
- *Implementation.* Carrying out the nursing care plan properly, skilfully and consistently.
- *Evaluation.* Revisiting the nursing outcomes, deciding on the extent to which they have been achieved and then adjusting the care plans as necessary.

Subjective and objective data

Assessment is the first and critical step of the nursing process. It should be as systematic, objective and 'scientific' as possible and aimed at obtaining as much accurate and relevant information or data about the individual as we possibly can, both on the initial encounter with the individual and also as a continuous process. Inadequate or inaccurate data may lead to omissions and/or incorrect judgements.

Two types of data are collected from the client: subjective and objective. *Subjective* data are obtained from the health history and relate to sensations or symptoms (e.g. pain, shortness of breath, anxiety). *Objective* data are observable data and relate to the signs of disease or disorder; they are obtained from physical examinations and measurements (e.g. blood pressure, urine output, aggression). Subjective and objective data complement and clarify each other. However, there may be situations when what you observe contradicts what the client is stating. This will necessitate further enquiries and investigations to understand the problem more fully.

Activity Subjective and objective data – scenario

Mr Ward is 68 years old. He is admitted to the ward with acute exacerbation of his chronic bronchitis. On assessment, Mr Ward states that he feels very breathless and finds it difficult to sleep because of persistent coughing. He also complains of feeling very tired and he is anxious about the outcome. His temperature is 39.5°C. His pulse is 110 beats per minute. Respiration is 22 and BP 140/90. He is producing copious greenish-coloured sputum. His chest X-ray reveals patchy consolidation of both lungs.

- List the subjective data noted in the scenario.
- List the objective data noted in the scenario.

In gathering assessment information, we may need to use several of the following approaches and techniques.

Interview the patient/client

Increasingly, nurses are being encouraged to take a person-centred approach to care planning (DoH, 1997, 2001a). This is particularly emphasised for learning disability through the White Paper *Valuing People* (DoH, 2001b) and for other patient groups through National Service Frameworks (DoH, 2001d). Ford & McCormack (2000) point out that although there is much progress to be made, a person-centred approach to nursing care is achievable provided that we seek to understand the individual's health aspirations and needs. Clearly, in order to do this we need to develop an empathic relationship based upon a therapeutic approach which entails more than a superficial encounter with the person (McMahon, 1998). Some of the questions that we might ask in our nursing assessment are likely to be searching and intimate and it may be difficult for the individual to disclose these details to a stranger in perhaps a strange environment. For some individuals the situation may be emotionally charged. They may be tearful, angry or anxious and in such a case, we would need to show that we appreciate and understand how they are feeling. Also see Chapter 5.

Interview the individual's relatives or a significant other person

In some cases the individual referred for healthcare may not easily be able to answer our assessment questions or may only be able to give partial answers. People in this category may include elderly confused people, very young children, people who have severe and profound learning disabilities, people with some mental illnesses and people whose consciousness is impaired (see Chapters 4 and 5). In such cases, you may need to interview another person on the individual's behalf. Such a person would need to know the individual well and would need to have the time and motivation to answer your questions. In some cases, the 'significant other' will be able to add to what the individual has told you but there may be some occasions where you have to rely entirely on this single source of information. At such times, you may need to remember that:

- the significant other is giving you their perception of the facts
- they may not know the answer and may guess, without telling you that they are doing so
- they may be unintentionally wrong in what they tell you
- they may have ulterior motives for giving you false information.

Relatives' and significant others' information therefore needs to be supported and triangulated by your own observations and/or written records if possible.

Collecting objective data

Collection of objective data takes place through the use of direct observation and the sense of touch. The use of most of the other senses, e.g. sense of hearing and smell, is however also important (see Chapter 5).

Use of measurement tools and scales or questionnaires

Dependent on the nursing specialty and the needs of the patient/client, the nurse may use a number of measurement tools that range from the simple to the complex, including the means to measure as objectively as possible psychosocial aspects of the individual's health. For instance:

- *'Low tech'*. Ruler or tape to measure the size of skin lesions, pupil gauge to measure relative pupil dilation, wristwatch to time pulse, breathing and other bodily events.
- *'Medium tech'*. Sphygmomanometer, electronic thermometer, auroscope, ophthalmoscope.
- *'High tech'*. ECG machine, TPR monitor, O_2 saturation monitor, glucometer.
- *Simple scales.* Height and weight charts for adults and children, BMI calculation, Glasgow Coma Scale.
- *Complex scales and questionnaires.* Pain assessment tools, anxiety scales, depression scales, psychiatric symptom scales.

Reference to medical and other records

Most individuals will be registered with a general practitioner (GP) and, with the increasing use of electronic data storage and access, these records may be easily accessible to the nurse. Some individuals will have been known to health services for a considerable time, especially if they have a chronic or complex health condition. It is likely in such cases that there will be records of previous consultations and admissions. Individuals who are in full-time care will have their own records, kept by their care organisation. If this organisation is a nursing home or NHS health trust, the records are likely to contain elements familiar to any nurse. In all cases, when accessing written past records remember that these may not necessarily be completely accurate and that what may have been recorded four or five years ago may not be true today. Again, there is a need to try to confirm or triangulate written data and to reassess as appropriate.

Use of the wider nursing and multidisciplinary team

Although the primary nurse will be chiefly responsible for the nursing assessment of the patient/client, the observations and skills of other members of the nursing and multidisciplinary team will be helpful. Indeed, the Nursing and Midwifery Council (NMC, 2004a) emphasises the need for nurses to work collaboratively with the patient/client and multidisciplinary team at all stages of the care planning cycle. This is reinforced and supported by the Department of Health papers *Making A Difference* (DoH, 1999) and *The NHS Plan* (DoH, 2001a), which discuss the need for nurses to 'work in new ways'. Such new working includes collaboration with other agencies and professionals and members of the public, as well as an extended assessment role for nurses. The National Service Framework for Older People (DoH, 2001d) requires a single assessment process of both health and social care needs (DoH, 2001c; Wild, 2002), the aim being to enable the exchange of confidential information and to avoid duplication of assessments.

The use of integrated care pathways by healthcare providers also enables a single record of assessment and care. An integrated care pathway (ICP) is a map or predetermined plan of care for a group of patients with a particular diagnoses or set of symptoms (e.g. ICP for acute myocardial infarction, hip replacement). Until integrated care pathways or single assessment processes become universal, it seems likely that nurses and other professionals will need to develop and maintain their own assessments and records. However, nurses may extend and consolidate their assessments by working collaboratively with other professionals. Rather than these professionals' assessments being alternative or parallel to nursing assessment, there is great opportunity for 'cross-fertilisation' and each professional is likely to learn from the other's perspective. The following are examples of ways in which the multidisciplinary team may help to provide extra layers of detail in nursing assessments and care planning:

- *Physiotherapists.* Assessment of movement, mobility and positioning.
- *Occupational therapists.* Assessment of the need for aids and adaptations to increase independence in activities of daily living.
- *Speech and language therapists.* Assessment of communication skills and needs, assessment of swallowing and dysphagia.
- *Psychologists.* Extensive assessment of emotional and cognitive elements of the individual's health.
- *Dieticians.* Detailed assessment of diet and nutritional status.
- *Social workers.* Housing, living circumstances, use of community facilities, benefits.

Validation, organisation and documentation of the data

Once the subjective and objective data have been collected, they need to be verified or validated to ensure that they are accurate and complete. Areas where data are missing are identified and remedied. The data are then clustered into groups of information, enabling you to get a clear picture of the health status of the client.

Nurses find it helpful to organise the data according to a nursing model to maintain a holistic approach and to enable the identification of nursing diagnoses and problems. If the aim is to identify a medical problem, then the body systems approach should be used as medical problems are often caused by malfunction of an organ or body system.

However, to obtain comprehensive information on both the medical and nursing problems, Alfaro-LeFevre (2002) suggests the use of both medical (body systems) and nursing models. Documentation of the data is a crucial step of assessment, forming the database required for analysis as well as continuity of care. Abnormal findings must also be reported to allow urgent problems to be dealt with appropriately.

Nursing diagnosis

The second stage of the problem-solving cycle is that of nursing diagnosis. Nursing diagnosis, which is different from medical diagnosis, aims to identify the problems that the individual is experiencing for which the nurse can offer interventions. Conversely, medical diagnosis aims to identify the individual's disease/disorder so that the doctor can treat it. The assessment stage of the cycle provides us with a potentially large amount of information about the individual. Gordon (2000, p29) argued that 'Collecting information is pointless if the meaning behind it is not derived'. To arrive at a nursing diagnosis or problem formulation, further steps such as clustering of the data, interpretation and analysis are required. The use of a conceptual framework or model enables the clustering of the data. The process of nursing diagnosis (shown in Table 2.1) enables a range of problems to be identified:

- *Actual problem*, i.e. the problem has already occurred. The patient/client is seeking help because of that problem. This includes their medical problem, such as asthma, and/or any nursing problem such as inability to wash themselves.
- *Potential problem*, i.e. the problem is not present yet but will occur if certain steps are not taken.
- *Collaborative problem*, i.e. a problem which requires the expertise of another member of the multidisciplinary team.
- *Social problem*, i.e. the individual's home circumstances may delay/prevent discharge.

Health assessment should not only be systematic, it should also be carried out in a holistic manner.

The holistic approach to assessment

Holism implies that for every human activity there are biological, psychological, social, cultural and spiritual influences. For example, Mary is 78 years old, recently widowed and living in her own home following rehabilitation for a minor cerebrovascular accident (stroke). She eats very little and is losing weight.

We might explain this behaviour by exploring a range of biopsychosocial, cultural and spiritual influences, as follows.

Table 2.1 Identification of problems and the range of actions to be taken.

Nursing diagnoses and actions		Shared problems and difficulties		Non-nursing problems and difficulties	
Type of problem	**Action**	**Type of problem**	**Action**	**Type of problem**	**Action**
• Actual problems and difficulties	• Plan to ameliorate or cure the problem as quickly as possible	• Actual or potential problems with activities of living that require the expertise of other professionals	• Refer to relevant professional and develop joint care plan	• Social difficulties that influence the individual's health	• Refer to social worker, spiritual advisor, voluntary organisation, housing office, etc.
• *Example:* the individual is unable to give himself drinks	• Write care plan with outcome 'John will be helped to drink at least ¼ litre of fluid at mealtimes'				
• Potential problems and difficulties	• Plan to prevent the problem actually occurring	• *Example:* the individual is underweight	• Refer to dietician and develop joint care plan with outcome 'John will maintain a body weight of . . . kg'	• *Example:* the individual will not be able to live independently after discharge	• Refer to care manager to arrange a place in residential care
• *Example:* the individual is at risk of developing a pressure sore	• Write care plan with outcome 'John will be free from pressure sores'				

Biological
- Is she in pain? Are there problems with chronic constipation, indigestion/dyspepsia, sore mouth, teeth/dentures?
- How physically able is she to take food from the plate and convey it to her mouth? Does she have the physical strength and co-ordination to carry out this activity?
- Does she experience dysphagia (difficulty in swallowing)?
- How hungry is she at mealtimes?

Psychological
- Does she enjoy her meals? Does she like the food?
- Is she able to choose the meals she eats?
- Is she motivated to eat or persist with meals?
- Is she low in mood, can't see the point in eating?
- Has she lost the will to live?
- Does she become confused and forget to finish meals?

Social
- Are there professional or family carers with the skills and time to help her with meals?
- Does anyone encourage her to finish meals?
- Is she able to produce appetising meals?
- Can she afford to feed herself properly?
- Is her home organised so that she can easily prepare meals?
- Is she able to shop for food?

Cultural
- What is her cultural background and what are her beliefs about illness?
- Is her behaviour influenced by her cultural beliefs, if any?

Spiritual
- Does Mary see herself as being at the end of her life and wanting to die?
- What gives meaning to her life?
- Who does she normally turn to when she is ill?
- Has she got any spiritual beliefs; If so, is her behaviour influenced by such beliefs?

Conceptual models of nursing

Clearly the range of biopsychosocial, cultural and spiritual questions one might ask in assessment is large and complex and there is a need for a systematic approach to the process of investigation into patients'/clients' health needs. Nursing models provide us with a structure for assessing and understanding individuals and their health and most are based upon a view of the individual as a holistic entity.

A nursing model helps in the generation of knowledge for use in nursing practice; the nursing process is a method of applying the knowledge. The range of nursing models is now very large and diverse.

Definition of conceptual models and components

> '*Conceptual models are made up of concepts, which are words describing mental images of phenomena, and propositions, which are statements expressing the relations between concepts. A conceptual model, therefore, is designed as a set of concepts and the statements that integrate them into a meaningful configuration*' (Fawcett, 1984: p2).

All nursing models, to varying degree, have similarities in terms of focusing on four common concepts, sometimes referred to as *meta-paradigms* (Fawcett, 1984):

- *Person.* The person is the recipient of care and has multidimensional needs, hence requiring an individualised approach to care.
- *Health.* This is subject to different interpretations by the client and healthcare professionals. The goal of nursing is to provide care that is individualised to the healthcare needs of the client.
- *Environment.* This refers to the social factors affecting the client as well as the setting in which care is delivered.
- *Nursing.* Nurses assess the impact of a disorder on a client and provide individualised care to meet the holistic healthcare needs of the client.

Types of conceptual model
There is a range of conceptual nursing models that can be used to organise (or cluster) data obtained from a nursing assessment. For instance, data related to a particular component of the model are grouped together, making it easier to interpret the data and establish relationships. Nursing models not only specify the focus of nursing but also identify areas where nurses can intervene independently with nursing interventions. Table 2.2 shows some components in three assessment frameworks or nursing models that can be used to organise (or cluster) the data obtained from a health assessment.

Nurses select models that best reflect their philosophy and the specialist needs of their client groups as follows.

Adult nursing
The range of conceptual models developed for use in adult nursing is potentially very large but in the UK, the most frequently used models include the following:

- *The Roper, Logan and Tierney model of nursing (2000).* This is by far the most widely used model in adult nursing in the UK. It has five components or concepts: activities of living (ALs) (as shown in

Table 2.2 Use of nursing models of care for organising assessment data.

Activities of Living (Roper et al., 2000)	Orem's Self-Care (Orem, 2001)	Health Functional Patterns (Gordon, 2000)
• Maintaining a safe environment • Communicating • Breathing • Eating and drinking • Eliminating • Personal cleansing and dressing • Controlling body temperature • Mobilising • Working and playing • Expressing sexuality • Sleeping • Dying	Universal self-care requisites • The maintenance of air, water, food, elimination, activity, rest and solitude, social interaction, prevention of hazards and promotion of human functioning Developmental self-care requisites • Promote processes for life and maturation • Prevent conditions that are deleterious to maturation Health deviation self-care requisites • Disease and injuries affecting structures and physiological and psychological mechanisms	• Health perception/health management • Nutritional/metabolic • Elimination • Activity/exercise • Sexuality/reproductive • Sleep/rest • Cognitive/perceptual • Role/relationship • Self-perception/self-concept • Coping/stress • Value/belief

Table 2.2), lifespan, dependence/independence continuum, factors influencing the ALs, and individuality in living.

- *Orem's (2001) self-care model.* This model emphasises the individual's need to care for themselves and the way in which illness or disability creates self-care deficits. It is particularly relevant for use in rehabilitation settings and has also been adapted for use by other branches of nursing.
- *Eshun–Smith model (1999).* This is an adaptation of a number of adult nursing models aimed at meeting the specific needs of elderly patients/clients during rehabilitation. Self-care is a core concept in this model, which will be discussed further later.
- *Standex assessment package.* This is an assessment framework based on the activities of living model (Roper *et al.*, 2000) and a psychological assessment. It is designed for use in nursing/care homes so that data can be collected and recorded in a methodical and structured manner, and to help practitioners to meet the requirements of the Care Standards Act 2003.

Children's nursing
There is a much smaller range of models that have been specifically developed for use in children's nursing and many nurses use

adaptations of adult nursing models. The following is of particular relevance:

- *Casey's (1993) partnership model.* This emphasises the way in which children's nurses work to support families in the care of the child. It is an adaptation of Orem's model (2001).

Mental health nursing
Roper *et al.*'s (2000) model or some adaptations of it are commonly used in mental health nursing. However, the following models have been developed with mental health nursing in mind:

- *Peplau's (1991) interpersonal model* explores the phases in the therapeutic relationship between the nurse and the patient and also analyses the different roles the nurse may play in that relationship.
- *Barker (2001)* put forward the concept of the tidal model, which explores the experience of the relationship between the nurse and the patient.

Learning disability nursing
Many practitioners in this branch of nursing tend to use an adaptation of Roper *et al.*'s (2000) and Orem's models of nursing.

- *The Ecology of Health Model* (Aldridge, 2003a, 2003b) deals with the biopsychosocial influences on health and specifically relates to the needs of people with learning disabilities.

The Eshun–Smith model for the older person
In this section, the Eshun–Smith model (1999) is described in some detail to demonstrate how it has been developed as a framework for specific assessment and care planning of the older person requiring rehabilitation. The overall aim of the model is to improve the quality of life of older patients by assisting them to regain the basic skills of daily living that may have been lost through illness. The central theme of the model is the self-concept or the ability to care for oneself and the promotion of a positive nurse–patient interaction, based on respect for the older patient and promotion of their dignity.

Figure 2.2 depicts the model and shows how patients are cared for from admission through the stages of assessment, planning, implementation and evaluation of care up to the time of discharge. It focuses on the importance of the nurse and patient working as partners in the belief that this encourages the patient to share in the desire for effective rehabilitation. The promotion of patient self-esteem is another focus and there is emphasis on the exchange of information, teaching and supervision as well as collaboration with the multidisciplinary team.

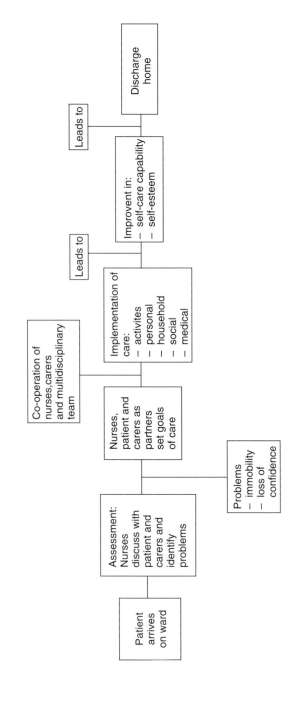

Figure 2.2 The Eshun–Smith model

Philosophy
The model has the following philosophical principles:

- Nurses need to empower patients by giving them information, involving them in their care, consulting them and giving respect to their opinions, beliefs and cultural values.
- There is a need for an ongoing involvement of carers in patient care as well as close multidisciplinary collaboration in the effort to help patients regain lost skills.
- Creating a stimulating ward environment should enhance the patients' potential for recovery.
- Continuing ability to undertake normal daily living activities implies continuing good health.
- Health promotion should be integral to any rehabilitation effort to improve the older patient's quality of life.
- Resources and facilities should be made available to enable nurses to create the opportunity and environment in which patients can relearn these self-caring skills.

Application of the model
The application of the model starts as soon as the patient is admitted to the ward. Nurses, patients and carers sit together in an admissions interview to assess and identify the patient's needs, set goals and plan how best these goals can be achieved. The role of the multidisciplinary team is important. Patients' need for their expertise is assessed during the admission interview. Nurses and therapists work together closely throughout the patient's stay. Issues affecting discharge are raised at this interview and reviewed regularly. Ward rounds and case conferences are held regularly with the medical staff to discuss and review patients' progress.

Care objectives
The principal means of assisting older patients to achieve the overall aim of improving their quality of life is to help them to regain as much as possible their ability to care for themselves. The approach for meeting this objective can be considered in two main parts: the promotion of self-care ability and the promotion of self-esteem. These two parts are interlinked. People will not aspire to become self-caring if they have no regard for their own self-esteem. By encouraging them to take care of themselves, they are by the same token being encouraged to take pride in themselves and regain their self-esteem. Figure 2.3 illustrates the care objectives of the model.

Promotion of self-care ability
The promotion of self-care ability is done mainly through the encouragement of patients to perform a variety of activities on the ward. Its

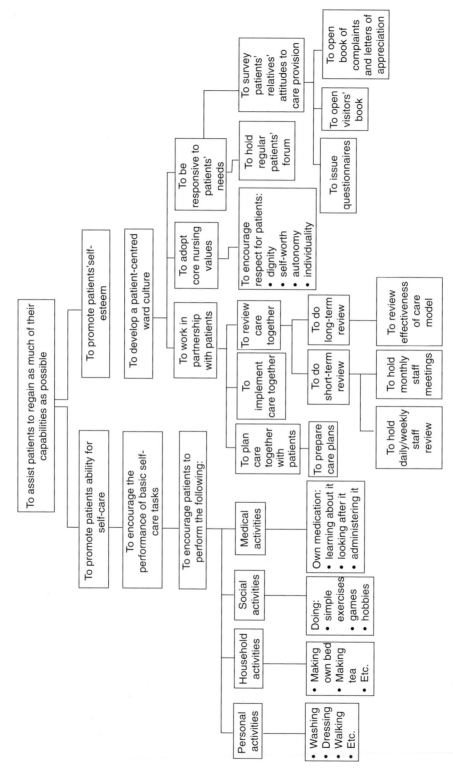

Figure 2.3 The care objectives of the Eshun–Smith model

purpose is to assist patients to regain any skills they may have lost through their illness and which they will require if they are to function independently when they are back at home. For that reason, the model focuses on patients who are clinically stable but have lost the motivation or ability to perform activities that will enable them to return home and cope safely. The activities involved are grouped into four categories: personal, household, social and medical/health-related problems:

- *Personal area of care.* Refers to activities like getting in and out of bed and washing and dressing independently.
- *Household area.* Patients are encouraged to do activities like making a cup of tea, toasting a slice of bread or reheating a frozen meal. How well patients perform these activities is assessed first on admission and then on a continual basis throughout their stay, as described below.
- *Social area.* Patients are encouraged to talk to other patients and participate in ward social activities like ward keep-fit exercises.
- *Medical area.* It is important that they understand their illness, how to cope with it and how to take their medication and the activities are meant to reinforce these skills.

Promotion of self-esteem
The second aspect of the model is the promotion of self-esteem. Self-esteem is achieved through positive nurse–patient interaction and the introduction of a patient-centred culture. For example, there is respect for the patient's autonomy as demonstrated by the way patients participate in assessment and care planning and by the consultations held with them regarding ward rehabilitation activities. Holding regular sessions of a patients' and carers' forum at which patients' concerns are discussed further promotes patient empowerment. Further, satisfaction surveys are carried out to obtain feedback on patients' and carers' experiences on the ward. Another facet of positive nurse–patient interaction is the way nurses relate to patients. For example, nurses make a point of asking patients how they wish to be addressed. They do not make the assumption that all patients wish to be addressed by their first names.

Assessment of self-care ability
Patients are assessed on rehabilitation activities that have been selected on the basis that they are important for the patient's well-being and that the ability to perform them independently will enable patients to cope better when they are discharged home. Some of the activities are considered to be critical and others desirable.

Critical activities are activities that patients should be able to perform independently if they are to be considered ready for discharge.

Table 2.3 Scoring of self-care activities (Eshun–Smith model of care, 1999).

Level	Level of dependence	Score
Level 1	• Total dependence – maximum assistance of 2. Requires help of 2 or more for all activities, e.g. lifting with hoist, washing, dressing	1
Level 2	• Assistance of 1–2. One or two people to help with everything, e.g. lifting, feeding, washing, dressing	2
Level 3	• Medium assistance of 1. Performs some activities with help of 1, e.g. stands, transfers, walks short distances with 1; washes, dresses top half	3
Level 4	• Minimum assistance of 1. Performs most activities with prompting/supervision, e.g. walks with zimmer plus standby; washes and dresses with minimum help	4
Level 5	• Independent with most activities. May still require supervision with medicine	5

These activities are: getting on and off a bed, eating and drinking, using the toilet independently, walking or wheelchair independence. Desirable activities are also important but they are such that even if the patient is unable to perform them completely on their own, assistance could be arranged for them at home. Desirable activities are: washing and dressing, using the kitchen safely, understanding own illness and medication required, and social interaction. Social interaction refers to the patient's ability to relate to people such as their own family, ward members and other patients. It gives an indication of the patient's mental and psychological status and is often helpful in gauging how much social back-up is required on discharge.

The Eshun self-care assessment chart (Table 2.3) is used to monitor how far the patient is progressing from dependence to independence within the identified activities. Both the critical and desirable activities are assessed once a week and scored to give an idea of how well the patient is doing. Scoring is based on five levels of achievement as shown in Table 2.3.

Scores depend on the reviewing nurse's judgement and it is not possible for it to be completely objective. However, it provides a measure of the progress being made and is taken into account when deciding whether or not a patient is ready for discharge. However, it is important to note that discharge is a professional decision for the medical and nursing staff and this measure is only one of a number of factors that are taken into account.

Care planning

Information obtained at the admission interview and from the assessment of self-care activities is fed into the patient's rehabilitation care plan. In carrying out the self-care assessment, the nurse identifies a number of factors that could act as barriers and interfere with the patient's progress. The aim of the care plan is to devise strategies that would enable the patient to overcome these barriers or problems. Nurses regularly review patients' progress and revise the care plans accordingly. Such revision is done in conjunction with the patient where possible.

Factors affecting the development of self-care ability
There are two main types of factors that hinder progress:

- *Physical factors*, e.g. lack of familiarity with the ward routine and staff, pain, breathlessness, dizziness, loss of appetite, loss of skill, loss of strength.
- *Psychosocial factors*, e.g. loss of motivation, apathy or lack of interest, loss of status, knowledge deficit, loss of insight, social, cultural or religious barriers. Assessment should include skilful interviewing in an attempt to identify the cause of the problem.

Some guidelines on completing the self-care assessment
It is useful to observe the following points when completing the assessment form.

Be precise
- Describe what the patient is capable of doing.
- Indicate how much help the patient needs.
- Indicate the nature of help the patient needs.
- Give some indication of the patient's mental or psychological state.
- Show how the patient is progressing from one level to another.

Discharge planning
This is another area where the application of the model is very important. Discharge plans are discussed at the admission interview and reviewed throughout the patient's stay. Patients are encouraged right from the beginning to start considering whether they want to return home after their hospitalisation, move in with family or go to residential or sheltered accommodation. This decision is by no means final; it simply provides an early indication of the patient's intention and serves as a guide to the level of performance to be achieved. Improvement in functional ability is followed by a home visit to assess home conditions and a series of meetings between patients, their families and members of the multidisciplinary team, including social workers, to discuss the type and amount of support needed on discharge.

From diagnosis to care planning
Once the client's problems have been identified, the nurse will plan in partnership with the client (as far as is possible) how the problems are

going to be addressed. This is the care-planning stage of the nursing process. A care plan is a statement of the outcomes of care and the methods that will be used to achieve them. The 'outcome' is what the intended result of the nursing intervention will be. The 'method' relates to the steps that need to be taken to resolve the problem in order to achieve the 'outcome'. The problem, outcome and planned action must be written clearly and unambiguously so that all staff will know exactly what they have to do, and also to enable evaluation of the care. Other essential characteristics of planning are setting priorities and ensuring that the plan is adequately recorded. Setting priorities is about deciding what problems need to be dealt with first and is paramount for client's safety. The record is important for communication between the caregivers, consistency of care, evaluation, audit and research, and legal reasons. Table 2.4 gives an example of a care plan.

The following issues need to be taken into account in care planning:

- *Evidence-based care.* The Nursing and Midwifery Council (NMC, 2004a) in clause 6.5 states that 'You have a responsibility to deliver care based on current evidence, best practice and, where applicable, validated research when it is available'.
- *Computerised, standard plans and care pathways.* These are pre-formulated plans or maps of care and may give abbreviated information. It is the responsibility of the nurse to 'individualise' the plan to meet the specific needs of the client. Any additional information is added in the appropriate sections of the plan.
- *Multidisciplinary plans.* All disciplines work from the same plan, enabling all information to be in one place. Where this is the practice, the nurse focuses on the human responses, i.e. how the client is responding to the 'whole' plan.

Table 2.4 Example of a care plan.

Problem/goal	Interventions	Expected outcome(s)
Risk of pressure ulcer **Goal:** John will be free from developing pressure ulcer	• Change position in bed 2–4 hourly • Change position in chair 2 hourly • Use pressure-relieving devices for bed and chair • Encourage gentle exercise and movement • Keep skin clean and dry at all times • Inspect pressure sites whenever giving care • Give nutritious balanced diet, fluid and supplements	• Skin is intact • Risk is managed

Implementation

Implementation is about putting the care plan into action. It encompasses various activities as follows:

- *Preparation for giving care*, e.g. looking at care plans, learning about the patient's problems and reading charts, receiving/giving reports and reading up on the management of problems.
- *Setting daily activities*, e.g. deciding how to organise the care for the shift or day.
- *Delegating care*, e.g. deciding how and when to delegate care to others.
- *Assessing and reassessing*, i.e. closely monitor physical and mental health responses to interventions.
- *Recording and reporting*, e.g. writing down what you have observed, status of patient's problems, interventions, patient's responses, ability of the patient to manage care needs, giving reports to others.

Evaluation

Evaluation is the process of ascertaining whether the care provided has been successful or not. It includes going through all the steps of the nursing process (assessment, diagnosis, planning and implementation) so as to decide whether to continue, modify or terminate the plan. For instance, if the outcome of the plan is 'free from pressure ulcer' and the patient has not developed an ulcer at the time of the evaluation or review, it suggests that the plan has worked and can be terminated. Conversely, if the risk factors are still present, you may decide to continue with the plan. If the patient has started to develop erythema at the pressure sites, you may have to modify the plan or write a new plan based on the changing situation.

Evaluation also provides data to assess the quality of the care delivery systems. Three types of evaluation are used to monitor healthcare practices (Alfaro-LeFevre, 2002):

- *Outcome evaluation.* Examine outcome of care, i.e. results. Ascertaining satisfaction with care.
- *Process evaluation.* Examine how the interventions were delivered.
- *Structure evaluation.* Examine setting in which interventions take place, such as resources, staffing level and skill mix, communication and management.

Advantages of using a conceptual model in assessment

Having used various examples to examine the concepts of nursing model and explored one model (Eshun–Smith) in some depth, we can now highlight some of the potential advantages of using conceptual models when assessing clients/patients. These are as follows:

- Provide a systematic approach to the collection and organisation of data.
- Provide a basis on which the nurse can make decisions about what types of information are essential to enable accurate evaluative judgements and making a diagnosis.
- Define what nursing is.
- Enable a consistent approach in the assessment and care of clients.
- Provide the theoretical framework for practice.

Key issues and developments

The context of care delivery and the practice of nursing are subject to diverse influences and changes. It is essential that nurses keep abreast of these changes and incorporate them in their practice. Some are listed below.

Confidentiality

The individual's right to confidentiality must be maintained. Any information that has been given by the client/patient is on the understanding that it will only be used for specific purposes and that only personnel with legitimate interest have access to it. Confidential information may be recorded on paper or on electronic media subject to the Data Protection Act 1988. The Access to Health Records Act 1990 gives patient/clients the right of access to manual health records and the Data Protection Act 1988 to their computer-held records. Nurses are professionally accountable for ensuring that security of patients' records is maintained regardless of the system used (NMC, 2004b).

Expanding nursing roles

Nurses are increasingly involved in advanced health assessment with the growth of advanced nurse practitioners to meet the changing demands of healthcare in various fields of nursing. These roles are associated with a higher level of education and practice. Advanced nurse practitioners may practise independently or in collaboration with physicians.

Computerised patient records

More documentation is being input directly onto computers. This involves new challenges. Nurses should be computer literate and able to use computers to access and enter information. New technology also facilitates diagnosis, decision making, research and immediate access to information by authorised personnel.

Integrated care pathways (ICP)

The use of integrated care pathways is becoming quite common in clinical practice. An integrated care pathway is a predefined plan of patient care relating to a specific diagnosis or operation (Burdis, 2005; Campbell *et al.*, 1998). It is evidence based and incorporates national and local guidelines to help organise and manage care more effectively. The ICP is used by all the multidisciplinary staff to record information about care and treatment for each patient. It promotes effective interprofessional working and ensures that important elements of care are not missed. Some of the key features of ICP are:

- improves multidisciplinary team working
- promotes review of current practice and application of evidence-based care
- reduces variation in treatment
- encourages active patient involvement in care
- useful tool for educating students and other staff
- possesses an integral audit mechanism
- improves resource utilisation
- provides a system of clinical record keeping
- identifies and manages risk.

Interprofessional working

Nurses meet patients with diverse needs. The need to address patients' problems effectively and in a timely fashion requires collaborative and flexible working with other disciplines.

Summary

Assessment is a critical stage of the nursing process and forms the basis for the care plan. If the assessment is inaccurate and inadequate, the standard of care given to the patient may be compromised and the patient may be put at risk; hence the need for assessment to be systematic and comprehensive. Assessment carries with it responsibility and accountability which means that nurses should keep up to date with expanded skills of assessment, current knowledge and research, relevant policies and professional and legal issues relating to their practice. The importance of clients' participation and involvement in their assessment and their rights to access to their records cannot be emphasised enough.

> ## Activity Problem identification/diagnosis and care planning
>
> - From the subjective and objective data you obtained on Mr Ward in the activity on page 54, identify and outline Mr Ward's actual problems.
> - Now give an outline of any potential problems that may develop for him.
> - Now for each actual problem and potential problem, try to set a goal.
> - For each goal set, identify strategies that could be taken/nursing interventions necessary to achieve that goal.

If you are able to carry out the above successfully, well done. If not, try again after you have had a chance to work in the clinical areas. Get your mentor to check your care plan.

References

Aldridge, J (2003a) The ecology of health model. In: Jukes, M & Bollard, M (eds) *Contemporary Learning Disability Practice*. Quay Books, Swindon.

Aldridge, J (2003b) Learning disability nursing: a model for practice. In: Turnbull, J (ed.) *Learning Disability Nursing*. Blackwell, Oxford.

Alfaro-LeFevre, R (2002) *Applying Nursing Process: promoting collaborative care*, 5th edition. Lippincott, Philadelphia.

Barker, P (2001) The tidal model: developing an empowering, person-centred approach to recovery within psychiatric and mental health nursing. *Journal of Psychiatric and Mental Health Nursing* 8 (3): 233–40.

Burdis, C (2005) Integrated care pathways in acute care. www.bcsnsg.org.uk/itin12/burdis.htm

Campbell, H, Hotchkiss, R, Bradshaw, N & Porteous, M (1998) Integrated care pathways. *BMJ* 316 (7125): 133–7.

Casey, A (1993) Development and use of the partnership model of nursing care. In: Glasper, E & Tucker, A (eds) *Advances in Child Health Nursing*. Scutari, London.

Department of Health (1997) *The New NHS – modern, dependable*. DoH, London.

Department of Health (1999) *Making a Difference*. DoH, London.

Department of Health (2001a) *The NHS Plan – an action guide for nurses, midwives and health visitors*. DoH, London.

Department of Health (2001b) *Valuing People: a new strategy for learning disability in the 21st century*. DoH, London.

Department of Health (2001c) *The Single Assessment Process Consultation Papers and Process*. DoH, London.

Department of Health (2001d) *National Service Frameworks*. www.doh.gov.uk/nsf/

Eshun, A B (1999) Effective rehabilitation for older people. *Nursing Standard* 13 (40): 39–43.

Fawcett, J (1984) *Analysis and Evaluation of Conceptual Models for Nursing*. F A Davis, Philadelphia.

Ford, P & McCormack, B (2000) Keeping the person in the centre of nursing. *Nursing Standard* 46 (14): 40–4.

Gordon, M (2000) *Manual of Nursing Diagnosis*, 9th edition. Mosby, St Louis.

Hogston, R (2002) Managing care. In: Hogston, R & Simpson, P M (eds) *Foundations of Nursing Practice: making the difference*, 2nd edition. MacMillen, Basingstoke.

McMahon, R (1998) Therapeutic nursing: theory, issues and practice. In: McMahon, R & Pearson, A (eds) *Nursing as Therapy*, 2nd edition. Stanley Thornes, Cheltenham.

Nursing and Midwifery Council (2004a) *Code of Professional Conduct: standards for conduct, performance and ethics*. NMC, London.

Nursing and Midwifery Council (2004b) *Guidelines for Records and Record Keeping*. NMC, London.

Orem, D E (2001) *Nursing Concepts of Practice*. Mosby, St Louis.

Peplau, H (1991) *Interpersonal Relations in Nursing: a conceptual frame of reference for psychodynamic nursing*. Putnam, New York.

Roper, N, Logan, W & Tierney, A (2000) *The Roper, Logan, Tierney Model of Nursing: the activities of living model*. Churchill Livingstone, Edinburgh.

Wild, D (2002) The single assessment process. *Primary Health Care* 12 (1): 20–1.

3

Concepts of health, illness and holism

C. Meurier

Learning objectives

- Discuss how health beliefs and perceptions of health may influence people's explanations of health and illness and the effects these may have on their health behaviour.
- Outline the components of a health history and their relevance in the collection of data.
- Explain what is meant by holistic assessment.
- Discuss the advantages and disadvantages of using a holistic approach in health assessment compared to the reductionist approach.

Introduction

In the previous two chapters, we looked at body functions and the process of health assessment. As explained, assessment is about collecting and interpreting data to identify a client's problems and needs so that appropriate interventions can be made. The questions that arise now are the what, why and how of assessment. To enable appropriate care to be given to the individual client, one needs to understand not only normal body functions but also in what way physical, social, psychological, cultural and spiritual factors may influence these functions and hinder or promote well-being.

This chapter will examine the concepts of health, illness and holism and their relevance to health assessment. By introducing and explaining these fundamental concepts, we hope that you will begin to appreciate the importance of considering the 'whole' person when assessing health needs rather than just focusing on the disease.

Being 'healthy'

In order to begin the process of health assessment, we need to clarify in our minds what health, being 'healthy' and being ill entail. At face value, this may appear simple enough. We all believe that we have a reasonably good idea about the meanings of these concepts. However, once we start discussing them and comparing our definitions with others, we begin to realise that our interpretations of these concepts may vary significantly and that in fact, these concepts are after all quite complex and multidimensional in nature. As health professionals, we are naturally concerned about how health is maintained, what causes ill health and what can be done for health to be restored. It is therefore imperative that we appreciate these variations in interpretations as well as their implications for practice so that we can be as effective as possible in our decision-making process during assessment and be able to provide appropriate interventions and advice, based on individual needs.

From a biological perspective, we know that a vast array of chemical reactions and physiological processes are responsible for normal body function, as discussed in Chapter 1. Any changes in physiological values and functions triggered by either internal or external factors are counteracted by the homeostatic system in order to restore harmony in body functions. Yet, these are not the only factors that influence body functions and health, although they are certainly very important. The contributions of external variables such as psychology, social relationships and environment (in its broadest sense) on health cannot be over-estimated. In practical terms, this means that in any comprehensive assessment of a client, we need to remember the dynamic nature of health and how various physical and psychosocial factors interrelate to maintain health or trigger illness. Before going any further, we need to start 'unpacking' the key concepts.

Defining health

As discussed, defining health is not as straightforward as one may imagine. We may define health as being free from disease or in terms of physical fitness. Indeed, views about health are not static and may vary from person to person. In no small measure, our life situation shapes our interpretations of health. For instance, age, gender, culture, spirituality, social background and emotional state all play a part in shaping people's views about health (Blaxter, 1990; Pender *et al.*, 2001).

The way an active child feels about health may be vastly different to an older person who may be afflicted by various impairments. Dossey *et al.* (2004) argue that people's perception about their own health influences the way they define health. For example, younger people may define health in terms of vitality and physical fitness whereas older people may view health more in terms of function and coping. In tandem with our lived experience, we frequently attach new meanings to health. Definitions and interpretations of health vary amongst health professionals too. Long (2001) found that health visitors emphasised the physical aspects in their definitions of health whereas community mental health nurses perceived health in a more 'holistic' manner, incorporating health into the wider domain of human relationship.

Thus, health is essentially a contested concept insofar as there is no complete agreement on its definition. Yet, for effective individualised care, we need to gain knowledge and understanding of the client's perspectives on health, illness and healthcare interventions.

Negative and positive definitions of health

To make some sense of the various interpretations of health, Blaxter (1990) has put forward the notion that definitions of health may be categorised as negative or positive. From this perspective, descriptions of health such as not experiencing signs and symptoms of disease (i.e. not having a swelling and pain) or simply being free of disease and disability (i.e. not having been diagnosed as having a disorder) will fall into the category of negative definitions of health. On the other hand, positive definitions of health will include statements linking health to feeling physically fit or, more generally, a condition of psychological and social well-being will be interpreted as positive (e.g. feeling able to cope with life).

In the Western world, the 'absence of disease' concept has been the most enduring and widely accepted view of health. It is considered as 'negative' because it focuses on an 'absence' of ill health rather than on the positive state. One is either healthy or has a disease; there is no in-between. Within this framework, health is considered as the direct opposite to disease. In this sense, it is a polarised view of health. Even if one feels unwell due to a disease process, one may be denied sympathy and may not be able to adopt the 'sick role' (Parsons, 1975) until such time as the disease has been formally diagnosed by the doctor. Conversely, people with chronic conditions and disabilities may be labelled as 'sick', although they themselves may otherwise feel healthy.

The 'absence of disease' definition of health is linked to what is called the 'medical model', in which disease is viewed as a pathological state or deviations of biological functions. Many people have embraced this view of health because of its apparent simplicity and the dominance of the medical view of health in Western societies. This view of health may sometimes have its benefits as people may at least regard themselves as healthy if they do not suffer from any diagnosed disease. Minor ailments can also be brushed aside because they may not be considered as 'real' disease.

In contrast to the medical model of health, other definitions of health project a positive image by equating health with all-round well-being. One typical example is the World Health Organisation's definition of health:

> 'Health is a state of complete physical, mental and social well-being, not merely the absence of disease' (WHO, 1958).

There is certainly an element of attractiveness in this definition of health, as it highlights health as a positive goal to aim for rather than focusing on 'absence of disease'. It fits in well with the philosophy of care of many health professionals who believe that their role is to enhance clients' health rather than just treating disease. However, one can also argue that it is far too idealistic and may well be an unrealistic aim for the majority of people. It also focuses too much on the individual's responsibilities for maintaining health and ignores the contributions of socio-economic factors in determining health and illness.

These apparent limitations in the definition of health have probably had a major influence on the WHO's subsequent ideas on health, as the following quote testifies:

> '. . . the extent to which an individual or group is able, on the one hand, to realise aspirations and satisfy needs and on the other hand, to change or cope with the environment. Health is therefore seen as a resource for everyday life, not the objective of living: it is a positive concept emphasising social and personal resources as well as physical capabilities' (WHO, 1984).

This revision of the WHO's definition of health addresses some of the problems inherent in the original definition, which was often seen as utopian. Health is now viewed as our ability to cope and adapt within a particular environment and as a 'resource for everyday life'. It also acknowledges individual and social responsibilities for health. This 'social model' of health proposes that it is too simplistic to blame ill health solely on personal and lifestyle factors; there is also a need to focus on broader variables which create obstacles to making healthy choices (WHO, 1986). For instance, the Black Report (Townsend et al., 1988) highlighted the importance of unemployment, social class, poverty and poor housing as detrimental to physical and emotional health. Thus there is a dynamic interaction between individuals and their wider environment and it is important that we consider the relative importance of behaviour and environment in creating health chances. The influences of these social variables on health will be discussed more extensively in other parts of the book. For now, we will concentrate on the factors that are thought to influence individual action.

Health beliefs and health behaviour

It is now accepted that differences in interpretations of health and health beliefs may influence health behaviour, in terms of whether or not one seeks help for a health problem and co-operates with advice and treatment. The effectiveness of health assessment and interventions is dependent on the extent to which we pay attention to these variables. To make it easy to understand how behaviour is influenced by multiple interacting attitudes and beliefs, a model may be used. Essentially, a model serves to simplify a complex phenomenon by focusing on those aspects that are in some sense fundamental. It helps to clarify our understanding of a complex concept or idea.

The health belief model

The health belief model (Maiman & Becker, 1974; Rosenstock, 1974) is a theoretical framework consisting of a number of key and interrelated concepts such as perceived susceptibility to and severity of a condition, behaviour efficacy, barriers to action and self-efficacy. The central tenet of the model is that people's conscious choices and behaviour are based on their health beliefs, i.e. their attitudes and ideas about health and illness. These beliefs are thought to influence health behaviour either positively or negatively, depending on the person's perceived vulnerability to a condition and the efficacy of a proposed action. According to Strecher & Rosenstock (1997), perceptions may range from total denial of susceptibility to perceptions of imminent risk. For instance, people without a family history of heart disease may not perceive themselves to be susceptible to the condition compared with those with a strong family history. The perceived consequences of contracting a disease or leaving it untreated are also thought to have an effect on health behaviour. Positive health behaviours are related to action that helps to maintain health, e.g. balanced nutrition, adequate exercise, immunisations and avoidance of risky behaviour. On the other hand, negative health behaviours are concerned with practices which may be detrimental to one's health, such as smoking, alcohol abuse and poor nutrition.

The health belief model enables us to trace the association between health beliefs and health behaviours (Figure 3.1). The model can also allow prediction of how a person will respond to potential risks to

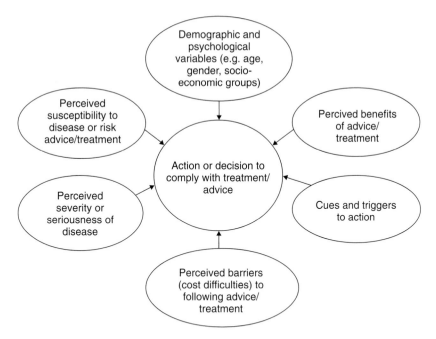

Figure 3.1 Factors that influence health behaviour, based on the health belief model

health, illness or healthcare interventions. Action cues and triggers are suggested to play a role in behaviour change. For example, hearing that a close relative has suffered a painful death from lung cancer as a result of excessive smoking may well be a trigger to quit smoking. However, the person may also choose to ignore this threat, depending on perceived barriers or the negative effects of a particular action.

The health belief model helps health professionals to understand more clearly why an individual is seeking help for a health problem or why the individual is not adhering to treatment or advice. This kind of examination enables the formulation of an effective care plan, based on individual needs and problems. It also enables us to take a holistic or biopsychosocial view of health. For instance, some people are more prone to illness because of their particular social circumstances and lifestyles (Whitehead, 1992). In others, genetic predispositions may play an important part in disease causation, although the influence of stressful environmental factors in drawing out the symptoms cannot be ignored (Senior & Viveash, 1998).

The key features of the health belief model can be summarised as follows:

- It is a framework for understanding people's health beliefs and health behaviours.

- It enables us to take our clients' perspectives into account when conducting a health assessment.
- It highlights the factors that may influence clients' decision making regarding the maintenance of their health and/or compliance with treatment.
- It allows us to target our intervention and health education in accordance with our clients' specific needs.

Illness, sickness and disease

As discussed, merely viewing illness or disease as the direct opposite of health provides an incomplete or even inaccurate picture of what health and illness are. It has also been seen that health is not a fixed point but fluctuates as the person adapts to changes in the internal and external environment. In this sense, health and illness should be seen as relative qualities and not absolute states. The use of a scale or continuum can vividly depict the potential movement between health and illness and vice versa (Figure 3.2).

As part of a comprehensive health assessment, you will collect data relating to symptoms and signs, which may count as illness. These symptoms can be physical (e.g. pain), psychological (e.g. feeling depressed) or social (e.g. feeling isolated). But usually there is some form of interaction between these three groups of symptoms, which you need to draw out when analysing and interpreting the data. Moreover, symptoms may interfere with every element or dimension of a person's life. For instance, a person who has persistent pain may not only become depressed but also may experience problems of social isolation. Symptoms are considered to be more than windows into a disease process and their assessment requires understanding of the person's experience and meaning relating to each symptom (Haworth, 2001).

The terms *illness*, *sickness* and *disease* tend to be used interchangeably. Although they may appear to refer to the same phenomenon, there is nonetheless a general acceptance that they not only describe different states but may also be subject to different interpretations. Like health, illness is essentially a 'contested' concept. People vary widely in their interpretations of what counts as illness. For instance, one person may report a particular set of symptoms to a doctor whereas

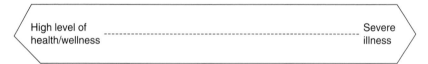

High level of .... Severe
health/wellness   illness

Figure 3.2   The health–illness continuum

another person might not. Illness may be regarded as perceptions of diminished or impaired functional abilities in one or more dimensions. Essentially, it is a subjective feeling, being concerned with how people feel. Sickness is reported illness. For example, someone may go to see a doctor or nurse because of feeling unwell. Disease refers to a special condition of ill health or pathological state in a patient.

Illness behaviour

Attitudes and beliefs about illness may influence the person's behaviour. This is referred to as 'illness behaviour'. The explanations or attributions that people make about an illness are also thought to influence their ability to cope and can also have a profound effect on their recovery. These explanations are known as 'illness attributions'. Illness behaviour and illness attributions influence how individuals describe, monitor and interpret symptoms as well as what types of actions are taken and whether or not healthcare facilities are used. It is common knowledge that not all people who develop symptoms of illness automatically react by visiting their doctor. The way they interpret the symptoms will influence whether they take action or not. A web of personal, family and sociocultural factors plays a major role in illness behaviour. Senior & Viveash (1998) found that not everybody with medical symptoms seeks medical advice. There are often differences in beliefs and attributions between doctors or nurses and patients as well. Unless these are explored, they may lead to barriers in communication, which could seriously affect the relationship between clients and healthcare professionals as well as the effectiveness of healthcare interventions.

Like health behaviour, illness behaviour is influenced by internal and external variables. *Internal* variables are concerned with the individual perceptions of the symptoms and the nature of the illness. Whether or not an individual seeks medical help will depend on how severe or disruptive the symptoms are perceived to be as well as the perceived seriousness of the symptoms. For instance, an individual is likely to view a crushing chest pain completely differently from mild flu symptoms. *External* variables, on the other hand, relate to the visibility of symptoms, social and cultural background, socio-economic factors and accessibility of the healthcare system. The visibility of symptoms will affect health behaviour in the sense that a person may react differently to symptoms of indigestion if they start passing large amounts of black stools. A person may also delay seeking medical help due to economic factors, such as not being able to afford to take a day off to see the doctor. These beliefs do not remain fixed but change in response to new information. For instance, if a particular symptom persists or changes in nature, the person's interpretation and consequent behaviour are likely to change too.

Understanding someone's beliefs and ideas about their illness or nature of their problems is important in health assessment. An assessment and subsequent care plan may contain serious omissions if the client's perspectives have not been taken into account. It may also cause difficulties in communication if clients feel that their problems have not been adequately understood by the health professional, affecting their response to treatment or advice. Thus assessment and intervention planning should be done in partnership with the client. In fact, it is now widely recognised that a person's ability to cope is influenced by their explanations and interpretations of their symptoms. This emphasises the importance of using the client's views as a starting point for exploring problems. With this approach, clients may feel more involved and willing to discuss their problems, hence enabling rich data to be collected. The focus in health assessment should be on the person as a whole.

Seeing the person as a whole

From the foregoing, it has become clear that health and illness are very complex concepts. We have to consider various perspectives when collecting and interpreting data during health assessment so that we can clarify as far as possible the nature of the client's health problems to enable appropriate interventions to be implemented. This approach could properly be termed *holistic*.

The holistic movement

Both holism and health have their roots in the concept of wholeness. The term 'holism' is derived from the Greek word *holos*, which means 'whole'. The South African philosopher Jan Christian Smuts (1926) first coined the word 'holism', although he was not the first one to use this concept. In fact, Florence Nightingale may have used the holistic approach, particularly in her advocacy of treatments that enhanced individuals' abilities to draw upon their own healing powers. Even in medieval European culture, illness was understood to be a disorder of the whole person in disharmony with inner and outer forces. Restoring the balance between these two forces would help the return of health.

With the rise of scientific medicine from the 18th century onwards, the 'absence of disease' model replaced this view of health. Increasing cultural value was placed on the scientific, material and rational and conversely, the metaphysical and religion were devalued. The application of scientific reasoning undoubtedly enabled medicine to make unprecedented technological advances. However, dissatisfaction with this mechanistic approach to healthcare gathered momentum around the 1950s, particularly in psychiatric healthcare settings. It was then

claimed that psychiatry was too focused on disease and medical interventions to the detriment of the social, psychological and behavioural
dimensions.

Soon, nurses from all fields of nursing started to embrace the holistic approach and this was evident in the philosophy of the nursing
models, which were being developed in the 1960s and 1970s. There was
also a concurrent surge in interest in alternative medicine, suggesting
that the biomedical approach was no longer considered as sufficient by
itself to effect healing.

Characteristics of holism

There are many definitions and interpretations of the term *holism*. It is
also often linked to alternative or complementary therapies, although
this is a rather narrow view of what holistic approaches in healthcare
entail. It has been suggested that holism cannot be defined but merely
interpreted in terms of what constitutes a 'whole' (Patterson, 1998).
Thus, it is generally accepted that the most useful way of interpreting
holism is that 'the whole is more than the sum of its parts' (Smuts,
1926), implying that people are interacting wholes.

In health assessment, it is important to take into account this multidimensional nature of people. This will help us to appreciate that a
person who has a *physical* illness may also be affected *psychologically,
socially* and *culturally*. In the holistic approach, the client's thoughts,
beliefs, attitudes and emotions are paramount. For instance, a medical
model will tend to emphasise the disease and its treatment, with the
practitioner usually taking the lead. In the holistic model, the client has
a central role in the care and will work in partnership with the health
professionals. It has also been suggested that *spirituality* forms an
intrinsic part of holism and that consideration of spiritual needs
enables a more comprehensive understanding of the whole person
(White & MacDougall, 2001). Some of the key components of the holistic approach are shown in Box 3.1.

Box 3.1 indicates that holism is concerned with all the factors relating to health and illness. There is also an implication that people can
influence health and illness through the life choices that they make and
in this sense, they have a degree of personal responsibility towards
their own health.

Reductionism in healthcare

A reductionist approach to healthcare is seen as the direct opposite to
holistic care. It is much criticised by proponents of holistic care. Within
the reductionist paradigm, the person is 'reduced to' the disease and it
is the responsibility of the doctor to diagnose the disease and initiate
treatment. Medicine is defined as the scientific study of the human
body. Within the framework of this definition, disease is understood to

---

Box 3.1 Components of the holistic approach.

- Searching for patterns and causes
- Considering the person as a whole with equal emphasis on the physical, psychosocial, cultural and spiritual aspects
- Viewing the body as an interactive system and not as a machine in need of repair
- Developing the ability to empathise
- Treating caring as a component of healing
- Emphasising human values
- Treating the client as an autonomous person
- Exploring the potential for growth, health and well-being
- Acting as a partner with the client
- Focusing on prevention and health education, not just on treatment of disease

---

be a breakdown in the functions of specific molecules, cells, tissues or organs. Patients are not expected to play any active role but are required to comply with treatment and advice.

A reductionist approach is not necessarily all negative. It needs to be recognised that reductionist science has enabled significant advances in the treatment of disease. For instance, scientific explanations of physiology by themselves may not tap people's inner subjective experiences but may become a powerful weapon in tackling health issues and promoting healing when combined with the holistic approach (Engebretson, 1997; Patterson, 1998).

The inclusion of holistic approaches in healthcare has made the client central to the caring process and has highlighted the need to consider a wide range of interventions in meeting health needs, involving various professionals working together within a multidisciplinary team. We need to acknowledge the respective contributions of both the holistic and reductionist approaches in healthcare. For instance, the physician's priority may be to look at the underlying cause of an illness and treat that. While this may be interpreted as a reductionist approach, it would be wrong to suggest that the physician is not interested in the personal factors. Realistically speaking, there are many situations in healthcare where a reductionist approach may be more appropriate in the initial stages. For instance, a nurse who is triaging in the accident and emergency department will focus primarily on the patient's medical needs in the initial stages. Within the hospital sectors, it is equally true to suggest that nurses and other health professionals are often pressured to achieve patient outcomes determined by the disease state and predetermined by lengths of stay (Jacobs, 2001). It has been argued that 'holism may be more appropriate as a final outcome than a stepping-off point' (Jacobs, 2001). Thus, while it is important for the

Box 3.2   Holistic approach principles.

- To focus on verbal and non-verbal interactions, enabling maximisation of client's self-discovery and enhancing decision making
- To establish a positive relationship
- To adopt a flexible approach
- To facilitate self-esteem, confidence and a positive outlook
- To use negotiating skills
- To encourage clients to participate fully and to develop self-responsibility
- To show empathy and respect
- To provide feedback
- To promote problem solving

nurse to consider all dimensions of an individual in health assessment and create conditions that promote optimal health, it is equally true that care must be prioritised according to the client's most immediate needs. It may not be in the best interests of the client to be a purist in either holistic or reductionist approaches. In some situations, we may initially have to focus on only a component of a person. But once this has been addressed, we have to place this component in the context of the 'whole'.

The holistic approach in health assessment

When using a holistic approach, the nurse considers all dimensions, with particular reference to the physical, psychosocial, cultural and spiritual aspects of the person. The relation between nurse and patient within a holistic approach is that of partnership and the nurse encourages collaboration and health-promoting behaviour. When practising holistically, nurses need to adopt particular communication types and techniques to obtain appropriate data to enable comprehensive assessment and care. These will be discussed in detail in Chapter 5. For now, the main principles of the holistic approach are listed in Box 3.2.

Assessment

Assessment was defined in Chapter 2 as the first stage of the nursing process. It is a systematic collection and interpretation of data relating to the client's health status. In holistic assessment, clients assume an active role by participating as much as possible. Information is sought about the client's health perceptions and beliefs, functional status and all other variables relevant to the client's health and illness. Information is obtained through history taking, physical assessment and diagnostic testing. Data obtained from these sources are organised in a clinical database and through critical thinking, appropriate judgements are made about the data, leading to the identification of the client's health needs and problems. The aims of holistic assessment are:

• to identify the client's health status
• to identify potential and actual health problems
• to evaluate the client's current knowledge
• to identify areas for health promotion and self-care
• to use the information gathered as a basis for care planning and delivery of holistic care.

Health history

The health history is taken by means of an assessment interview. It is a method of gathering subjective data about the health status of the client. The data are called subjective because they relate to what the client has said rather than what is observed independently. The information obtained through the health history can subsequently be validated by the physical assessment. In fact, the health history provides a focus for the physical assessment. The source of data for the health history is from primary sources and/or secondary sources. Primary sources data are obtained directly from the client and/or the client's family whereas secondary sources data are obtained from other health professionals or from the clinical record. The data obtained from the health history are used to identify the client's health problems and develop an individualised plan of care.

The types of health history taken will depend on a number of factors, such as the client's condition, the client's concerns and problems, the goals of assessment, the healthcare settings and the time available for the interview. A new client would merit a 'complete health history' on admission to establish a comprehensive database. However, in some situations, a shorter and more focused interview may be more appropriate. For instance, in an emergency situation, only information required immediately to treat the life-threatening condition is collected. A longer and more comprehensive history can then be taken when the client's condition has stabilised. It must also be emphasised that assessment through health history is an ongoing process and does not occur just on admission.

Components of health history

In most healthcare settings, standardised forms are used to document the data gathered from the health history. These forms may be based on a model of nursing, e.g. activities of living model (Roper *et al.*, 2000) or Orem's self-care model (2001) (see also Chapter 2). In some clinical areas, proformas or integrated care pathways are used for specific conditions whereby statements relating to the condition already exist and the nurse is required only to confirm that assessment relating to various items has taken place and any variances are noted. Regardless of the types of documentation used when assessing clients, it is important for the nurse to individualise the care plan to the client's specific needs by incorporating data from the health history.

The health history must be as comprehensive and holistic as possible. It should not focus purely on the medical dimension but also on the more holistic aspects, such as the client's feelings about the condition, its effects on the client's life and functional abilities. Conventionally, the health history addresses the following components:

- biographical data
- reason for seeking health evaluation or chief complaint(s)
- current health status or current illness
- previous experience of illness/past history
- personal and social history/lifestyles
- cultural and spiritual history
- family health history
- patterns of daily living/functional abilities
- review of systems.

Biographical data
Biographical data provide the information to identify the client as a person and to anticipate the special needs of the client. The biographical data include personal details such as the client's name, address, phone number, gender, date of birth/age, marital status and next of kin or significant others (see also Chapter 8).

As part of the process of gathering biographical data, nurses will also pay attention to sociocultural variables. For instance, information about ethnicity, level of education, employment and socio-economic status will also be collected. This information is important for understanding the client's health beliefs and attitudes as well as identifying other social factors that may determine the client's response to health, illness, interventions and health education advice. This will enable an individualised care plan to be developed for the client.

Reason for seeking health evaluation/chief complaint
After establishing the initial rapport from gathering biographical data, the nurse will pursue the reason for healthcare evaluation, or chief complaint. The client is encouraged to talk freely about their health concerns, using appropriate communication techniques as discussed in Chapter 10. This will not only enable the main problem to be identified but will also give cues to what further assessments and investigations may be required.

Current health status or current illness
Once the reason for seeking healthcare or the chief complaint has been established, the nurse will guide the client into elaborating on the characteristics of the health problem or symptom. The context, associations

and chronology of the health problem are explored. It is important to focus on the patient's perspective of the problem and not to introduce technical language, which may confuse the client. The essential characteristics of the problem need to be fully understood. For instance, the client will be asked to focus on the following key characteristics of the complaint:

- *Location.* Where is it? Does it radiate?
- *Quality.* What is it like?
- *Quantity or severity.* How bad is it?
- *Onset, progression and duration.* When did it start? How often is it experienced? How long does it last?
- *Context and setting.* What the client perceives as the cause of the problem. What circumstances may have contributed to it?
- *Exacerbating or remitting factors.* What makes it worse? Does anything make it better? Which treatments have been tried?
- *Associated problems.* Has the client noticed anything else that accompanies it?

Information obtained from the above characteristics will help the nurse to build a picture of the client's problem and its impact on daily activities of living, including the client's feelings about the problem and expectations of healthcare. This will suggest what further evaluations and investigations are required as well as enabling decisions on the most appropriate plan of care.

Previous experience of illness or past medical history
Information about the client's past history may shed light on the current problem or may highlight other problems and risk factors as well as the client's reactions to illness and treatment. The types of data collected will relate to birth, growth, development, childhood diseases, allergies, previous health problems, hospitalisations, surgical history, medications, history of blood transfusions, accidents and injuries.

Personal and social history
As stated earlier, social and lifestyle variables play an important role in health and illness (see also Chapter 8). It is therefore important to collect data relating to the client's personal habits (e.g. lifestyle, smoking, alcohol intake, use of drugs, hobbies), nutritional habits, exercise patterns, sleep/rest patterns, relationships, occupation, financial status, housing and sexuality). Gathering data in these areas will give insight into how the client lives and may explain some of the factors that may be contributing to disease and illness.

Cultural and spiritual history
It is also important to find out about the cultural and spiritual beliefs and practices of the patient. These are personal to each patient and may

directly affect or be affected by the patient's health status. These are discussed in more detail in Chapter 10.

Family health history
Some health problems seem to run in families. This may be due to genetic predisposition, although environmental factors may also play an important part. Sharing the same environment and culture would have exposed the client to similar health risks or socialisation. The client will be asked about occurrences of illness and genetic conditions in the family, including at the least the immediate blood relatives. Information about family illness can provide evidence about the client's current problems. It is now widely accepted that there are some familial tendencies towards heart disease, hypertension, cancer, diabetes and obesity.

Patterns of daily living/functional abilities
Data need to be collected about the client's daily routine not only to establish a baseline but also to explore the client's perception of any difficulties with activities of daily living such as mobility, eating, elimination and dressing. It is important to find out whether these difficulties existed before or were triggered by the present health problem. The nurse will also need to assess the level of dependence or independence in these activities and whether supervision and assistance will be required. Information on functional abilities will help to identify any risk factors or areas that will require further evaluation by physical assessment.

Review of systems
In this component, the nurse will ask the client a series of system-related questions as a way of checking that no vital information has been overlooked. In the review of systems, both positive and negative findings should be recorded. This part of the health history can be combined with the physical assessment. The types of symptoms or diseases that can be ascertained by review of system are shown in Table 3.1.

Documenting and using data from the health history

The nurse is required to keep an accurate record of the health assessment (NMC, 2005). Date and time of the assessment interview will be noted, and the name and signature of the nurse who has taken and recorded the health history must be included in the documentation or any institutional policy adhered to. Data from the health history will be sifted and analysed to identify any potential or actual health problems. However, some of the data will need to be validated by physical assessment and diagnostic tests. Health interventions will be based on the problems identified from the health assessment.

Table 3.1 Review of systems (see also Chapter 6).

Systems	Checklists
• Integumentary (skin, hair, nails) system	• General state of health. History of skin diseases, changes in skin colour, rashes, bruises, moles or lumps, pruritus, abnormal growth of hair (hirsutism). Loss of hair (alopecia), changes in nails, dry or moist skin
• Musculoskeletal system	• Joint stiffness/pain, back pain, limitation of movement, arthritis, fractures and swelling
• Nervous system	• History of altered consciousness, headache, convulsions, speech problems, inco-ordination, weakness or paralysis, loss of memory, head injury, change of sensation, irritability, mood changes, depression, anxiety and sleep disturbances • *Ears*: Hearing deficits, use of hearing aid, vertigo, tinnitus, infection, discharge and earaches • *Eyes*: Wearing spectacles. History of eye problems
• Endocrine system	• Endocrine problems: diabetes, hypothyroidism, thyrotoxicosis
• Respiratory system	• *Nose*: Epistaxis, sinusitis, allergies, frequent colds and obstruction • *Throat*: Hoarseness, frequent sore throats, pain/stiffness, goitre and tonsillectomy • Dyspnoea, sputum, cough, wheezing, asthma, haemoptysis
• Cardiovascular system	• Chest pain, hypertension, dyspnoea, oedema, anaemia, myocardial infarction and varicose veins
• Immune system	• Vaccination history • Infections
• Gastrointestinal system	• Bleeding/swollen gums, mouth sores, dentures, toothache and sore tongue • Nausea or vomiting, loss of appetite, loss of weight, diarrhoea, constipation, usual bowel habits and blood in the stools
• Urinary system	• Frequency, urgency, nocturia, haematuria, changes in urine colour, incontinence, dribbling and suprapubic pain
• Reproductive system	• *Female*: Menstrual history (e.g. last menstrual date, regularity, menorrhagia), bleeding following intercourse, last smear test, vaginal pruritus, discharge, number of pregnancies, number of children, type of contraception, menopause, hormone replacement therapy. Breast disease, etc. • *Male*: History of erectile dysfunction, prostate problems, infections, etc.

Summary

In this chapter, concepts of health, illness and holism were examined in detail to provide background knowledge to enable health assessment to be carried out knowledgeably, comprehensively and effectively. In particular, it has been emphasised that considering the client as a 'whole' or 'holistically' will enable a more individualised and systematic assessment, taking into account the biopsychosocial and spiritual factors. The components of the complete health history were presented. It was pointed out that a comprehensive health history will normally be taken on admission or first encounter while also emphasising that on occasions it may not be possible to take a complete history because of the client's condition or other circumstances. In these situations, it was suggested that the minimum information may have to be taken to decide what care and treatment are immediately required. As assessment is an ongoing process, a more holistic assessment may follow once the client's condition has stabilised.

Activity

- Discuss the relevance of the concepts of health, illness and holism in health assessment.
- Discuss the strengths and weaknesses of the holistic and reductionist approaches.
- Describe the purpose of a health history.
- List the components of the health history and state what information will be collected for each component.

References

Blaxter, M (1990) *Health and Lifestyles.* Tavistock, London.

Dossey, A M, Keegan, L & Gazzetta, C E (2004) *Holistic Nursing: a handbook for practice,* 4th edition. American Holistic Association, Aspen Publishers, New York.

Engebretson, J (1997) A multiparadigm approach to nursing. *Advances in Nursing Science* 20 (1): 21–33.

Haworth, S K (2001) Holistic symptom management: modelling the interaction phase. *Journal of Advanced Nursing* 36 (2): 302–10.

Jacobs, B B (2001) Respect for human dignity: a central phenomenon to philosophically unite nursing theory and practice through consilience of knowledge. *Advances in Nursing Science* 24 (1): 17–35.

Long, A (2001) Functionalism and holism: community nurses' perceptions of health. *Journal of Clinical Nursing* 10 (3): 320–9.

Maiman, L A & Becker, M H (1974) The health belief model: origins and correlates in psychological theory. *Health Education Monographs* 2: 336–53.

Nursing and Midwifery Council (2005) *Guidelines for Records and Record Keeping*. NMC, London.

Orem, D E (2001) *Nursing: concepts of practice*. Mosby, St Louis.

Parsons, T (1975) The sick role and the role of the physician reconsidered. *Millbank Memorial Fund Quarterly* 53 (3): 257–77.

Patterson, E F (1998) The philosophy and physics of holistic health care: spiritual healing as a workable interpretation. *Journal of Advanced Nursing* 27 (2): 287–93.

Pender, N J, Murdaugh, C L & Parsons, M A (2001) *Health Promotion in Nursing Practice*, 4th edition. Appleton & Lange, Stamford, Connecticut.

Roper, N, Logan, W & Tierney, A (2000) *The Roper, Logan and Tierney Model of Nursing*. Churchill Livingstone, London.

Rosenstock, I M (1974) The health belief model and preventive health behaviour. *Health Education Monographs* 2: 354–86.

Senior, M & Viveash, B (1998) *Health and Illness*. Palgrave, Basingstoke.

Smuts, J C (1926) *Holism and Evolution*. Macmillan, New York.

Strecher, V J & Rosenstock, I M (1997) The health belief model. In: Glanz, K, Lewis, F M & Rimer, B K (eds) *Health Behavior and Health Education: theory, research, and practice*, 2nd edition. Jossey-Bass, San Francisco.

Townsend, P, Davidson, N & Whitehead, M (1988) *Inequalities in Health. The Black Report and the health divide*. Penguin, Harmondsworth.

White, B F & MacDougall, J A (2001) *Clinician's Guide to Spirituality*. McGraw-Hill, Boston.

Whitehead, M (1992) The health divide. In: Townsend, P, Davidson, N & Whitehead, M (eds) *Inequalities in Health*. Penguin, Harmondsworth.

World Health Organisation (1958) *Constitution of the World Health Organisation*, Annex 1. WHO, Geneva.

World Health Organisation (1984) *Report of the Working Group on Conception and Principles of Health Promotion*. WHO, Copenhagen.

World Health Organisation (1986) *The Ottawa Charter*. WHO, Copenhagen.

Factors to consider when assessing patients

A. Crouch, G. Rumbold, M. Thompson and W. Turner

Learning objectives

- Discuss the principle of 'respect for persons' and its implication for practice.
- Identify and discuss some of the key ethical aspects related to the assessment of patients/clients.

Section 1: Introducton

Prior to and during health assessment of patients, factors such as ethical issues, the health status of the patient/client, the age and cognitive ability of the patient, learning disability as well as gender issues need to be considered as these can have an impact on the assessment process. The aim of this chapter, therefore, is to discuss these factors. Issues and documents referred to in sections 1 and 3 relate mainly to adults so particular reference will be made to the assessment of children in section 2 of this chapter.

Ethical aspects of assessment

In this section we will explore some of the essential ethical aspects of the process of completing a patient assessment. Clearly, it is not possible to fully discuss all the ethical issues involved so four key aspects will be discussed: privacy, confidentiality, respect for dignity and truthfulness. All these aspects can be subsumed under the principle of respect for persons and it is this principle which we will explore first.

Respect for persons – definition

The phrase 'respect for persons' is frequently used by philosophers and ethicists, but what is meant by it? It has generally been held to mean that each person should be treated as being of equal value regardless of his or her achievements or status. Rumbold (1999: p241) expands this definition to say that 'not only is a person of worth or value irrespective of their achievements but also irrespective of their lack of achievements or lifestyle, and that therefore in our dealing with patients we should treat them all equally as having intrinsic worth and value'.

In the process of taking a nursing history, a nurse will learn much about a patient. Some of this will be information which we might describe as 'clinical'; that is, information that is directly pertinent to their health status. However, much of the information gleaned will be related to the patient's lifestyle.

Some of this latter information may have a bearing on the client's condition and treatment, while some of it may be irrelevant. However, whichever the case, the nurse should refrain from making any judgement about the rights or wrongs of the person's lifestyle.

Application of the principle of respect during assessment

The NMC (2004, clause 2) states that 'As a registered nurse or midwife, you must respect the patient or client as an individual' and, expanding on this, goes on to state:

> *'You are personally accountable for ensuring that you promote and protect the interests and dignity of patients and clients, irrespective of gender, age, race, ability, sexuality, economic status, lifestyle, culture and religious or political beliefs' (NMC, 2004, 2.2: p3).*

This statement concurs with the principle of respect for persons, which holds that each individual is of the same intrinsic worth as any other regardless of their beliefs, values and customs. Thus, for example, if the way in which a person conducts their life has contributed to their condition, the nurse should not condemn their behaviour, nor express a personal view about the morality of that behaviour. The nurse would, however, be quite justified in providing the patient/client with the relevant information as to how they might improve their health status by changing their behaviour. Thus, informing a patient/client about the dangers to health of, for example, smoking, overeating, excessive alcohol consumption or sexual promiscuity is justified. But, and it is a very important but, the nurse should not in any way allow knowledge of the client's lifestyle to affect the way in which she or he interacts with them.

Autonomy

An intrinsic element of the principle of respect for persons is respect for autonomy. 'The requirement to respect autonomy is a major part of the core rationale of health work . . .' (Seedhouse, 1998). And in the context of assessment, this means that the patient has the right to divulge as little or as much information as they wish. This can obviously confront the nurse with something of a dilemma, for if there is information which the nurse considers pertinent to the patient's condition and treatment but which they are reluctant or even refusing to divulge, then what should the nurse do? Clearly, she cannot insist that the patient provide that information. All she can do is point out to the patient the importance to the healthcare team of having the information in order to give appropriate care and treatment. The same applies if the patient refuses to undergo any form of examination as part of the assessment process. Patients have the right to refuse any form of treatment be it curative or exploratory. However, having entered the healthcare system, whether as an inpatient or in a clinic or health centre, if they refuse to undergo the examinations necessary for health professionals to make a diagnosis and determine the appropriate treatment options, they do lose their right, both in law and morally, to such examinations and treatment. From an ethical stance, patients cannot expect health professionals to give them the most appropriate treatment if they do not provide all the relevant information, be this verbally or by allowing the appropriate examinations.

One of the essential elements to the exercising of any rights is the acknowledgement that this imposes duties. First, the possession of rights implies that others have duties (Rumbold, 1999). Thus, if clients have rights, then nurses and other healthcare workers have duties to ensure that those rights are met. Second, the person exerting their rights has a duty to ensure that the providers of the treatment have all the information they need in order to provide the most appropriate treatment. The right to autonomy is not therefore any more absolute than any other right. A client cannot say 'I want you to treat me, but I'm not going to give you access to all the information you need in order to do so'. Such refusal, we would argue, negates their right to treatment.

What to do when a patient needs treatment but refuses to give all the necessary information

The dilemma for the nurse (or any other healthcare professional) is that they are presented with a person who is clearly in need of treatment but who is refusing to allow them to obtain the information they need in order to give that treatment. The professional has two options: either to provide care and treatment on the basis of the limited information they have or to refuse all treatment. Either option could be detrimental to the patient. The principle of respect for autonomy would suggest that the way forward is to leave the decision to the patient. To explain to them that one can either treat them on the basis of the limited information they have made available, which may have detrimental consequences, or not to treat them at all, which will certainly have detrimental consequences. Either action is likely to contravene clauses 1.2 and 1.4 of the Code of Professional Conduct (NMC, 2004). To leave the decision to the client would comply with clauses 2.1, 3.1 and 3.2.

Activity

Please refer to the Nursing and Midwifery Code of Professional Conduct (2004), clauses 3.1 and 3.2.

- Consider the statement in each of those clauses and reflect on how it could be applied in practice during health assessment.

It should now be obvious that there are no clear-cut answers to ethical or moral dilemmas. For the nurse these largely arise when there is conflict between the stipulations of the Code of Professional Conduct, standards for conduct, performance and ethics, and the actions of the client, or when there is a conflict between two or more clauses of the Code. This being said, there are certain principles to which the nurse should adhere within the assessment process, and these we will now begin to explore.

Privacy

> *'It is one of the first rules of nursing which all* student *nurses learn that at all times they must ensure the patient's privacy when carrying out nursing procedures'* (Rumbold, 1999: p132).

This is fundamental and an essential aspect of care (DoH, 2000). There is an assumption, as Rumbold (1999) points out, that pulling screens or curtains around a patient ensures privacy. Nothing is further from the truth. Yes, curtains or screens ensure that others cannot *see* what is going on but they do not ensure that others cannot *hear*. A major part of the assessment process is the asking and answering of questions. In terms of ensuring privacy – that is, ensuring that others cannot hear what is being discussed – the use of curtains or screens becomes irrelevant. If patients have a right to privacy – and the right to privacy is a basic human right – then they have the right to assume that all conversations between them and the nurse will be undertaken in conditions that prevent others from overhearing them. There is no justification for nurses obtaining a nursing history in situations in which other patients and/or their visitors can overhear what is being said if they are to comply with the patient's right to privacy or indeed, clause 5 of the Code of Professional Conduct (NMC, 2004).

The point is that 'out of sight' does not equal 'out of mind' and certainly does not equal 'out of hearing'. Conversations between nurse and client, particularly during the history-taking process, need to be conducted so that no one else (be they other patients/clients or their visitors) can hear what is being discussed. Unfortunately, the way in which most hospital wards in the NHS are arranged, this is often not a possibility. In doctors' consulting rooms in health centres and outpatient departments and in accident and emergency departments, this is generally not a problem given that patients are interviewed in individual rooms or cubicles. But in hospital wards the situation is very different. All that divides one patient from another is usually a curtain, which means that whoever is on the other side of the curtain may hear what is being said. Nurses need to be aware of this and at least take steps to ensure that conversations are kept at a lower level and at best, fight for separate interview rooms in which such conversations can take place. For, as the Code of Professional Conduct states, 'Where you cannot remedy circumstances in the environment of care that could jeopardise standards of practice, you must report them to a senior person . . .' (NMC, 2004 8.3; p9). To interview clients in a situation in which the conversation can be overheard is clearly to jeopardise standards of practice.

Confidentiality

One aspect of ensuring confidentiality in the assessment process has become self-evident, inasmuch as the environment in which it is undertaken should be such that no others can overhear what is being said. But the principle of maintaining confidentiality goes further, covering to whom any information obtained should be divulged. The Code of Professional Conduct (clause 5) states that:

'You must protect confidential information', and 'You must treat information about patients and clients as confidential and use it only for the

purposes for which it was given. As it is impractical to obtain consent every time you need to share information with others, you should ensure that patients and clients understand that some information may be made available to other members of the team involved in the delivery of care' (NMC, 2004 5.1: p7).

Two questions immediately arise. First, to whom, if anyone, should the nurse divulge the information obtained when taking a nursing history? And second, what information is confidential? In some ways the first question is more easily answered, at least in theory. When a person enters into the healthcare system, they enter into a relationship not with just *one* professional but with the healthcare team who will be caring for and treating them. Although clinical information is of a confidential nature, it may be legitimately shared by members of the healthcare team involved in the care of the patient (Rumbold, 1999). Patients have no right to expect that relevant information will not be shared among those who have responsibility for their care and treatment – how else could they do their job? And, I suspect, most clients would expect this to be the case and consequently become very frustrated when several individual practitioners ask them the same questions.

The principle of confidentiality means two things. First, that information shared between client and a health professional is confidential between them and those health professionals who need to know the information. Second, that no health professional has the right to impart that information to anyone else other than when required to do so by law.

What is confidential?

The second question, 'What information is confidential?', is less easily answered. As has already been stated, some of the information obtained by a nurse when taking a nursing history will be directly relevant to the patient's care and treatment, whereas some of it will have little or no relevance at all. The questions then are 'What information is relevant and what is not? And, of that which is not relevant, how much is confidential?'.

The question of what is relevant or not is perhaps reasonably easily answered. For all the nurse has to decide is whether the information is pertinent to the patient's treatment and care. Thus information about their symptoms or drugs they have been taking, for example, is clearly relevant and, whilst confidential, might rightly be shared with other members of the healthcare team. Information about their lifestyle may be relevant; for example, if a patient has been admitted with breathing difficulties and they admit to smoking 40 cigarettes a day, this is clearly relevant. But if they say they have never smoked but enjoy visiting a public house on a regular basis, is that relevant? That they do not smoke clearly is. Does the information that they frequent a public house have any relevance and should it be shared with others? Public houses do tend to have smoky atmospheres. Such information could be relevant. If, on the other hand, to take an extreme example, they say they have never smoked, do not live or work in a smoky environment but enjoy scuba diving, how much of that is relevant? The fact that they are not a smoker, nor likely to be a passive smoker, is relevant. The fact that they go scuba diving is not. There is then no need for the nurse to share this information with others.

To what extent is irrelevant information confidential?

If a patient says they enjoy scuba diving or that they have recently been on holiday to Tenerife, assuming this has no relevance to the cause of their condition, this clearly does not fall within the category of information which can justifiably be passed on to other members of the team. The question is, should it be treated as confidential?

> '. . . some information is clearly not of a confidential nature. Patients will tell nurses things about themselves which they do not expect to be held in confidence, things which would form part of normal social intercourse (Rumbold, 1999: p154).

Information such as an interest in scuba diving or having holidayed in Tenerife falls into this category. There is therefore no reason for the nurse to hold such information in confidence. On the other hand, there is no requirement to pass it on to others or record it in the nursing notes since it is not relevant to the client's care. Nevertheless, as a rule of thumb, the nurse should be advised to obtain the client's permission before passing such information on to others, be they other staff or patients/clients.

Respect for dignity

One of the most common phrases used by nurses is that they will 'respect the patient's dignity'. But what is meant by dignity? And is there a difference between what nurses mean when they make such a statement and the real meaning of dignity? Essentially the dignity of any individual is about how they see themselves. More than anything else, a person's dignity is about his or her self-respect.

At a conference, Edgar (2003) suggested that 'The concept of dignity is complex, as it embraces aspects of human behaviour and physical autonomy; the mutual recognition and respect of human beings; and the capacity of humans to construct a sense of their own identity and worth'. This then means at least two things. First, that we treat each individual patient as being of worth in themselves. In other words, that we respect them as a person. Second, it means that we afford them the appropriate circumstances and conditions to allow them to retain that sense of identity and self-worth. But is this not exactly what we fail to do when people come into hospital?

One of the first things patients are generally asked to do when admitted to hospital (be it an elective or emergency admission) is to get undressed and change into bedclothes. Patients are vulnerable not only because of physical or mental impairment. Sadly, health professionals, including nurses, frequently increase the patient's vulnerability by reducing rather than enhancing their dignity. Having placed the patient in unfamiliar surroundings such as 'a hospital or clinic, they are then required to dress in nightclothes even though it is daytime and even if they are able to be up and about' (Rumbold, 1999: p81).

What effectively we do to people, whatever their age, when they come into hospital is to reduce them to infancy. We create a parent–child relationship in which the nurse (or other health professional) is parent and the client a child. Immediately the client suffers a loss of dignity, a loss of self-worth. They cease to feel that others value them for what they are and consequently feel themselves to be of less value. To know and understand this is essential for nurses when carrying out an assessment. They need to be aware that the system has placed the client in a position where they feel degraded (i.e. from adult to child) or at the very least put into an inferior position to those around them (doctor or nurse) in uniform.

Assessment involves more than a conversation between nurse and client (important though that is); it also involves making observations and examining the patient. In assessing a client's needs, the nurse has to undertake a number of observations, including the recording of vital signs (see Chapter 5), which is relatively innocuous. She also needs to examine the client in order to record, for example, observations of skin colour and condition, mobility and so on. Such observations require the client, at times, to remove what little clothing they have left. While such an examination may be undertaken in a setting that ensures privacy, it still nevertheless increases the affront to dignity felt by the client. This affront to dignity cannot be totally overcome but it can be reduced. What is essential is that nurses are aware of the effects of their actions and do their best to minimise their effects.

Truthfulness

As has already been noted, the process of assessment involves a conversation between the nurse and the patient and/or the patient's guardian, advocate or partner, where appropriate. It is a dialogue in which the nurse asks the questions and the patient provides the answers. However, as with any conversation, it is a two-way process (see Chapter 5). Both participants ask and answer questions and both present points of view. What concerns us here is how the nurse responds to the patient and the nature of the information they give.

As has already been intimated, it is not a conversation between equals. The nurse, rightly, is legitimately allowed to ask questions of a personal nature of the patient. She can ask the patient to divulge their age, marital status and, if relevant, their sexual orientation. Such questions the patient may not legitimately ask of the nurse. If they do so, the nurse is justified in refusing to answer. But if they ask questions about their condition, treatment or prognosis, the nurse is bound to answer truthfully.

Immanuel Kant, the 18th century German philosopher, argued that there is no justification for telling an untruth and that there is a moral duty to tell the truth. Thus, if a patient asks questions pertaining to their condition, the nurse must answer truthfully. Now the truthful answer to any question may be 'I don't know' and if that is the case, it is a perfectly legitimate answer. However, what Kant said was that 'In every utterance one should be truthful. This implies that while one should never tell an untruth, it is acceptable to withhold the truth – to say nothing' (Rumbold, 2002). There is therefore no requirement to voluntarily divulge the truth. In other words, if the patient does not ask, then there is no necessity to provide the answer. But a word of warning: just because a patient does not ask does not necessarily mean they do not want to know. It may be they do not know how to ask, may feel that they are not allowed to or may be too frightened to ask. It is therefore incumbent on the nurse to both create an atmosphere of openness and trust in which patients feel able to ask questions and to provide the opening for them to do so.

Section 2: The environment, health status, age and cognitive ability of the patient, learning disability and health assessment

The need to take into account ethical issues has been highlighted in section 1. The environment within which assessment takes place could also impact on the assessment process. As stated in section 1, the assessment process also involves a dialogue. Where necessary, it should be taken directly from the patient as it is more likely to be accurate than if it were taken from a third person (see Chapter 5). This is, however, not always possible due to poor health status of the patient.

Age as well as the cognitive status of individuals may also influence the way in which assessment is carried out. Children, for instance, go through different stages of physical and psychosocial development. These mean differences in behaviour and understanding of what is being said at the different stages which could impact on the health assessment process. There are also clinical differences between adults and children, which affect how children may be assessed. Therefore the aim of this part of the chapter is to discuss these factors.

Learning objectives

- Discuss the need for a health assessment to be carried out in a conducive environment.
- Explore how the health status of a patient may impact on the health assessment process.
- With particular reference to children, discuss how age and cognitive ability of the patient may influence the assessment process.
- Give an outline of the aspects of children that need to be assessed.

Environment

The use of the correct environment helps to facilitate the assessment process. To encourage a meaningful assessment, for example, the nurse needs to be able to engage with the patient in an environment which is free from distractions.

Assessment is sometimes carried out in the patient's home with family members around (ENB, 1999). Good interpersonal skills are needed to ensure that confidentiality is also maintained in such surroundings.

The Department of Health (2004, Standard 7: p20) advocates the use of an environment 'that is safe and well-suited for the age and stage of development of the child and young person'. The room or the area where the assessment takes place should thus not be too hot or cold but must be kept warm. This is particularly important when assessing babies, younger children and the elderly, to avoid excessive heat loss.

The decor of the room should also be suitable. An adult environment, for example, can be frightening for a child. For an adolescent, a room decorated with teddies may make them feel that they may be treated as a child. Care should therefore be taken to ensure that the environment is suitable and appropriate for the age of the patient.

The time when an assessment is carried out with a patient is also important. Sometimes a patient is brought into hospital during the night and might be feeling tired. This could affect the information-gathering process since the patient is less alert and may not co-operate fully. The patient's wishes should be respected at all times and the assessment should be carried out with sensitivity. Some of the necessary information may have to be collected from the next of kin or other appropriate person, e.g. one who accompanies the patient to the hospital and who is able to give the necessary information but with the patient's consent where possible.

Health status of the patient

The client's physical and/or mental health status should also be taken into account prior to and during the assessment process because any form of disability will impact on their responses to holistic health assessment. A patient, for example, might be brought into hospital in an unconscious state and unaccompanied, in which case close nursing observations will be relied upon during assessment until the patient is able to contribute fully. The activities below should help you identify how other medical conditions might impact on the assessment process.

Activity

- A patient is admitted to the ward with right-sided paralysis following a cerebrovascular accident (stroke). Can you determine how this condition might affect the assessment process?
- Can you identify any other medical condition that may affect the client's ability to give information or co-operate fully in the assessment process?
- How may this impact on the assessment process?
- How could the assessment be adapted to ensure effectiveness?

Having a disability does not mean that the patient cannot fully participate in their holistic health assessment but rather that the assessing nurse will adapt the assessment to meet the person's disability needs. A partially or non-sighted person, for example, may need help that is tactile and expressive in touch. Please also see Chapter 5.

The following activities should give you some idea how the mental health status of a patient may affect the assessment process.

Activity

(1) Please reflect on the following condition/situation and outline how each of them may affect the assessment process.
- A patient who is very withdrawn due to severe depression
- A patient who has sustained injuries in a fight but who is very drunk and needing assessment and treatment.

(2) What could be done by the healthcare professional to enable and enhance a holistic assessment of the patients referred to?

Anxiety and nervousness

Uncertainty about what is going on, and what is going to happen to one, could also lead to anxiety and fear irrespective of age. Nervousness and the need for 'everything to be all right' can also cause the patient to give the answers that they think you want to hear, rather than how they actually feel (Adam *et al.*, 2002). To avoid any anxieties, the patient should be given informed choices at all times. It will also be useful to reassure the patient by spending time and explaining clearly:

- how long the assessment may take
- the way in which the assessment will be carried out
- where the assessment will take place
- who will be involved in carrying out the assessment
- the outcomes of the assessment.

Such explanation can help reduce psychological anxieties surrounding the assessment. This could reinforce a mutual partnership between the healthcare professional and the patient and allow the patient a level of control.

Children's health status can change very rapidly (Hockenberry *et al.*, 2003). However, children and adolescents need time and use of adapted tools (Duff, 2000; Hockenberry *et al.*, 2003) in order to carry out a full holistic assessment.

The patient's age

During the assessment process the patient's age and level of understanding also tend to determine what type of information needs to be gathered, what assessment tools and methods need to be employed, as well as what documentation needs to be considered. When assessing older people, for example, the current NHS documentation that directly relates to their management, such as the National Service Framework for Older People (NSF: DoH, 2001), should be taken into account. Legal issues related to adults (part 1) are also different to those of children. Children also differ from many adults in their dependent status (Whalley *et al.*, 2002). Thus, when dealing with children, the Children Act of 1989 (DoH, 1991) as well as the National Service Framework for Children, Young People and Maternity Services (NSFCYPMS: DoH, 2004) must be taken into account. Some of the main points related to the Children Act and the NSFCYPMS will therefore be discussed below.

Children – legal issues

The Children Act, which took effect from 1991, aims to protect the welfare of the child. It is also designed to ensure that parental responsibility is maintained and necessary support is provided (DoH, 1991). The nurse needs to establish, before the assessment takes place, if the parent or carer has responsibility for the patient and is in a position to give the best support. If not, the assessment may be delayed until the responsible parent or carer is able to support the patient. Children, young people and their parent or guardian should be provided with appropriate information, as well as be listened and responded to (DoH, 2004).

For a child under the age of 16 years in England and Wales, the right of the parents to give consent to treatment ceases if and when the child is 'Gillick competent' (Jones, 2003; Tingle & Cribb, 2002). Although the right of a child under 16 to consent to treatment in the Gillick Report (Tingle & Cribb, 2002) is in relation to decisions about contraceptives, it is also central to decision making about other healthcare treatments (Hoyte, 2002). In Scotland, the Age of Legal Capacity Act (1991, section 2.4) states that a child under the age of 16 may give consent to examination and treatment where, in the opinion of a medical practitioner, she or he understands the nature, reasons for and possible consequences of that examination or treatment.

Child protection

The Children Act 1989 (DoH, 1991) and the NSF for Children, Young People and Maternity Services (DoH, 2004) also advocate the protection of children through effective intervention if they are in danger. Thus, staff who come in contact with and who assess children following accidents must be able to recognise possible signs of physical or sexual abuse. Where there are reasonable grounds to suspect any form of child abuse but where the child is not in immediate danger, a child assessment order may be used. In urgent cases, emergency protection orders may be used. In such cases, the court is empowered 'to give directions about medical or mental health examinations or other assessments when making an interim care order, an interim supervision order, a supervision order, child assessment order or an emergency protection order' (DoH 1991, 7.2, 8.41: p32, 42). Staff should also be aware of and must follow local as well as national policies and procedures for child protection (NMC, 2004a 5.4: p7) should the need arise.

Children should be kept informed of what happens to them (DoH, 1991, 2004). They should be listened to and involved in decision making and their feelings and wishes taken into account. Healthcare professionals are required to work with parents to enable them to provide adequate care for their children. Parents should therefore be given the information and guidance necessary for such care. The older child and/or a child with a suspected non-accidental injury should, however, be given the opportunity to speak to staff in confidence, preferably in a soundproof room.

Differences in information required and clinical differences

The information that one needs to gather during holistic assessment also varies according to the age of the patient. The plan of care and treatment is usually dependent on the child's age and weight, with particular reference to the administration of medicines, for example. Recording of the age and weight of a child during health assessment is therefore important.

Apart from their dependent status, another way in which children differ from adults clinically relates to their developmental vulnerability. Growth and developmental processes in individuals are very complex. Although children follow the same pattern of development and maturation, they differ in their growth rate, size and capabilities. Growth results in changes in external dimensions and is accompanied by corresponding changes in the structure and functions of internal organs and tissues (Whalley et al., 2002). They are also 'characterised by cycles of accelerated and slow development, which vary from organ to organ and from system to system' (Whalley et al., 2002). These changes in the body also result in changes in normal body function values (Cox, 2004), examples of which are given in Table 4.1. These values are different from those of adults.

Changes in the body also occur rapidly in size and shape in the adolescent and this may be accompanied by a period of clumsiness in an attempt to adapt to the changes. The body also alters in function: a girl's first menstruation may be a worrying physical experience that needs to be taken into account.

The type, prevalence and intensity of conditions also vary from those that occur in adults. Children, for instance, often present with relatively rare but serious genetic and congenital abnormalities and relatively common but low-severity conditions such as otitis media and asthma (McGlynn et al., 1995). In contrast, morbidity in adults is characterised by conditions that are common and severe. Conditions such as gastroenteritis and diabetes (type 1) are also more common in children but a disorder such as dementia is more likely to occur in the elderly.

Cognitive development and ability

Children also go through different stages of psychosocial development, outlined by Erikson, and cognitive development, as studied by Piaget and Inhelder (Mooney, 2000; Smith et al., 2003). A thorough knowledge of basic child developmental theories is necessary for the assessment of the well-being of children and adolescents. The stages as explained by Piaget and Inhelder (Mooney, 2000: Table 4.2), for example,

Table 4.1 Vital signs: normal range for different age groups.

Age	Respiration rate (per minute)	
• Newborn	30–40**	
• 6 wks–6 months	28–40*	
• 6–12 months	24–40	
• 12–24 months	20–40	
• 2–6 years	20–30	
• 6 years +	15–25	
	Heart rates/pulse	
	Resting	**Active**
• Newborn	100–120	120–160
• 6 wks–6 months	100–120	120–150
• 6–12 months	90–120	120–140
• 1–2 years	90–110	110–130
• 2–6 years	90–100	100–120
• 6–10 years	80–90	90–110
• 10–14 years +	70–85	85–100

Temperature			
• 0 months/ children	36–37.5°C	Core = 37°C	(Variations depend on route used – see further reading)
• Adults	36.2–37.3°C	Mean 36.8°C	(depends on route used – as above)

Further reading

Carroll, M (2000) An evaluation of temperature measurement. *Nurs Stand* 14 (44): 39–43.

Craig, J V, Lancaster, G A, Willamson, P R & Smyth, R L (2000) Temperature measured at the axilla compared with rectum in children and young people: systematic review. *BMJ* 320: 1174–8.

	Blood pressure	
	Systolic	**Diastolic**
• Newborn – 1 year	60–78	40–45
• 1–2 years	90–106	50–70
• 3–7 years	90–120	60–66
• 8–12 years	100–120	70–78
• 13 years + /adult	100–120	70–80

Reproduced with permission from Kelley, 1994; *Glen & Colson, 1995; **Gill & O'Brien, 2003; Hockenberry *et al.*, 2003.

Table 4.2 Overview of psychosocial and cognitive development stages (Mooney, 2000; Phillips, 1998; Whalley et al., 2002).

Age of child	Psychosocial stages (Erikson)	Cognitive stages (Piaget)	Understanding (Piaget)
0 year 1 year	**Infancy** Birth • Trust vs mistrust ----------18 mths	**Sensorimotor stage** (0–2 years)	• Learning and knowledge are gained mainly through the senses. Everything seems to centre on immediate need. Words may not be understood but child responds to tone of voice.
2 years 3 years	**Toddlerhood** • Autonomy vs shame and doubt ------------3 yrs	**Preoperational stage** (2–7 yrs)	• Language development is rapid. Egocentric at this stage; does not understand rules and only sees things from their point of view. Deals with one aspect at a time.
4 years 5 years	**Early childhood** • Initiative vs guilt ------------5 yrs		Every operation is flexible and can be reversed. Associates words with objects.
6 years 7 years	**Middle childhood** • Industry vs inferiority	**Concrete operational stage** (7–11 yrs)	• Now thinks concretely. Able to adopt the viewpoint of others. Can concentrate on more than one aspect. Rules become important.
8 years 9 years 10 years 11 years 12 years 13–19 years	------------12 yrs **Adolescence** • Identity and repudiation vs confusion	**Formal operational stage** (12 years +)	• Deductive and abstract reasoning. Time of great change and anxiety.

highlight the differences in the cognitive development of humans from age 0 through to that of the young adult.

Such differences affect behaviour and understanding of what is being said or done and have implications for practice. Hamers *et al.* (1994), for example, found that the vocal and verbal expressions of a child are what influence the assessment of pain the most. Crying was found to be the most reliable source but this militates against a child who is silent (Simons & Robertson, 2002). Secondly, the egocentric nature (preoperational stage: Table 4.2) of children under age five means that they expect the nurse to know that they are in pain without expressing it (Bee, 2004; Simons & Robertson, 2002). They may also think that the nurse feels they deserve not to have any analgesia when no pain relief is forthcoming, because pain is usually 'perceived as punishment' (Liossi, 2002: p24); they thus suffer in silence (Bee, 2004). It is therefore important to have some understanding of the thought processes which affect a child's communication, as well as considering their cognitive and language abilities, as this is likely to affect the means by which information is gathered during assessment.

In adults, cognitive ability may be affected by a blow on the head or by a medical condition such as dementia or brain tumour. Information may thus need to be sought from the patient's partner, relative or friend during health assessment. Little or no education (Stevens et al., 1999) or the use of a language that may be foreign could also create barriers to cognition. At the other end of the scale, physical changes, including slow articulation rate and a restricted range of expression, might also make it difficult for one to identify how an elderly person is feeling (Biggs, 2000). Very good observation and interviewing skills are therefore vital in the assessment of the older person.

Research findings also suggest that decrease in encoding speed is associated with ageing (Kline & Schieber, 2001). Evidence suggests that memory also tends to decline with age (Stevens et al., 1999) and that younger adults tend to retain and recall more information and events than older adults (Poon, 2001). The loss of efficiency in memory may underlie cognitive changes. This means that the ability of an older person, for example, to remember events surrounding their illness might be affected. In such situations, patience is required when obtaining data from the client. Information also needs to be presented slowly and clearly, and repeated where necessary, to enhance the assessment process. Studies on memory also suggest that older adults tend to perform better in familiar surroundings. The assessment of older people should thus be carried out at home if at all possible, as they are more likely to remember events surrounding their illness. The adaptation of the assessment to meet the needs of individuals is also necessary.

Learning disability

A client whose cognitive ability is severely impaired may be unable to respond directly to the assessment. This may be because they have a learning disability, physical disabilities or mental health problems.

Activity

- Find out what is meant by the term 'learning disability'.
- Are there any parliamentary Acts in relation to learning disability and healthcare?
- Reflect on how any such Acts may impact on the health assessment process of someone with learning disability.

People who have learning disability should be treated with respect and the assessment carried out with dignity. The use of child-like language and child-like non-verbal communication should be avoided when talking to adults with learning disability. Holistic assessment might be problematic but it is still necessary to try to ascertain the client's wishes and needs by using information gained from a carer, an advocate or other responsible adult or recorded information (Tippett, 2001). Care should, however, be taken to ensure that the assessment is not based on the opinion and needs of the carer, advocate or other person accompanying the client. Cognitive appropriate tools can also be used (Duff, 2000) to assist in the gathering of information. The use of other non-verbal communication tools (Gates, 2003), such as Makaton, Sign-a-long or picture exchange communication systems (PECS), may be complemented with different approaches to the assessment.

The assessment of children

The clinical differences between adults and children and the different levels of cognition in children at various stages of development also affect how children may be assessed. First, a child's height is disadvantageous to any sense of power, so to enhance the assessment process, every attempt should be made to meet the child at eye level (Glen & Colson, 1995).

The use of play (DoH, 2004) might also be employed with the preschool child but a school-age child or an adolescent needs to be spoken to directly, along with their parent/s. A pictorial questionnaire such as DOMINIC-R designed for the assessment of the mental health of children aged 6–11 (middle childhood), has also been shown to be useful (Valla *et al.*, 2000).

Early identification of any deviations from normal through 'integrated diagnosis and assessment processes' is essential (DoH, 2004: p21). It is, however, important that 'each assessment builds on earlier ones', 'to avoid the child's story having to be repeated', as advocated by the DoH (2004: p20). The assessment of children may also be completed in three parts. The first part is referred to as the 'across-the-room assessment' (Thomas, 1996: p39) and only involves close observation of the child, whilst talking to the parent or whoever is with the child about the complaint or reason for admission. This should give some clues about the child's general appearance and the seriousness of the condition or injury.

Health history includes:

- biographical data
- reasons for admission
- chief complaint.

This should be followed by a head-to-toe (physical) examination with emphasis on ensuring a clear airway is maintained and accurate assessment of vital signs (Thomas, 1996). The ongoing growth and development of children forms part of the physical assessment. A health history should then be taken. Events that occurred during pregnancy (MacLennan, 1999; Tookey & Peckham, 1999), labour and the perinatal period may have significant effects on a child's future development. The health history therefore includes the child's prenatal, birth and developmental history, as outlined below.

Prenatal history

- Any viral infections.
- Drugs (including alcohol) taken by the mother during pregnancy.
- Any pre-existing maternal condition such as phenylketonuria.

Birth/postnatal history

- Mode of delivery, e.g. normal delivery, forceps delivery or birth by caesarean section.
- Condition at birth; Apgar scores.
- Birth weight, length, head circumference measurements.
- Any congenital abnormalities.
- Feeding method – breast or bottle fed.
- Any neonatal difficulties.
- Maternal history of postnatal depression (Murray & Cooper, 1997).

Developmental history

Developmental history helps to determine the physical growth, motor development and milestones, as well as the cognitive and psychosocial development of the child. It also allows any deviations from the norm to be identified, treated and/or managed. The information gathered at birth forms a baseline for comparison. The assessment of physical growth involves serial assessments and recordings of the child's weight, head circumference (for infants), height, nutritional assessment and general review of systems (Whalley et al., 2002).

The following factors should also be recorded:

- accidents
- illnesses/childhood diseases
- surgical history
- allergies
- immunisation (types and dates received; any adverse reactions)
- quality of sleep and rest.

There are also certain questions that need to be borne in mind when gathering developmental history:

- Does the child demonstrate physical growth within the normal range for his/her age?
- Are vital signs within normal range for the child's age?
- Are the child's vision and hearing abilities within normal range?
- Does the child perform gross and fine motor milestones within normal range for age?
- Is the child able to demonstrate psychosocial developmental milestones for age?
- Does the child demonstrate cognitive development for age?

Current daily activities of living such as eating and drinking habits, elimination and developmental issues such as sexuality should be explored as appropriate.

Like the adult patient, health assessment of the child is an ongoing process. However, the assessment tools used for different age groups do vary. It is thus important for nurses to familiarise themselves with the different assessment tools. In all cases, however, any documentation of information gathered on the patient should be accurate, legible, comprehensive, clear, contemporaneous, signed and dated on the appropriate forms (DoH, 2004; NMC, 2004b).

Section 3: Gender and health assessment

The health of men and women living in Britain has improved over the past century and life expectancy has risen (Social Trends, 2003). This has been attributed to improvements in the standard of living, especially in relation to the nation's diet and housing, and advances in medical science and technology.

However, according to the Secretary of State for Health (1999), there is inequality in health between men and women related to their social groupings, which persist throughout life. Several factors contribute to these inequalities, relating to the biological, socio-economic, psychological and environmental aspects of adult life in the United Kingdom today.

Certain illnesses, such as those related to the reproductive organs, are gender specific. Research also suggests that certain illnesses are more prevalent not only in certain age groups but also in men than in women and vice versa. The aim of this section therefore is to discuss some of the gender issues that need to be considered during health assessment.

Learning objectives

- Identify and discuss the prevalence of certain conditions in men and women.
- Discuss the reasons for the differences in the health patterns of men and women.
- Discuss some of the health-related behaviours for men and women.
- Consider gender differences and be sensitive when assessing the health of patients.

Trends and patterns of health and disease among men and women

Type 1 diabetes mellitus is more common in children and young people (Whittaker, 2004). Type 2 diabetes mellitus is, however, more common in people aged 40 years and above but it is disproportionately higher and usually diagnosed before age 40 in ethnic minority groups (Diabetes UK, 2000). It is also more prevalent in men than in women. However, obese women are more prone to developing type 2 diabetes than obese men (Chambers *et al.*, 2004; Garrow & Summerbell, 2002). Women with diabetes also have a greater risk of dying from it (DoH, 2001).

In England and Wales, the prevalence of asthma and chronic obstructive pulmonary disease (COPD) is also currently higher in females than in males (Whittaker, 2004). This latter condition appears to be strongly linked to socio-economic states and with the prevalence of cigarette smoking (Social Trends, 2004). It has also been related to poor housing conditions and poor ventilation (Stobbart, 1999).

Coronary heart disease (CHD), although seen as a male problem, is the single leading cause of death amongst women in the UK. CHD has been linked to smoking, obesity and high cholesterol levels in men, high blood pressure, premature menopause, diabetes (Pennel Initiative, 1998) and poverty (Payne, 1991) in women.

Osteoporosis is more common in women, particularly following menopause. Since osteoporosis is a major cause of fracture, the incidence of fractures, especially after the age of 40, is also higher in women than in men (Pennel Initiative, 1998).

Sexually transmitted disease has been increasing in recent years among young people under the age of 25. The number of cases diagnosed in young women rose from 11 800 in 1995 to 28 900 in 2001 (Social Trends, 2003).

A survey of psychiatric morbidity in the year 2000 identified mental health problems affecting people aged 16–74. A higher proportion of women were reported to be suffering from symptoms of fatigue, sleep problems, stress and anxiety (Clarke, 2001). This higher reported rate of mental illness among women reflects differences in the way men and women are socialised. Women are more likely to talk openly about their feelings, anxieties and illnesses. Men are often expected to display independence and self-reliance and are less inclined to admit to having psychological problems (Clarke, 2001).

Health issues and dilemmas for men and women

A report of the National Audit Office (2001) concluded that there is a problem with obesity among the British population. According to this report, using the Body Mass Index scale, 1:5 adults are described as obese and if this ratio is added to those described as overweight, then nearly 60% of the population needs to lose weight. Over half of all women and two-thirds of all men are described as either obese or overweight (Denscombe, 2004). In a more recent national study, however, the Office for National Statistics (OFNS, 2004) found that 42% of men and 32% of women are overweight. Ruxton (2004) links the rise in adult obesity to the increasing prevalence of childhood obesity. Trends in adult obesity suggest that more men are overweight and more women are obese. The picture in childhood and adolescence is less clear-cut.

The potential health risks associated with overweight include cardiovascular disease, diabetes, gallstones and varicose veins (OFNS, 2004: p17). Assessment of weight and body mass among male and female members of the population should therefore consider gender and age differences.

Activity

Using the Body Mass Index assessment scale, work out your own health status in relation to your weight and height (see Chapter 7, p. 254).

- Compare your results with those of other men and women who would describe themselves as having a healthy body.
- Also note their perceptions and views.
- Consider how you can use the information from the Body Mass Index to promote health.

The Department of Health (1993) noted that gender differences in mortality also exist. Currently, the life expectancy at birth for a boy is about five years less than for a girl born at the same time. According to the Chief Medical Officer's 1992 annual report (DoH, 1993), the male death rate is higher than the female death rate in all age groups. The difference in life expectancy, morbidity and mortality between men and women has been described by some as in 'crisis' and has led to growing interest (Luck & Bamford, 2000).

There is also growing concern about the gap that exists between the healthcare of men and women in the UK (Clarke, 2001). In the year 2000 the Department of Health estimated that eight times as much money was spent on female health issues as on male health issues. There is screening for breast cancer and cervical tumours but no equivalent screening for prostate cancer. Testicular self-examination should, however, be encouraged (see Chapter 6).

Men and health-related behaviour

There is evidence to suggest that some of the differences in trends and patterns in men's health stem from their health-related behaviour. This may be influenced by their knowledge, attitudes and health beliefs. Men are less inclined to visit their family doctor (Pennel Initiative, 1998) and, more importantly, they are shy about seeking health assessment related to their personal problems. As a result they tend to have poor health outcomes, including a higher incidence of deaths from heart attacks (Discovery Health, 2003).

Women and health-related behaviour

Women tend to visit their doctors twice as often as men, according to NHS official figures. It has been pointed out that women often become the 'health keeper' in their households (Clarke, 2001), suggesting that women's frequent visits to their doctors may often be on behalf of their family members.

Described as the 'ladettes', some young women have taken to binge-drinking, heavy smoking and girls' nights out. Denscombe (2004) also indicates that this lifestyle can be seen among women in their 30s, with women aged 30–45 smoking and drinking more heavily than in the past, which could explain why the incidence of COPD is higher in women than in men. Women of this age group also tend to undertake little exercise.

Activity

Readers may familiarise themselves with the following theories which may help to explain clients' health-related behaviour:

- The health belief model formulated by Rosenstock in 1966 and developed by Becker in 1987 (Naidoo & Wills, 2004).
- The theory of reasoned action by Fishbein and Ajzen (Naidoo & Wills, 2004).

The differences between men and women in relation to health and disease should be taken into account prior to and during health assessment in order to provide a sound basis for action planning.

A health assessment approach: some practical aspects to consider

Privacy, confidentiality and dignity

These have been discussed already but other points to consider include personal and cultural preferences. The patient may or may not wish their spouse/partner to be present so they should be asked about this discreetly.

Male clients from other cultures may not want to be examined by a female and religious and cultural beliefs may deter some men from exposing their physical bodies. Similarly, some women may not wish to be examined by a male.

Consent

Informed consent should be obtained. Therefore the man or woman should be made aware of the extent and duration of any procedures involved in the assessment.

Differing health beliefs between the client and the assessor

There may be distinct differences in the clients' perspectives on health when compared to those of the healthcare professional. Carter & Green (2002) emphasised the importance of assessing how people perceive their bodies and how this influences their self-image and self-esteem.

Effective listening skills and the principles of empathic understanding should be employed (see Chapter 5). Convey (1999), in his text on the habits of highly effective people, describes empathic listening as a skill which suggests that the assessor should seek first to understand the client and his beliefs about his health, before attempting to change his health-related behaviour.

The client's perception of their body image

Price (1999) defines body image as a concept that involves three areas: body reality, body ideal and body presentation.

Body reality
A man may perceive his weight, height build and posture as being within 'normal' range. This influences how he sees himself, and his masculinity. In reality, the male client may be overweight, have a problem with hair loss and excessive fat around the abdominal area. The assessor should be aware of this discrepancy and demonstrate sensitivity when discussing issues to do with a man's or woman's body.

Body ideal
People often have definite beliefs about how their bodies should look and perform. This is often influenced by the society and also ethnic and cultural values. The assessor should be aware of this and again show sensitivity.

Body presentation
This relates to how the man or woman presents their body to others socially. This includes dress, use of make-up, jewellery, hairpieces, wigs and dentures. The assessor should observe how clients present themselves, without being judgemental about their appearance. Often ill health, pain and disease can affect a person's body image.

Aim of assessment

To obtain a health history from the client in an attempt to determine his or her background, lifestyle, family history and the presence of illness or injuries. The assessment should form the basis for the development of an action plan. The process may be divided into categories.

Pre-assessment interview

The assessor should arrange a short chat with the client and those accompanying him or her to explain the assessment process, obtain his or her consent and determine the conditions under which the assessment will be undertaken, as discussed earlier in this chapter. This preinterview will enable the client to express their wishes, ask questions and voice concerns.

The client's personal and social history

Family history

The assessor should discuss the following with the client:

• health status of immediate family members
• medical problems affecting male and female family members
• the person's perceptions of their roles and responsibilities, including occupation, family and responsibility for significant others such as elderly or disabled relatives.

Physical examination

An appropriately qualified nurse, midwife or doctor may carry out this aspect of the assessment. Physical examination can be quite detailed and sensitive so this should be explained to the client in the pre-assessment interview. Some men may request a male doctor. Physical examination of a man may involve the following:

• a head-to-toe examination of the man's body including examination of the male genitalia (see Chapter 6).
• rectal examination, recommended to men over 50 or those with a family history of prostate cancer
• men can develop breast lumps, which may be benign or malignant. This should thus be taken into account.

It is important to note that the assessor must have a sound rationale for carrying out these tests. The use of pathological testing must relate to the personal health history, physical examination and family history of the client. Other specific pathological tests may be carried out where indicated, examples of which are given in Box 4.1.

Box 4.1 Pathological tests

• Resting electrocardiograph (ECG) recording
• Stress ECG testing
• Urine testing
• Sputum analysis
• Blood tests – to measure cholesterol, triglycerides, glucose, liver and kidney function tests, red and white blood cell count, clotting times

Activity	
Condition	**Find out and list some specific tests that may be carried out for each of the conditions listed**
• Bowel cancer	
• Gastric ulcers	
• Tuberculosis	
• HIV testing	
• Hepatitis A,B,C	
• Prostate and testicular cancer	
• Lung cancer	
• Sexually transmitted infections	

Activity

- The reader may wish to consider the gender-specific pathological tests which may be carried out on a male or female client. Refer to Social Trends (2003) and Chapter 7.

Physical assessment of the female client

Physical examination of a woman may involve many of the points already mentioned in this section of the chapter. However, there are specific aspects related to the female client which need to be considered:

- *Breast and pelvic examination*. Clinical breast and pelvic/vaginal examination should be carried out sensitively by a qualified health-care professional.
- *Cervical smears*. Women aged 18 years and over should have a smear taken every three years as part of the screening process for cervical cancer.
- *Sexually transmitted infection (STI) screening*. Women who are sexually active may require screening for STIs such as gonorrhoea, syphilis, genital herpes and HIV.
- *Bone density/bone mass measurement*. This should be offered to women over the age of 50 and those who are at risk of osteoporosis or fractures.

Assessment and sexual orientation

The client's concept of sexuality and their sexual orientation also need to be considered in the assessment process. The Royal College of Nursing (RCN, 1994) issued a statement in an attempt to alleviate discriminatory practice and address the needs of lesbian and gay clients. This statement requires nurses to ask themselves the following questions:

- Do I know much about gay, lesbian and other alternative lifestyles?
- Do I know how I feel about people whose perception of sexuality differs from my own?

The PLISSIT model (Fogel & Lauver, 1999) is an example of an assessment tool that healthcare professionals can use to address issues of sexuality with their clients during assessment. The model suggests four possible levels of intervention:

(1) *Permission*. During the assessment of the client's personal history, a sexual history should form part of the basic questions. This allows the client permission to ask questions and express their wishes relating to their own care, e.g. clients may be asked about their gender and how they would describe their sexual orientation.
(2) *Limited information*. If the client wishes to discuss this further, the healthcare professional should be prepared to listen and question with sensitivity and empathy.
(3) *Specific suggestions*. Appropriately trained healthcare professionals may need to be involved at this level to work in partnership with the client to further assess their specific needs.
(4) *Intensive therapy*. The client may need to be referred to a specialist for further assessment and support.

Post-assessment interviews

The findings of the assessment should be discussed with the client by an appropriately qualified healthcare professional, in a private and confidential environment. In the case of medical assessment, the doctor should discuss the findings and outcomes of medical investigations.

According to Clarke (2001), a medical diagnosis can create a label for the man or woman, which may be seen as a stigma. An example of this might be when a doctor breaks the news of a sexually transmitted infection (STI) or malignant disease to a client. Healthcare professionals need to appreciate this when discussing findings of their assessment with the client.

Post-assessment interviews should include:

- identification of risk factors and health behaviours associated with disease

- abnormal findings and what these may indicate
- health issues for discussion, including diet, exercise and lifestyle
- health education and health promotion
- self-help strategies.

Questions to consider prior to and during assessment

All the points made in this chapter imply the need to consider the following questions prior to and during health assessment.

- Who is being assessed?
- In what environment is the assessment taking place?
- Where is the assessment taking place? (Hospital, home, workplace)
- Are there appropriate facilities to carry out the assessment, e.g. a private room or area to ensure privacy and confidentiality?
- What resources does the assessor require?
- What information needs to be collected and why?
- What skills does the assessor need? (See Chapters 2 and 10)
- Who needs the information?
- What are the implications for the client?
- How can the assessment form the basis for action planning, health promotion and healthcare delivery?

Summary

Holistic health assessment cannot be based on assessment of the patient in isolation. As discussed in this chapter, ethical considerations, the environment in which the assessment takes place, health and disability status, age, cognitive ability and gender of the patient are all factors that need to be considered during health assessment. The need for sensitivity and adaptation of the assessment process to meet individual needs has been emphasised.

Activity

- What is meant by 'respect for persons' and how might this impact on the assessment process?
- Ensuring a patient's privacy and dignity is a fundamental and essential aspect of care. Discuss.
- Identify and discuss some of the main factors that need to be considered before and during a health assessment, with particular reference to children.
- Explore some of the main gender issues that need to be considered during health assessment.

References

Section 1

Department of Health (2000) *Essence of Care: patient focussed benchmarking for healthcare practitioners*. HMSO, London.

Edgar, A (2003) *Dignity and the Elderly: issues in the ethics of healthcare practice*. Paper given at Ethics in Healthcare Practice Conference, University College Northampton, December 3rd, 2003.

Nursing and Midwifery Council (2004) *Code of Professional Conduct: standards for conduct, performance and ethics*. NMC, London.

Rumbold, G (1999) *Ethics in Nursing Practice*, 3rd edition. Baillière Tindall, Edinburgh.

Rumbold, G (2002) Ethical issues in cardiac care. In: Hatchett, R & Thompson, D (eds) *Cardiac Nursing – a comprehensive guide*. Churchill Livingstone, Edinburgh.

Seedhouse, D (1998) *Ethics – the heart of health care*. John Wiley, Chichester.

Section 2

Adam, L, Amos M & Munro, J (2002) *Promoting Health: politics and practice*. Sage, London.

Bee, H (2004) *The Developing Child: a journey through childhood and adolescence*, 9th edition. Longman, New York.

Biggs, S (2000) *Understanding Ageing: images, attitudes and professional practice*. Open University Press, Buckingham.

Cox, C L (2004) *Physical Assessment for Nurses*. Blackwell Publishing, Oxford.

Department of Health (1991) *The Children Act* 1989. HMSO, London.

Department of Health (2001) *National Services Framework for Older People*. HMSO, London.

Department of Health (2004) *National Service Framework for Children, Young People and Maternity Services. Executive Summary. Change for children – every child matters*. www.dh.gov.uk/PolicyAndGuidance/HealthAndSocialCare-Topics/ChildrenServices/fs/en.

Duff, L. (2000) All about pain. *Paediatric Nursing* 12 (7): 5–6.

English National Board for Nursing and Midwifery (1999) *Researching Professional Education. Preparation for the developing role of the community children's nurse*. ENB, London.

Erikson, W W (1963) *Childhood and Society*. Norton and Company, London. Cited in Whalley, F, Wong, D L & Hockenberry M (2002) *Wong's Nursing Care of Infants and Children*. Mosby, St Louis.

Gates, B (2003) *Learning Disabilities*, 7th edition. Mosby, London.

Gill, D & O'Brien, N (2003) *Paediatric Clinical Examination Made Easy*, 4th edition. Churchill Livingstone, Edinburgh.

Glen, S & Colson, J (1995) The care of children. In: Hinchliff, S, Norman, S & Schober, J (eds) *Nursing Practice and Health Care*. Edward Arnold, London.

Hamers, J P H, Abu-Saad, H H, Halfens, R J G & Schumacher, J N M (1994) Factors influencing nurses' pain assessment and intervention in children. *Journal of Advanced Nursing* 20: 853–60.

Hockenbery, M, Wilson, D, Winkelstein, M & Kline N (2003) *Wong's Nursing Care of Infants and Children*, 7th edition. Mosby, St Louis.

Hoyte, P (2002) Medico-legal aspects of child health surveillance. In: Harnden, A & Sheikh, A (eds) *Promoting Child Health in Primary Care*. Royal College of General Practitioners, London.

Jones, B (2003) The interests and rights of the patient. In: Jones B (ed.) *Childhood Disability in a Multicultural Society*. Radcliffe Medical Press, Oxford.

Kelley, S J (1994) *Pediatric Emergency Nursing*, 2nd edition. Appleton and Lange, Norwalk, Connecticut.

Kline, D W & Schieber, F (2001) Vision and ageing. In: Birren, J E & Schaie, K W (eds) *Handbook of the Psychology of Aging*. Academic Press, New York.

Liossi, C (2002) The nature of paediatric procedure-related cancer pain. In: Liossi C (ed.) *Procedure-Related Cancer Pain in Children*. Radcliffe Medical Press, Oxford.

MacLennan, A, for the International Cerebral Palsy Task Force (1999) A template for defining a causal relationship between acute intrapartum events and cerebral palsy: international consensus statement. *BMJ* 319: 1054–9.

McGlynn, E, Halfon, N & Leibowitz, A (1995) Assessing quality of care for children: prospects under health reform. *Archives of Paediatrics and Adolescent Medicine* 149 (4): 359–68.

Mooney, C G (2000) *Theories of Childhood: an introduction to Dewey, Montessori, Erikson, Piaget and Vygotsky*. Redleaf Press, St Paul, Minnesota.

Murray, L & Cooper, P J (1997) Effects of postnatal depression on infant development. *Archives of Disease in Childhood* 77: 99–101.

Nursing and Midwifery Council (2004a) *Code of Professional Conduct: standards for conduct, performance and ethics*. NMC, London.

Nursing and Midwifery Council (2004b) *Guidelines for Records and Record Keeping*. NMC, London.

Phillips, S (1998) Infancy through late childhood. In: Kozier, B, Erb, G, Blais, K et al. (eds) *Fundamentals of Nursing: concepts, process and practice*. Addison-Wesley, New York.

Poon, L W (2001) Differences in human memory with ageing. Natural causes and clinical implications. In: Birren, J E & Schaie, K W (eds) *Handbook of the Psychology of Aging*. Academic Press, New York.

Simons, J & Robertson, E (2002) Poor communication and knowledge deficits: obstacles to effective management of children's postoperative pain. *Journal of Advanced Nursing* 40 (1): 78–86.

Smith, P K, Cowie, H & Blades, M (2003) *Understanding Children's Development*. Blackwell Publishing, Oxford.

Stevens, F C J, Kaplan, C D, Ponds, R W H M, Diederiks, J P M & Jolles, J (1999) How ageing and social factors affect memory. *Age and Ageing* 28: 379–84. http://ageing.oupjournals.org/cgi/reprint/28/4/379.pdf.

Tingle, J & Cribb, A (eds) (2002) *Nursing Law and Ethics.* Blackwell Science, Oxford.

Tippett, A (2001) All about me: documentation for children with special needs. *Paediatric Nursing* 13 (10): 34–5.

Thomas, D (1996) Assessing children – it's different. *RN* April: 38–44.

Tookey, P A & Peckham, C S (1999) Surveillance of congenital rubella in Great Britain, 1971–96. *BMJ* 318: 769–70.

Valla, J P, Bergeron, L & Smolla, N (2000) The Dominic-R: a pictorial interview for 6- to 11-year old children. *Journal of the American Academy of Child and Adolescent Psychiatry* 39 (1): 85–93.

Whalley, F, Wong, D L & Hockenberry, M (eds) (2002) *Wong's Nursing Care of Infants and Children.* Mosby, St Louis.

Section 3

Carter, S & Green, A (2002) Body image and sexuality. In: Hogston, R & Simpson, P M (eds) *Foundations of Nursing Practice.* Palgrave, Basingstoke.

Chambers, R, Wakley, G & Jenkins, J (2004) *Demonstrating Your Competence 2: women's health.* Radcliffe Medical Press, Oxford.

Clarke, A (2001) *The Sociology of Health Care.* Pearson Education, Harlow.

Convey, S (1999) *Seven Habits of Highly Effective People.* Simon and Schuster, London.

Department of Health (1993) *On the State of the Public Health. Annual Report of the Chief Medical Officer.* HMSO, London.

Department of Health (2001) *National Service Framework for Diabetes Standards.* DoH, London.

Denscombe, M (2004) *Sociology Update.* Olympus Books, UK.

Diabetes UK (2000) *Understanding Diabetes.* www.diabetes.org.uk/diabetes/under.htm.

Discovery Health (2003) *Health Risk Assessment.* http://health.discovery.com.

Fogel, C & Lauver, D (1999) *Sexual Health Promotion.* WB Saunders, London.

Garrow, J & Summerbell, C (2002) Obesity. In: DoH (eds) *Health Needs Assessment.* Radclifffe Medical Press, Oxford.

Luck, M & Bamford, M (2000) *Men's Health Perspectives: diversity and paradox.* Blackwell, Oxford.

Naidoo, J & Wills, J (eds) (2004) *Practising Health Promotion: developing practice.* Baillière Tindall, Edinburgh.

National Audit Office (2001) *Tackling Obesity in England.* National Audit Office, London.

Office for National Statistics (2004) *The National Diet and Nutrition Survey: adults aged 19 to 64 years.* Stationery Office, London.

Payne, S (1991) *Women and Poverty.* Harvester Wheatsheaf, London.

Pennel Initiative (1998) *The Pennel Report on Women's Health. Positive steps for later life.* Lawrence Cheung Limited in partnership with Wyeth. Health Service Management Unit, University of Manchester.

Price, B (1999) *Altered Body Image (NT clinical monographs).* Emap Healthcare, London.

Royal College of Nursing (1994) *The Nursing Care of Lesbians and Gay Men: an RCN statement.* RCN, London.

Ruxton, C (2004) Obesity in children. *Nursing Standard* 18 (20): 47–52.

Secretary of State for Health (1999) *Saving Lives: our healthier nation.* Stationery Office, London.

Social Trends (2003) *No 33.* Stationery Office, London.

Social Trends (2004) *No 34.* Stationery Office, London.

Stobbart, M J (1999) Prevention and management of COPD. *Professional Nurse* 14 (4): 241–4.

Whittaker, N (2004) *Disorders and Interventions.* Palgrave, Basingstoke.

Communication skills for holistic health assessment

A. Crouch

Learning objectives

- Define the term 'communication'.
- Describe the main aspects of the communication process.
- Identify and discuss factors that facilitate effective communication.
- Identify and discuss communication skills needed for the gathering of subjective and objective data during holistic assessment.
- Discuss barriers to communication and how these may affect the information-gathering process during holistic assessment.

Introduction

The importance of holistic assessment has been highlighted in the previous chapters. Not only are the patient's biographical data required but physical, psychological, social, cultural and spiritual data are also needed. The gathering of such data requires optimal communication skills on the part of the health professional carrying out the assessment. Information-gathering processes could, however, be quite challenging for some (Attree *et al.*, 1994). Evidence does also suggest the lack of effective communication between healthcare workers and patients (Audit Commission, 1993; Cantwell & Ramirez, 1997; Simons & Robertson, 2002). It is also evident that blocking behaviours are sometimes used by nurses during health assessment to avoid distress in having to deal with psychological issues that may arise (Wilkinson, 1991; Wilkinson *et al.*, 2002).

Registered nurses and midwives are, however, required by the Nursing and Midwifery Council (2002: p13) to 'engage in, develop and disengage from therapeutic relationships through the use of appropriate communication and interpersonal skills'. This requires knowledge of the barriers to and boundaries of effective communication and embraces the use of effective and appropriate communication skills (NMC, 2004: pp12–13). This chapter is therefore aimed at discussing some of the communication skills needed for effective gathering of data during holistic health assessment. Some of the main barriers to effective communication will also be identified and discussed.

Definition and classification

Communication can be defined as a two-way process in which information is transmitted and received. It also involves feedback between the recipient and the transmitter of information. The main elements involved in the process (Figure 5.1) therefore include the:

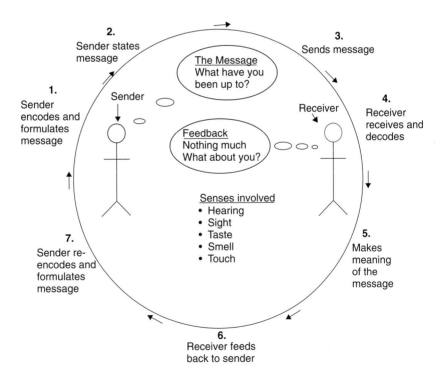

Figure 5.1 The process of communication

- sender/transmitter (encoder)
- message
- receiver (decoder)
- feedback.

The content of the message is important but unless the process of communication is right, the understanding of the message could be adversely affected. Effectiveness of the communication process is therefore of vital importance. Effective communication could be defined as the process of transmission and reception of information, in which an understanding of what is transmitted is achieved by the receiver. This means that communication involves both the activity of sending and receiving messages, and the interpretation of the messages.

All the special senses of both the transmitter and the receiver of the message, which are the senses of hearing, sight, smell and touch, are involved in the process of effective communication (Figure 5.1). The sense of taste might also be involved as appropriate.

Verbal communication

Communication can be classified into two categories: verbal and non-verbal. The verbal category includes speech; that is, oral communication that may be direct and personal and in which facial expression and gestures can be used to give impact. It may also be communicated indirectly as in the use of a telephone, an interpreter or a messenger.

The verbal category also includes written messages. As with the use of telephone, one must compensate for the lack of face-to-face contact with a written message and it does not have the same impact.

Non-verbal communication

General behaviour and attitudes are referred to as non-verbal communication. The tone of voice, gestures, listening, head nodding, facial expression, eye contact and the use of touch come under this category. Other forms of non-verbal communication include orientation, which refers to the body's position and the angle at which one person interacts with another. It is usually referred to in conjunction with physical proximity, which is the distance between two people. This distance is sometimes referred to as territorial or personal space (Atkinson, 2003a). Each of us appears to have our own idea of personal space which is a form of private territory and if someone gets too close, we tend to move backwards in order to re-establish the space. Certain procedures involve the invasion of the patient's space so the nurse needs to be self-aware during the health assessment process.

Other behaviours such as the type of clothes we wear and how we wear them, for example, tell others more about us than we realise. On a typical hot summer's day, for instance, it might be assumed that someone wearing a woollen jumper and a coat is unwell and perhaps feeling very cold. Many tend to wear dark-coloured clothes during winter in England but the use of dark-coloured clothes, in particular black, brown, red or a mixture of those colours, by some West Africans (Ghanaians, for instance) denotes mourning for the dead. Although the examples given may reflect individual preferences or cultural variations in the choice of clothing, they are behaviours that communicate some form of message to us.

Generally, non-verbal communication can substitute for and reinforce other forms of communication, as well as helping to convey a message. Relationships are also established and maintained mainly by the use of non-verbal signals (Argyle, 1990).

Factors that facilitate effective communication

Certain factors related to the sender, the message and the receiver of the message are necessary for effective communication. When in a dialogue with someone, it is important for the *sender* of the message to:

- speak clearly and loudly
- use understandable language
- use face-to-face (two-way/direct) communication where possible
- pace the speech appropriately (not too fast or too slow)
- maintain eye contact
- use gestures appropriately, e.g. for emphasis, but avoid mannerisms that are distracting
- use correct non-verbal behaviour to support the spoken words
- use readable written words (easy to read).

The *message* should be:

- goal directed or purposeful
- understandable
- clear
- unambiguous
- relevant
- accurate
- precise but sufficient.

The *receiver* of the message should:

- face the sender if possible
- be very attentive
- listen carefully and actively
- use questions, gestures, pictures, etc. to clarify what has been said where necessary.

According to Argyle (1990), 80–90% of communication is non-verbal and head nodding, facial expression and the tone of voice are more important than verbal messages. On taking a patient's pulse, for instance, where the pulse rate is very slow and irregular, the patient might pick up non-verbal clues from the nurse that something is wrong. When the patient asks if all is well, the response might be 'yes' but the anxious look and the rechecking of the pulse could negate the reassurance given. Thus, congruence between the verbal and the non-verbal message is also important if the message being conveyed to an individual is to be interpreted correctly and meaningfully.

All verbal and non-verbal behaviour appears to have, and could be interpreted as having, meaning. If all behaviour is accepted as having meaning, then it could be said that all life is indeed enriched and is dependent on communication, and all nursing and midwifery activities could be described as communication. This stresses the importance of effective communication during holistic health assessment of patients and clients.

Skills needed during holistic health assessment

Subjective data

Free expression by the patient with little or no inhibition is important during holistic health assessment. Hence before and during a health assessment, one needs to take into account factors that could affect the communication process as discussed in Chapter 4. Very good interviewing techniques are essential for the gathering of the general health history. This encompasses the biographical data and subjective data on the patient's physical, sociocultural, spiritual and psychological state, which involves the use of a combination of verbal and non-verbal skills.

Having obtained consent where possible, the use of a private room for taking the health history could help put the patient at ease and avoid inhibition (Audit Commission, 1993). Some explanation should then be given to the patient as to what the health assessment will involve, why it is necessary and who will be involved in the process.

Body messages are of great importance when carrying out a health assessment. For example, if the nurse looks in the opposite direction whilst the patient or client is expressing how they are feeling, the patient would probably assume that the nurse is not interested in what they are saying, and is therefore not listening. Burnard (2004), Duxbury (2000) and Egan (2002) advocate the use of attending skills, which have the acronym S O L E R, which stands for:

- Sit squarely
- Open posture to be adopted

- Lean slightly towards the patient
- Eye contact should be maintained
- Relax.

The employment of such non-verbal skills implies that one is interested and is paying attention to what is being said. As mentioned, however, we tend to function within an invisible distance around us, which is known as personal space (Atkinson, 2003a). Care should thus be taken to avoid sitting too close or too far away.

According to Nelson-Jones (2004), the face is the main part of the body used for sending messages and so the nurse needs to demonstrate interest through a friendly, relaxed facial expression and smiling. Smiling also conveys warmth and caring (Carcio, 1999; Lichtman, 2005), so the adoption of the SOLER position and the expression of a smile as and when appropriate could encourage the establishment of good rapport, as well as encouraging the client to talk.

Eye contact is also suggestive of the nurse's intention to engage with the patient but care should be taken not to overuse it. Eye contact is also used to gain the patient's attention. It should, however, be borne in mind that it is not acceptable in every culture. For instance, eye contact is interpreted as confrontational and adversarial by some Japanese patients (Lester, 1998; Rajan, 1995). Cultural variations in the use of eye contact during communication should therefore be taken into account.

Having adopted an appropriate position, we then need to use both closed and open questions to elicit data.

Closed questions

Closed-ended questions are questions that require short answers (Box 5.1). Such questions begin with what, who, which, when and are particularly useful when collecting biographical data such as the patient's name, address and telephone number. Closed questions may also be used to elicit specific answers and facts.

Although the use of such questions saves time, they do not allow for exploration. They do, however, allow patients with conditions such as breathlessness, severe pain or depression, for example, to give 'yes or no' answers. During the interview, questions must be designed to elicit the necessary information from the patient where possible.

Box 5.1 Examples of closed questions.

- **Example 1:** The question 'what is your name?' requires only a short answer.
- **Example 2:** Do you smoke? The answer to this is likely to be 'yes' or 'no'.

Box 5.2 Examples of open questions.

- **Example 1**: Tell me what happened.
- **Example 2**: How are you feeling about the treatment?
- **Example 3**: How are you feeling right now?

Box 5.3 Example of paraphrasing.

- **Patient:** Passing water is rather painful and worrying because the urine looks darkish in colour.
- **Nurse:** It has been uncomfortable to pass urine; you are also concerned about the colour of it?

Open-ended questions

Open-ended questions (Box 5.2) are those that require more than one or two words or a short answer from the patient. They begin with how, when, where and what. Open questions can also be in the form of a statement.

Example 1 (Box 5.2) is likely to encourage the patient to give a full description of what happened. The questions should not be rushed. They should also be stated clearly and tactfully, especially when interviewing about sexuality or private parts of the body, to avoid any embarrassment.

It is important for the patient to feel that they would be listened to, if they were to continue talking. This could be achieved by the use of the following skills.

Minimal prompts

The use of minimal prompts such as 'uh huh', 'yes', 'OK', also suggests that you are listening which could encourage the patient to talk, but care should be taken to avoid the overuse of such prompts. It is also important to check for understanding in order to ensure the accuracy of the information being gathered.

Paraphrase

A paraphrase is the restatement of what someone has said, in your own words, without changing the meaning (Box 5.3). The appropriate use of paraphrases should not only help to move the interview forward but also help the sender of a message to listen to what they have just said and allow any correction to be made where necessary (Egan, 2002). Paraphrases are therefore useful in checking for understanding.

Silence/close observation

The use of the above skills on their own might not be enough to gain full information. The use of silence gives one an opportunity to listen, as well as observe for clues such as the client's body movements, gestures, facial expressions and posture. The client's non-verbal expressions, such as a smile, the use of gestures, body movements and eye contact, for example, are all helpful in the gathering of information during holistic health assessment (Workman, 2003). For example, although individuals react differently to pain, in some cultures it is quite normal for a patient to express pain by groaning loudly. Other behaviours such as frowning, muscle tension, grimacing and moaning have also been observed in patients who complained of pain (Mateo & Krenzischek, 1992). Since pain causes discomfort, people in pain also tend to adopt a more comfortable position. Depending on the intensity or nature of the pain, one might place one's hand on the area affected. Mobility might also be restricted, especially if the pain is located in a limb or lower abdomen. Such non-verbal expressions should reinforce what the patient is saying verbally. Thus, whilst interviewing a patient, close observation of their non-verbal expressions, apart from listening actively (Chuk, 2002) could help gather important information.

Even when the patient's verbal and non-verbal expressions appear to be congruent, the nurse should be careful to avoid misinterpretation of behaviours, which might be acceptable in certain cultures. In Lester's study (1998), for example, Blanter expressed regret after observing the admission and treatment of a Haiti woman who was apparently speaking to 'spirits' whilst waiting to be seen for an abdominal pain. The Haiti woman was diagnosed as having a psychological illness because she was heard speaking loudly to the 'spirits', a behaviour that was apparently normal within her culture.

Other non-verbal aspects of the patient, such as the length and state of the finger and toenails, as well as the clothes worn, could help gather information. It could, for instance, be assumed that the patient's personal hygiene is probably neglected where the nails are long and dirty and the clothes appear very dirty, with an offensive smell.

Empathy
During health assessment, it is also vital to demonstrate empathic understanding through active listening skills, some of which have been discussed above. The word 'empathy' is defined as the ability to enter another's world, to see the world as they see it (Burnard, 1999). It is debatable whether this could ever be achieved but Burnard (1999: p75) advocates that, in order to enter the world of the patient, one must be willing 'to explore and intuitively allow the patient to express themselves fully'. This means listening carefully and responding in a way that indicates an understanding of what the patient said from their own perspective, which involves the use of attending, listening, observation and reflective skills (Egan, 2002). In the process, the nurse reflects back to the patient facts and feelings. An example of this is shown in Box 5.4.

Box 5.4 Example of empathic reflection.

- **Nurse**: What I've picked up from this discussion is that you have difficulty in passing urine. You feel tired and have difficulty in coping with household chores. You are also worried because your urine seems to be darkish in colour. Is that right?
- **Patient**: Yes. That is right.
- **Nurse**: It would be useful then if you could please give us a urine sample for examination. Following that, I would also like to check your pulse and blood pressure to help give a better picture of what is happening. How does that sound?

Summarising

A summary is the restatement of the main points of what has been said. Where an assessment tool in the form of a questionnaire is being used, a summary may be used to check understanding of main points of discussion at the end of a section within it. The technique is also used at the end of an interview to clarify and review main and relevant points, at the same time acting as an introduction to a physical examination where appropriate (Box 5.4), or goal setting and care planning.

Objective data

In order to get more detailed information, objective data are required. This encompasses a physical examination. As stated in Chapter 6, certain techniques such as inspection (looking, observation), palpation, auscultation, etc. may be used for this assessment. These techniques imply the use of communication skills such as observation, touch and listening, respectively. Although some examples of how close observation might be used for assessment have been given above, a more specific example of how it might be employed for gathering objective data is given below.

Close observation

As already stated, close observation is a form of communication involving the sense of sight and which is essential during holistic health assessment. A head-to-toe examination, for instance, forms part of a physical examination. As an example, the skin should be closely observed for pallor, redness, jaundice and cyanosis (Chapter 6). The skin should also be observed for any rash, scars, oedema and elasticity (Chapters 6 and 7). The upper and lower limbs should also be observed for symmetry, physical deformities and for any dysfunction.

During close observation, other senses may be employed. Following urine collection, for example, it is closely observed for colour, amount and for any odour. A scanty amount of urine which also smells fishy, for example, denotes infection and needs to be sent to the pathological laboratory for further investigation, culture and sensitivity to antibiotics. A dark-coloured urine, on the other hand, may be indicative of haematuria (blood in the urine), which also requires further investigation.

Close observation could also be useful in the assessment of a client's mental state. It is, for example, important for the verbal expression of the patient to be congruent with their non-verbal expression, otherwise the message being conveyed may be misinterpreted. Occasionally a patient may claim to be feeling fine but looks very tense and not relaxed which could mean that the patient is anxious about something. In such a case, a catalytic intervention may be necessary. This means the ability to draw the patient 'out and encourage them to discuss issues further' through the use of questions (Burnard, 1999: p29). Cathartic interventions, that is, enabling the patient or client to release any pent-up feelings, may also be useful (Burnard, 2004). These are counselling skills which could facilitate better communication during holistic assessment, but their use requires training.

Auscultation (involves listening)

Physical assessment of the patient also involves listening. Although, for example, electronic devices for the measurement of the patient's blood pressure are now in use (Chapter 6), the nurse needs to know how to use the sphygmomanometer and the stethoscope. Their use involves auscultation (listening – Chapter 6), which is a communication skill. Other procedures that involve listening include the use of the stethoscope to auscultate the chest for crepitus and heart murmurs and in the assessment of a child, for the assessment of the apex beat. The nurse should therefore not only be familiar with assessment procedures which involve the use of instruments but must also know how to use instruments as well as have very good hearing.

Touch

Touch could be used to share warmth, provide reassurance and help increase self-esteem. There are also certain assessment procedures, such as taking a patient's pulse, temperature or blood pressure, which involve the use of touch. The employment of touch is also essential during physical assessment, including palpation (Chapter 6) of a tender or painful area of the body, assessment of pressure sores or an invasive procedure such as a vaginal examination, all of which involve the invasion of the patient's personal space. Such procedures should therefore be carried out with consent.

There are also cultural and individual preferences in relation to the use of touch. According to Rajan (1995), for instance, the French tend to touch others when talking but English people prefer to maintain a certain distance. Touch should therefore be used with caution and with consent.

Barriers to communication during holistic assessment

There are factors that could affect the effective transmission and receiving of information, examples of which are highlighted in Figure 5.2. These include environmental and cultural factors, the mental state of the people involved in communication, the subject being discussed and age-related barriers. Since all the senses might be involved in the process of effective communication, impairment of any of these senses, and other physical disorders, could also affect the interaction, some of which will be discussed in more detail. Such barriers should therefore be taken into account during a holistic health assessment since they could affect the amount as well as the quality of the information being gathered.

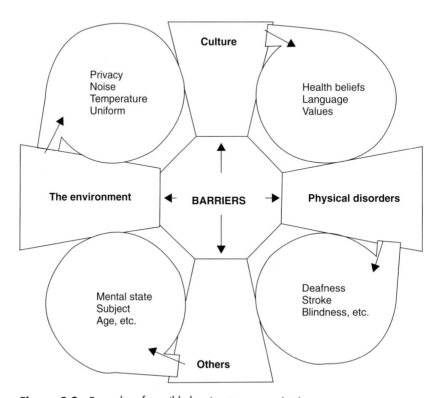

Figure 5.2 Examples of possible barriers to communication

Environmental factors

The context within which the assessment takes place is important. A room that is too hot or too cold, for instance, could hinder the communication process. The white coats of doctors and the nurses' uniforms could also be intimidating to some patients who then might feel unable to express themselves freely.

Noise

When children accompany adults, this could result in the parent or guardian not being able to concentrate fully on the questions being asked. This could in turn lead to the parent or guardian giving brief answers in order to complete the interview as quickly as possible (Whalley *et al.*, 2002). Thus, important information needed to aid diagnosis and/or care planning might be forgotten or withheld. Where possible, children could be engaged in some form of play to help minimise or avoid interruptions.

Interruptions by noisy ward bells, alarm bells and the ongoing ringing tone of the ward telephones could also occur. This could be avoided through the use of an admission room.

Cultural factors

Since the main means of communication is through the use of language, it is essential for the healthcare professional and the client to understand each other's language. Evidence from the Audit Commission (1993) suggests that language difficulties can lead to poor-quality assessment and management. The use of jargon by healthcare professionals should also be avoided.

On occasions, difficulties are experienced during communication even between people from the same nationality due to differences in local accents and expressions. It is therefore important for healthcare workers to speak clearly and slowly where necessary.

Language barriers also occur where either the healthcare professional or the patient does not speak English at all or speaks little English. The use of friends and relatives (Robinson & Phillips, 2003) or interpreters as translators for non-English speaking patients appears to be normal practice in some hospitals. The use of interpreters, in general, does help in the gathering of information during health assessment but it is time consuming. The use of family members as interpreters also helps to reduce the cost of professional interpreters but this could mean poor quality in the translation, as reported by Robinson & Phillips (2003).

There may also be issues that the patient would like to discuss but which they do not want the family member or the interpreter to know about. The translation of personal and confidential issues could cause embarrassment for either the patient or the translator. Thus, important information, necessary for correct diagnosis or identification of the patient's problems, might be held back. Moreover, some interpreters might not understand the medical jargon used so the message being conveyed could be misinterpreted (Audit Commission, 1993). In some instances, some of the detailed information given may be omitted or altered by the translator (Farooq *et al.*, 1997). Hornberger *et al.* (1996) also reported that some translators do sometimes add to the information given by the patient.

According to Robinson & Phillips (2003), misunderstanding on the part of the health professional could lead to stereotyping which could in turn affect diagnostic skills. They reported, for instance, that a lady who presented with 'multi-specific pains' was thought to be 'making more of her usual gut pain, but it was later on proven that that pain was due to a myocardial infarction'. Thus the use of family members as interpreters is not always helpful and interpreters should be trained for the role they play. In their study, Robinson & Phillips (2003) also found that many patients felt a bilingual liaison service accessible from home would be beneficial, so this should be considered.

Where there are no interpreters of any kind, communication may be even more difficult and the use of open questions may prove to be a hindrance rather than helpful (Robinson & Gilmartin, 2002).

Different cultural groups also tend to behave in certain ways because of their health beliefs. Vietnamese, for example, do not encourage the expression of strong emotion. Consequently, the verbal expression of Vietnamese clients might not always be congruent with their non-verbal behaviours and could lead to misinterpretation of the message being conveyed. This is because even when in pain, a Vietnamese patient may or may not admit that they are in pain and may put on a smile (Shanahan & Brayshaw, 1995). This could make it difficult for the healthcare professional to make a proper assessment and diagnosis of the patient's problem. This emphasises the need for one to have some knowledge and understanding of these important cultural differences.

Physical disorders

Certain physical disorders are associated with communication difficulties. A patient who has right-sided paralysis following a stroke, for example, is likely to have difficulty in speaking. Such difficulty occurs not just because of muscular paralysis but also because the speech centre in the brain is usually affected. Assessment of a patient with such a condition can therefore be frustrating for both the patient and the healthcare professional. The use of a close relative to help gather the necessary information initially may be helpful.

Conditions associated with the heart, such as chronic heart failure, and with the lungs, such as chronic obstructive pulmonary disease (COPD), tend to produce breathlessness. Patients with such conditions tend to have difficulty in talking so patience is needed when assessing such patients. The use of closed questions for such patients if they are on their own during assessment could help minimise the amount the patient has to say and avoid further respiratory harassment.

Chronic heart failure is also associated with memory loss and confusion, both of which are barriers to communication (Rogers *et al.*, 2000).

Deafness and blindness are also examples of physical disorders that could affect the communication process. It is often suggested that Braille should be used for blind people during health assessment. However, it needs to be borne in mind that being blind does not necessarily mean one is also deaf although this might be the case for some patients. Braille should be used only when necessary, such as for patients who have a combination of blindness and deafness, to enhance the communication process.

Activity

• What other physical conditions might impede the communication process?
• What could be done to minimise the effects of such conditions on the communication processes?

Age

Older people

Studies have shown that there are high levels of hearing loss among residents in nursing homes (Stumer *et al.*, 1996; Tolson & McIntosh, 1997). This could be attributed to the ageing process since it is accompanied by changes in the body. Changes in the quality of speech (Dreher, 2001), restricted range of expression, the gradual decline in visual acuity and a reduction in hearing tend to affect the ability to give and receive information correctly (Biggs, 2000). It is therefore important for the healthcare professional to face the patient to allow for lip reading, speak slightly louder than normal and in good lighting conditions to help improve communication with the elderly (Dreher, 2001). Where a client is known to use a hearing aid, it is important to ensure that they are wearing it and that it is turned on.

Disorientation in the elderly could also occur when they are not in their own surroundings and particularly following an admission to hospital or to a nursing home. This could in turn lead to fear and anxiety and could further influence the communication process during holistic assessment. At all times the nurse should remember to be sensitive to the needs of the elderly, avoid discrimination (Doh, 2000; Moore, 2001) and communicate respect, acceptance, warmth and empathy to enhance the information-gathering process.

Children

Depending on the age, it needs to borne in mind that different methods might be employed for the gathering of information. The main form of communication of a baby or a toddler, for example, is crying. Some parents get to know their babies well and are able to tell why their baby is crying, with particular reference to hunger or the need to be winded or for a change of nappy. Although a baby might cry when in pain or when unwell for any reason, one needs to be aware that an infant with blocked airways is usually unable to cry. In either case, the baby requires a thorough head-to-toe physical examination. A very close observation of the child's reactions to stimulus and to touching parts of the body is also of crucial importance. For older children, the use of play and pictures can be effective in the holistic health assessment. Like adults, a child is unlikely to communicate with someone who does not respect their worries and concerns (Glen & Colson, 2003). Acceptance, respect and empathy should therefore be shown during the assessment of children.

Following phenomenological research, Simons & Robertson (2002) reported that parents could be left feeling anxious about pain and unwilling to express their concerns where communication between nurses and parents is poor. In order to avoid parental anxiety, a competent assessment of a child's pain and its management is necessary and parental involvement in holistic assessment of all children is of particular importance (RCN Institute, 2001).

Other possible barriers to communication

Emotion

The mental state of an individual could also affect the effectiveness of communication. According to Heron (2001), for instance, emotions such as anger, fear, grief and embarrassment could be suppressed or bottled up. Anger, for example, might be expressed as loud sounds, whilst fear might be expressed as trembling, grief as tears and embarrassment as laughing. A person who is anxious, upset or frightened for some reason might not be able to speak freely. Hence some vital information necessary for diagnosis might be withheld. Exploration of how the client is feeling through the use of open questions (see Box 5.2) and close observation could be useful in eliciting any pent-up emotions.

Enabling the release of emotions through tears or anger through sounds (catharsis) could prove helpful as this seems to allow the person to think more clearly after expressing it (Burnard, 2004; Heron, 2001). Active listening skills and the demonstration of empathy could also help allay fears and enhance the communication process during health assessment.

Learning disability
Most people tend to develop cognitively along predictable lines but there are wide variations in the population. Some people are unable to learn to read and write due to cognitive impairment (Atkinson, 2003b). Patients with learning disability do therefore have difficulty in communicating. The use of diagrams, videos and special communication techniques such as Makaton could help enhance the assessment process. Demonstration of patience, respect and warmth by the nurse is also required.

Subject
Sometimes the subject being discussed, such as issues related to sexuality, genitalia and personal issues in general, could cause some embarrassment. In such cases the healthcare professional needs to be sensitive during the assessment process.

Patient unable to ask questions
Research findings suggest that sometimes patients have questions to ask but do not do so (Porter & Macintyre, 1991; Rogers et al., 2000). Those who manage to ask questions are sometimes met with a hostile reception and, unbeknown to them, labelled as trouble makers (Porter & Macintyre, 1991). For the patient to be able to give information freely, an atmosphere which encourages questions from the patient should be fostered.

Use of computer-mediated communication
Currently, a common workplace practice is computer-mediated communication. Information on the patient is stored on the computer in practically every department, including the general practitioner's surgery. There is also exchange of information on clients between members of staff and departments via email (Torrance et al., 2002). These systems increase the potential for a breech in privacy and confidentiality. Patients who are aware of such systems may withhold important information about themselves during holistic health assessment (Torrance et al., 2002). Staff should therefore be sensitive in the use of computers. Moreover, there should be policies in place to ensure maintenance of confidentiality.

Activity

- Can you think of other barriers of communication that could affect the assessment process? How could these barriers be minimised or avoided?
- The next time you go to your placement area, make a note of the different communication skills used during holistic assessment of patients.
- Find time to discuss the skills observed in practice with your mentor.

Record keeping

Having obtained the information required, accurate and legible records need to be kept to enhance care planning, implementation and evaluation, as well as continuity of care. The characteristics of the written communication should also include the following (NMC, 2004):

- clearly written
- easily understood
- unambiguous
- precise but sufficient
- preferably written in black
- indelible.

Summary

The examples given above confirm that a great deal of information can be gathered through behaviours such as the spoken word, facial expressions, head nodding, voice tone, touch, gestures, posture and the general appearance. Thus all verbal and non-verbal behaviours seem to have meaning and all life is indeed enriched by and is dependent on communication. All nursing and midwifery activities could also be described as communication. Since all the senses are involved in the communication process, holistic health assessment of the patient could be greatly enhanced where all senses are consciously engaged in the gathering of information and care is taken to minimise or avoid the barriers to communication.

Activity

- Outline and discuss the factors that facilitate the communication process.
- Examine the factors that can hinder communication and explain how these could be minimised or avoided.
- Discuss the communication skills needed for holistic health assessment of a patient.

References

Argyle, M (1990) *Bodily Communication*, 2nd edition. Routledge, London.

Atkinson, L (2003a) Caring, comforting and communicating. In: Kozier, B, Erb, G, Berman, A J *Fundamentals of Nursing: concepts, process and practice*, 7th edition. Prentice Hall, New Jersey.

Atkinson, L (2003b) Teaching. In: Kozier, B, Erb, G, Berman, A J, Snyder, S (eds) *Fundamentals of Nursing: concepts, process, and practice*, 7th edition. Prentice Hall, New Jersey.

Attree, M, Button, D & Cooke, H (1994) Students' evaluation of the process of conducting a patient assessment. *Nurse Education Today* 14: 372–9.

Audit Commission (1993) *What Seems to Be the Matter: communication between hospitals and patients*. HMSO Publications, London.

Biggs, S (2000) *Understanding Ageing: images, attitudes and professional practice*. Open University Press, Buckingham.

Burnard, P (1999) *Counselling Skills for Health Professionals*, 3rd edition. Stanley Thornes, Cheltenham.

Burnard, P (2004) *Acquiring Interpersonal Skills: a handbook of experiential learning for health professionals*, 3rd edition. Nelson Thornes, Cheltenham.

Cantwell, B M & Ramirez, A J (1997) Doctor–patient communication: a study of junior house officers. *Medical Education* 31: 17–21.

Carcio, H A (1999) *Advanced Health Assessment of Women: clinical skills and procedures*. Lippincott, Philadelphia.

Chuk, P (2002) Determining the accuracy of pain assessment of senior student nurses: a clinical vignette approach. *Nurse Education Today* 22: 393–400.

Department of Health (2000) *The NHS Plan*. HMSO, London.

Dreher, B B (2001) *Communication Skills for Working with Elders*. Springer, New York.

Duxbury, J (2000) *Difficult Patients*. Reed Elsevier, Oxford.

Egan, G (2002) *The Skilled Helper: a systematic approach to effective helping*. Brookes Cole, California.

Farooq, S, Fear, C & Oyebode, F (1997) An investigation of the adequacy of psychiatric interviews conducted through an interpreter. *Psychiatric Bulletin* 21 (4): 209–13.

Glen, S & Colson, J (2003) Nursing processes in health promotion. In: Hinchliff, S, Norman, S & Schober, J (eds) *Nursing Practice and Health Care*. Hodder Arnold, London.

Heron, J (2001) *Helping the Client: a creative practical guide*, 5th edition. Sage, London.

Hornberger, J, Gibson, C, Wood, W *et al.* (1996) Eliminating language barriers for non-English-speaking patients. *Medical Care* 34 (8): 845–56.

Lester, N (1998) Cultural competence. Nursing dialogue. *American Journal of Nursing* 98 (8): 26–34.

Lichtman, R (2005) *Gynaecology: well women care*. Appleton and Lange, Norwalk, Connecticut.

Mateo, O M & Krenzischek, D A (1992) A pilot study to assess the relationship between behavioural manifestations and self-report of pain in post anaesthesia care unit patients. *Journal of Post Anaesthesia Nursing* 7: 15–21.

Moore, A (2001) Champion for older people. *Nursing Older People* 12 (10): 10–11.

Nelson-Jones, R (2004) *Introduction to Counselling Skills: text and activities*, 5th edition. Sage, London.

Nursing and Midwifery Council (2002) *Requirements for the Pre-registration Nursing Programme*. NMC, London.

Nursing and Midwifery Council (2004) *Guidelines for Records and Record Keeping*. NMC, London.

Porter, M & Macintyre, S (1991) Psychosocial effectiveness of antenatal and postnatal care. In: Robinson, S & Thomson, A M (eds) *Midwives Research and Childbirth*, vol 1. Chapman and Hall, London.

Rajan, M F J (1995) Transcultural nursing: a perspective derived from Jean-Paul Sartre. *Journal of Advanced Nursing* 22: 450–5.

Robinson, M & Gilmartin, J (2002) Barriers to communication between health practitioners and service users who are not fluent in English. *Nurse Education Today* 22: 457–65.

Robinson, M & Phillips, P (2003) An investigation into the perceptions of primary care practitioners of their education and development needs for communicating with patients who may not be fluent in English. *Nurse Education Today* 23: 286–98.

Rogers, A E, Addington-Hall, J M, Abery, A J *et al.* (2000) Knowledge and communication difficulties for patients with chronic heart failure: qualitative study. *BMJ* 321 (7261): 605–7.

Royal College of Nursing Institute (2001) *Clinical Practice Guidelines for the Recognition and Assessment of Acute Pain in Children: implementation guide.* RCN, London.

Shanahan, M & Brayshaw, L (1995) Are nurses aware of the differing health care needs of Vietnamese patients? *Journal of Advanced Nursing* 22: 456–64.

Simons, J & Robertson, E (2002) Poor communication and knowledge deficits: obstacles to effective management of children's postoperative pain. *Journal of Advanced Nursing* 40 (1): 78–86.

Stumer, J, Hickson, L & Worrall, L (1996) Hearing impairment, disability and handicap in elderly people living in residential care and in the community. *Disability and Rehabilitation* 18 (2): 76–82.

Tolson, D & McIntosh, J (1997) Listening in the care environment: chaos or clarity for the hearing-impaired elderly person. *International Journal of Nursing Studies* 34 (3): 173–82.

Torrance, R J, Lasome, C & Agazio, J (2002) Ethics and computer-mediated communication: implication for practice and policy. *Journal of Nursing Administration* 32 (6): 346–53.

Whalley, F, Wong, D L & Hockenberry, M (eds) (2002) Wong's Nursing Care of Infants and Children. Mosby, St Louis.

Wilkinson, S M (1991) Factors which influence how nurses communicate with cancer patients. *Journal of Advanced Nursing* 16: 677–88.

Wilkinson, S M, Gambles, M & Roberts, A (2002) The essence of cancer care: the impact of training on nurses' ability to communicate effectively. *Journal of Advanced Nursing* 4 (6): 731–8.

Workman, B (2003) *Key Nursing Skills*. Whurr, London.

Physical assessment

C. Meurier, J. Brown and A. Crouch

Learning objectives

- Outline the purposes of physical assessment.
- Relate physical assessment to the appropriate stages of the nursing process.
- Describe the techniques of inspection, palpation, percussion and auscultation and identify aspects of these techniques that are relevant for undergraduate pre-registration nurses.
- Describe the preparation of a client for physical assessment.
- Discuss the purpose of a general survey and observations of vital signs in physical assessment.
- Discuss the use of the body system approach in the physical assessment of the patient.

Section 1: Introduction

In this chapter, the principles of physical assessment will be explained. Physical assessment allows the collection of objective data. This, together with the subjective data collected from the health history discussed in Chapter 3, will enable identification of the client's problems and serve as the foundation of the individualised care plan discussed in Chapter 2. This chapter is divided into several sections. The first section is concerned with how to conduct a physical assessment, the techniques of physical examination, general survey and observation of vital signs. The remaining sections will look at assessment of particular body systems.

Undergraduate pre-registration nurses will not be expected to carry out some of the more advanced physical assessment discussed in this chapter, but it is covered here not only to provide a 'holistic' view of physical assessment but also to follow recent trends for nurses to take on more advanced roles following qualification and further training. Core competencies that should be possessed by nurses working at an advanced level are well documented in the literature (Hamric, 2000; Rolfe & Fulbrook, 1998). The Code of Professional Conduct (NMC, 2004a) allows nurses to undertake many enhanced roles provided they are adequately trained and competent.

The NHS Plan (DoH, 2000) identifies ten key roles for nurses, including ordering diagnostic investigations such as pathological tests, making and receiving referrals direct, admitting and discharging patients for specified conditions and within agreed protocols, and prescribing medicines and treatment. The Department of Health (DoH, 2001) has also circulated a strategic plan of action to develop nurses in the acquisition of knowledge, skills and competencies to meet the needs of patients with acute and critical illness wherever they are nursed. These trends imply the need for nurses to develop their assessment skills. A more patient-centred and holistic approach to nursing care would result if nurses were equipped with the skills to work within this climate of change (Carroll, 2004).

In a physical assessment, the nurse uses the senses of sight, hearing, touch and smell for gathering objective data on the client. The skills of physical assessment are used by the nurse in a variety of situations from admission to discharge. A physical assessment on admission allows the nurse to identify the client's problems. Subsequent physical assessments are used to detect changes in the client's health, to monitor the effects of interventions and to identify new problems, whether actual or potential. Thus, physical assessment is a continuous process and is integrated in the day-to-day care of the client, e.g. inspection of the client's skin during a bed-bath. Nurses not only need to understand the principle of physical assessment but also be able to perform relevant aspects of it competently in their field of practice. Some post-registration nurses as well as nurses doing advanced postregistration courses will also be engaged in advanced health assessment.

Nurses and physicians have different reasons and goals in performing a physical assessment. The Royal College of Nursing (RCN, 1997) believes that nurses offer a complementary source of care to that offered by the physicians. Physicians collect and analyse data obtained from a physical assessment in order to arrive at a clinical diagnosis and initiate treatment. Nurses use data from a physical assessment in order to assess the client's functional abilities and plan nursing care (see Chapter 2). Undoubtedly, some overlaps are inevitable and in some settings (e.g. GP practice and other specialist/advanced nursing practice), the nurse practitioner has responsibilities for physical assessment of the undiagnosed client.

The purpose of physical assessment

Physical assessment serves a number of purposes:

- to obtain information on the client's overall health status
- to enable additional information to be obtained about any symptoms reported by the client
- to detect changes in a client's condition
- to evaluate how the client is responding to interventions.

Approach to physical assessment

It is essential for a systematic approach to be used in physical assessment. The most common approaches are head to toe and the body systems approach. In the head to toe approach, the nurse systematically assesses every part of the body, beginning at the head and progressing to the toes. The body systems approach focuses on the cardio-vascular, respiratory, digestive and nervous systems, as discussed in Chapters 1 and 3. Both of these approaches are based on the medical model and will lead to the identification of medical problems. Nurses also need to identify the data according to a holistic nursing model for the purpose of nursing diagnoses and problems. For instance, Gordon (2000) suggests that data obtained from the physical assessment should be organised and interpreted in line with a holistic nursing framework, such as the Functional Health Patterns (FHPs). In the UK, nurses are familiar with using the Activities of Living (Holland *et al.*, 2003) framework for organising and interpreting data.

Preparation for physical assessment

Good preparation is essential for a competent physical assessment. All necessary equipment (e.g. stethoscope, sphygmomanometer, thermometer, penlight, gloves) is assembled in the room where the assessment will take place. The type of physical assessment that a nurse may perform will be in congruence with the nurse's educational and clinical preparation and job responsibilities, the client's chief complaint and the protocol of the clinical setting in which the nurse works. According to Bickley & Szilagyi (2003), a new client requires a comprehensive physical assessment whereas a more focused examination may be more appropriate when a problem needs to be assessed as precisely and carefully as possible, and after taking into account the client's health history and disease patterns. On the other hand, Norman & Cook (2000) suggest that nurses should perform an initial mini assessment comprising a brief history, quick visual inspection and quick physical assessment in order to obtain a snapshot for further investigation of the patient's condition. It is important for nurses to follow the protocol that is applicable to their clinical setting.

Clear explanation will be given to the client regarding what is involved in the procedure. Concurrent health education is also given as required. When performing a comprehensive physical assessment, the client will be asked to undress and wear a gown. As the physical assessment is an anxious time for the client, it is important for the nurse to take time to make the client comfortable and relaxed. The physical assessment should be performed in a quiet environment where possible as noise may interfere with the procedure. Before starting the examination, nurses should wash their hands in the presence of the client in order to demonstrate that the client's welfare is paramount. Standard infection control precautions are taken, particularly when handling body fluids or dealing with wounds.

It must be noted that much of the physical assessment performed by nurses is incorporated into their day-to-day work. Because nurses are with the patients 24 hours a day, they are in a unique position to assess the patients' condition and responses to treatment on a continuous basis.

Techniques of physical assessment

Four basic diagnostic assessment techniques are used to collect objective data (Estes, 2002):

* inspection
* palpation
* percussion
* auscultation.

These techniques are used to assess body systems and are usually performed in this order, with the exception of examination of the abdomen. In abdominal examination, auscultation is used before palpation and percussion as the latter two can alter bowel sounds (Estes, 2002). Undergraduate pre-registration nurses will focus primarily on inspection and only perform limited aspects of the other three techniques (e.g. palpation in assessing the pulse, oedema and temperature; percussion to assess tenderness; auscultation when taking the blood pressure and recording apical pulse). However, full details of all four techniques are covered in this chapter to enable undergraduate pre-registration nurses to understand the total context of physical assessment in the diagnosis and monitoring of patients' conditions in line with the 'holistic' approach taken in this book. Undergraduate pre-registration nurses will work within the multidisciplinary setting where they will observe doctors and advanced nurse practitioners performing these physical assessment techniques.

Bickley & Szilagyi (2003) recommend that physical examination be performed from the right side of the client (even for left-handed practitioners) as certain examinations and measurements are more reliable when performed from that side. Good lighting is also required to inspect a number of body structures.

Inspection

Inspection is the process of systematic observation, using the senses of sight and smell. For instance, sight is used to assess the client's respiratory status (e.g. respiratory rate, cyanosis). The olfactory sense can provide important information on the client's health status, e.g. fruity breath odour from diabetic ketoacidosis and fishy smell of urine in urinary tract infection. Inspection begins from the moment the nurse encounters the client and is an ongoing process. The nurse will begin with an inspection of the client as a whole, which is referred to as a general survey. Then each body part is inspected thoroughly and systematically to determine normal and abnormal findings. Comparisons are made between the left and right sides to evaluate symmetry. Only the area being examined must be exposed. The nurse will also apply this technique whenever nursing care is given as part of an ongoing assessment.

Palpation

In palpation, the sense of touch is applied to elicit specific information regarding the following:

- texture (is the skin rough or smooth?)
- moisture (dry or wet)
- temperature (hot or cold)
- accumulation of fluid (oedema)
- pulses
- size and shape
- motion (movable, still, vibrating)
- tenderness or pain.

The hands are the tools used in palpation and they need to be warmed before beginning. Different regions of the hand are used to assess different structures, applying varying degrees of pressure. This is shown in Table 6.1.

There are two main types of palpation: light and deep. Light palpation involves using the finger pads to apply gentle pressure on the skin to a depth of 1 cm, and it is used to assess skin texture, tenderness and masses. In deep palpation, the skin is depressed to a depth of 4–5 cm to detect masses. It is used in assessment of the abdomen and reproductive system.

Percussion

Percussion is the technique of tapping the body with short, sharp strokes to generate sound waves, enabling information to be obtained on the location, size and density of underlying structures. Five percussion sounds can be heard (see Table 6.2), depending on the density of underlying structures:

- flatness
- dullness
- resonance

Table 6.1 Types of structures assessed by different parts of the hands.

Parts of the hands	Structures examined
• Finger pads	• Skin texture, moisture, oedema, swelling, pulses, lumps, consistency of organs
• Dorsum (back) of the hand	• Body temperature
• Palm of the hand	• To discriminate vibrations (e.g. cardiac thrill, fremitus)

Table 6.2 Percussion sounds.

Percussion sounds				Normal and abnormal findings	
Sound	Intensity	Pitch	Quality	Normal location	Abnormal location
Flatness	Soft	High	Flat	Bone (sternum), muscle (thigh)	Lungs (severe pneumonia, collapsed lung)
Dullness	Medium	High	Thud	Liver, diaphragm	Lung (pleural effusion, atelectasis)
Resonance	Loud	Low	Hollow	Lungs	No abnormal location
Hyper-resonance	Very loud	Very low	Booming	Child lungs	Emphysema
Tympany	Loud	High	Musical	Gastric air bubble	Air-distended abdomen, severe pneumothorax

- hyper-resonance
- tympany.

Different parts of the body will emit their own distinctive sounds. An unexpected sound may indicate an abnormality, which needs to be investigated further.

There are two principal types of percussion: direct and indirect. In direct percussion, one or two fingers are used to tap directly on the body part. This can elicit areas of tenderness and is used, for example, to assess the sinuses for tenderness. Indirect percussion is a two-handed technique. The distal part of the middle finger of the non-dominant hand is pressed firmly against the skin. The middle finger of the dominant hand is then used to strike this finger and the sound produced is evaluated. Indirect percussion is used to obtain information on the underlying structures.

Auscultation

Auscultation involves listening to the sounds produced by the body (e.g. breath, heart and bowel sounds), using a stethoscope with a diaphragm and a bell. The diaphragm is used to listen to high-pitched sound whereas the bell is used for low-pitched sound.

The general survey and vital signs

The first step in a comprehensive physical assessment is to perform general observations of the client and obtain the vital signs. The general survey provides information on the client's general state of health and observations of the vital signs gives information about the client's baseline physiological status and the functioning of a number of systems.

General survey

The general survey is essentially about gaining a first impression of the client as a whole. It begins as soon as one encounters the patient and will include observations of general appearance (Table 6.3), mental status and posture.

Mental status, speech and behaviour
It is important to note the level of consciousness and orientation such as state of alertness and responsiveness. The client's neurological status should be promptly assessed if any changes in the level of consciousness are observed.

Speech should be clear and understandable. Slurred speech may indicate neurological disorders or excessive alcohol intake. Stroke can

Table 6.3 General physical appearance assessment.

Components	Assessment and rationale
• Age	• Compare chronological age with apparent age. Chronic disorders, chronic alcoholism, manual labour and genetic syndromes may make clients look older. Endocrine disorders may cause dwarfism or delayed puberty, which may make clients look younger
• General state of health	• Does the client appear well, acutely ill or chronically ill? This may help to decide on the immediate needs of the client
• Signs of distress	• Any evidence of cardiac or respiratory distress, pain, anxiety or depression
• Height and build	• Is the client tall or short, slender or muscular? Does the body appear symmetrical? Very short stature is seen in Turner's syndrome, childhood renal failure, achondroplastic and hypopituitary dwarfism
• Nutritional status and body build	• Is the client emaciated, thin, plump or obese? Changes in weight may provide important diagnostic data. Calorific intake, changes in body fluid, body fat and muscle mass may all influence weight. Cachexia may result from cancer or advanced cardiac or pulmonary disorder. Cushing's syndrome causes abnormal distribution of fat in the face, trunk and posterior neck. Psychological disorders such as anorexia nervosa may cause severe emaciation
• General appearance of skin	• Observe the skin for pallor, cyanosis, jaundice, rashes and bruises. The skin may be a 'window' for a number of systemic disorders
• Facial features	• Observe facial expression when the client is at rest, smiling, talking and during physical examination. Facial features are symmetric with movement. In Parkinson's disease, the face is expressionless. Stroke and Bell's palsy may cause weakness on one side of the face. A depressed person has a flat or sad affect. The person may have a starry eye in hyperthyroidism. Decreased eye contact may be observed in depression, anxiety or in certain cultural groups
• Dress, grooming and hygiene	• Are the clothes clean, well-fitting and appropriate for weather? How do they compare with clothing worn by people of comparable age, culture and socio-economic status? Note any body odour or odours of urine or faeces. These observations may provide clues to the client's mental state, changes in weight, signs of neglect or incontinence

result in dysphasia. Hearing difficulties may be associated with loud speech.

The client will usually be co-operative and pleasant. In certain psychiatric conditions, there may be distortion of reality, affecting behaviour patterns. Intoxication may also cause disturbance in behaviour.

Besides organic brain syndromes, confusion may be secondary to some physical disorders.

Posture, gait and mobility

The client should be observed while walking, sitting and changing positions. Abnormal posture, gait and mobility may be associated with bones, muscles and neurological disorders. Curvatures of the spine such as scoliosis, lordosis and kyphosis cause abnormal posture. In Parkinson's disease, the gait is typically shuffling. Stroke may cause weakness or paralysis of one side of the body. In arthritis, movement can be slow and difficult due to stiffness and pain in the joints.

Assessment of the vital signs

Physical examination of the client usually begins with assessment of the vital signs. Findings from vital signs assessment give clues on how the body systems are functioning as well as providing a baseline. Deteriorating or critically ill patients may also be identified which may in some instances prevent cardiorespiratory arrest or prompt admission to critical care (Alcock *et al.*, 2002). Traditionally, assessment of vital signs includes temperature, pulse, respiration and blood pressure. When dealing with an unconscious patient, however, attention must be paid first to the assessment and maintenance of breathing before anything else. The nursing management of patients has also become more complex (DoH, 2000). This, together with advances in medical technology, requires nurses to use a wider range of tools (e.g. glucometer, pulse oximetry) in the physiological assessment and monitoring of patients' condition (Trim, 2005).

Temperature

Optimal cell functions are dependent amongst other variables on the core body temperature being maintained at a relatively constant level within a range of 36–37.5°C (Childs *et al.*, 1999). Because of the influence of the circadian rhythm on body temperature, the optimal time to detect an abnormal temperature is 6 pm (Carroll, 2000). There are various anatomical sites that are used to measure core body temperature. However, it must be noted that there may be a variation of as much as 0.6°C according to the site of measurement (Jamieson *et al.*, 2002). It is important to minimise factors that can decrease the accuracy of the reading even further.

Aims of recording body temperature
The aims of recording body temperature are to (Jamieson *et al.*, 2002):

- establish a baseline temperature
- monitor fluctuations in temperature (e.g. temperature fluctuations in the postoperative period may indicate infection or development of deep vein thrombosis)

- monitor for signs of incompatibility from a blood transfusion
- monitor the temperature of a patient being treated for an infection
- monitor the temperature of patients with hypothermia.

Measurement of body temperature: equipment, routes and method
Body temperature is measured by one of the following types of thermometers:

- disposable thermometer
- electronic thermometer
- tympanic thermometer.

To comply with health and safety guidelines to reduce exposure to mercury, the mercury-in-glass thermometer should not be used in clinical settings (Jamieson *et al.*, 2002).

Bernando (1999) makes the following recommendations for safe and accurate measurement of temperature:

- Only one site should be selected for monitoring temperature trends, although the site may have to be changed in response to changes in the patient's condition.
- Scheduled calibration and testing of the thermometers should be carried out to avoid drift in measurement reading.
- Selection of a site that enhances the comfort of and co-operation from the patient.

Oral route This is a common mode of monitoring temperature. However the accuracy of the measurement depends on which site in the oral cavity is used and it is recommended that the posterior sub-lingual sites are best (Carroll, 2000). Other factors such as mouth breathing, intake of food and drink, smoking and oxygen therapy have been found to influence the accuracy of oral temperature measurement. This route may also be unsuitable for some groups of patients such as the confused, young children and patients who are prone to seizures (Carroll, 2000). Many clinical areas have now stopped using this route.

Temporal route The temporal artery thermometer is used in some clinical areas for monitoring core body temperatures. In an evaluation of its use, it was found that it could give erroneously low temperatures and the error was attributed to poor operator technique and lack of cleaning/maintenance of the thermometers (Ostrowsky *et al.*, 2003).

Axillary route This route is thought to poorly reflect the core body temperature because it is not close to any major blood vessels and the thermometer is exposed to environmental temperature (Carroll, 2000).

Tympanic route The tympanic mode of monitoring body temperature has become popular, particularly because of the safety and speed with which a measurement can be made (Childs *et al.*, 1999). It has been found to correlate well with core body temperature (Jamieson *et al.*, 2002). However, operator technique, size of ear canal and metabolic occurrences have been found to affect the accuracy of the measurement (Knies, 2003). Tympanic devices work by inserting into the ear canal a probe that picks up the infrared radiation emitted from the tympanic membrane (Carroll, 2000). If the probe is incorrectly inserted, the final measurement may be different from the true tympanic membrane temperature (Childs *et al.*, 1999).

Rectal route This route is used only as a last resort, i.e. when the other routes are not practical. It is considered to be uncomfortable, embarrassing and unnecessary as other routes can provide equally accurate measurement of temperature (Carroll, 2000).

Palpation The peripheral skin temperature can be gauged by palpation of the skin (Trim, 2005). The skin may feel cool to touch due to potential vasoconstriction or poor perfusion. The skin may feel hot to touch in infections. However, Singh *et al.* (2003) found that clinicians' use of touch in monitoring temperature is sensitive but not specific. Its use is essentially to alert nurses to do a further investigation if an abnormality is suspected from the palpation.

Abnormal findings from temperature assessment
Hyperthermia, pyrexia or fever When the body temperature exceeds 38°C, it is termed as hyperthermia, pyrexia or fever. An excessively high body temperature is known as hyperpyrexia. Pritchard & Mallett (2001) identify three grades of pyrexia: low-grade (normal to 38°C), moderate to high-grade pyrexia (38–40°C) and hyperpyrexia (40°C and above). Raised body temperature is seen in:

- viral or bacterial infections
- inflammatory conditions
- damage to the hypothalamus.

Hypothermia Hypothermia is a body temperature of below 35°C. It can be caused by prolonged exposure to cold. Older people are particularly prone to hypothermia due to disturbances of homeostatic temperature control.

Pulse
The stretching of arteries during systole and recoiling during diastole result in a palpable pulse in the arteries (Jamieson *et al.*, 2002). These may be palpated where the arteries come close to the skin surfaces, e.g. carotid, femoral, brachial, radial, popliteal, posterior tibial and dorsalis pedis (Figure 6.1). Assessment of the pulse is performed to determine

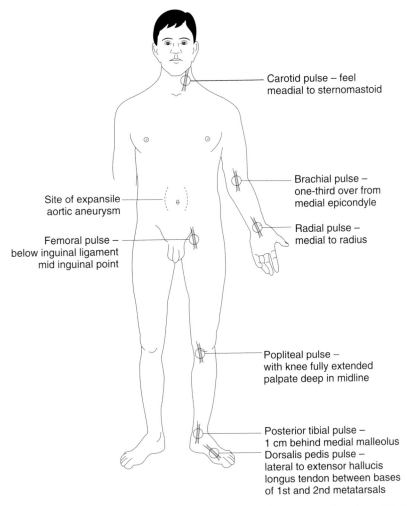

Figure 6.1   Sites of peripheral pulses (reproduced with permission from Cox, 2004)

heart rate, rhythm and volume of blood being pumped out by the heart. It can also be used to check the patency of the blood vessel. The pulse is felt by the technique of *palpation*, using the pads of the first three fingers.

Pulse oximetry
The pulse oximeter is now routinely used in clinical practice to measure the oxygen saturation level in peripheral (capillary) blood (SpO_2) (Woodrow, 2004) as well as obtaining a pulse rate. However, like other electronic forms of pulse monitoring, it only gives an average value of the pulse rate and does not provide any information on the pulse

rhythm and volume, for which a manual evaluation by palpation is necessary (Trim, 2005). Therefore, it should be used primarily for assessment of oxygen saturation (O'Neil & Legrove, 2003).

Pulse oximetry works by transmitting red and infrared light through the tissues, which indicates the percentage of oxyhaemoglobin present in the capillaries. A good knowledge of respiratory physiology is required for nurses to critically evaluate the readings from the pulse oximeter (Casey, 2001). The pulse oximeter is used to determine how well oxygen is being transported to the cells of the body but the reading should be interpreted in association with other related clinical signs (Casey, 2001). The normal oxygen saturation values are 95–98%. Although a value of 90% or less may be indicative of respiratory failure, it is usual for patients with chronic obstructive pulmonary disease to have oxygen saturations of 85–90% and giving these patients a high percentage of oxygen may reduce their hypoxic drive (Trim, 2005).

Pulse rate and rhythm

Pulse rate is calculated by counting the number of pulse beats per minute, starting from zero. A watch with a second hand is required. The radial pulse is commonly used to assess the pulse rate but in a cardiorespiratory emergency, the carotid or femoral artery is palpated as they more accurately reflect cardiac activity. If the rhythm is regular, the pulse rate can be calculated for 30 seconds and then multiplied by 2. If the rate is unusually fast or slow or appears irregular (arrhythmia), the pulse rate is counted for the full minute. If the pulse rate is irregular, it is recommended than an apical and radial check is taken and the pulse deficit (i.e. difference between the apex beats and radial pulse) noted (Docherty, 2002).

The normal pulse rate for an adult is from 60 to 100 (mean 70) beats per minute. A pulse rate of over 100 beats per minute is termed *tachycardia* and *bradycardia* is a pulse rate of under 60 beats per minute (Trim, 2005). Some of the causes of tachycardia are hypovolaemia, stress or anxiety, pyrexia, pain, myocardial ischaemia, sympathetic stimulation, respiratory distress and arrhythmia such as atrial fibrillation. Bradycardia may occur in ischaemic heart disease, vagal stimulation, hypoxia, nausea and vomiting caused by parasympathetic stimulation (Docherty, 2002) and cardiac medication (e.g. beta-blockers).

Pulse amplitude (volume)

Pulse volume is the strength of the pulse which reflects the stroke volume and peripheral resistance. It is felt by palpating the artery with the finger pads using moderate pressure. A normal pulse will be easily palpable and obliterated by strong finger pressure. The following descriptive terms are used to refer to changes in pulse volumes:

- absent pulse (not palpable)
- weak or thready (easily obliterated with light pressure)
- bounding pulse (readily palpable and forceful; not easily obliterated by finger pressure).

Breathing

Assessment of breathing includes observations of respiratory rate, rhythm, depth and oxygen saturation. The measurement of oxygen saturation level by the pulse oximeter has already been covered. Knowledge of normal breathing patterns is important to understand and detect abnormalities. *Inspection* of the chest should reveal bilateral, equal and symmetrical movements (Ahern & Philpot, 2002), and a pause between inspiration and expiration (Bennett, 2003).

Respiratory rate
The respiratory rate is counted by observing the rise and fall of the chest wall during inspiration and expiration over one minute. The following must be observed:

- rate, rhythm and depth of respirations
- symmetry of chest wall.

The normal respiratory rate for an adult is 12–18 breaths per minute (Ahern & Philpot, 2002).

Altered breathing
A respiratory rate of less than 12 breaths per minute is called *bradypnoea* and a rate of over 20 breaths per minute is *tachypnoea* (Bennett, 2003). Bradypnoea occurs in respiratory depression, hypothermia, opiate ingestion and central nervous system depression whereas tachypnoea is associated with restrictive lung disease (Chestnutt & Prendergast, 2004), anxiety and hypercapnia (raised CO_2 level). *Kussmaul* breathing is deep and rapid respiration associated with metabolic acidosis. *Cheyne–Stokes* breathing is described as irregular rate and depth of breathing with alternating periods of apnoea (absence of breathing) occurring in left ventricular failure, cerebral injury and imminent death.

Blood pressure

Blood pressure (BP) assessment is performed to evaluate cardiac output, fluid and circulatory status, and arterial resistance. Blood pressure is the force exerted by the blood through the wall of blood vessels and is a product of cardiac output and peripheral resistance. The systolic arterial BP is the pressure exerted on the arterial wall during systole, i.e. contraction of left ventricle. Diastolic arterial BP is the pressure in the arteries during relaxation (diastole) of the heart. Blood pressure is recorded as a fraction in mmHg, with the top number representing systolic BP and the bottom number diastolic BP. BP is usually measured at the arm (Figure 6.2).

Measurement of blood pressure

Adequate blood pressure is essential to maintain the flow of blood and hence oxygenation to the tissues. Accurate measurement of blood pressure is essential to ensure correct medical management (McAlister & Straus, 2001). Stevenson (2004) identifies three factors that may affect accuracy of blood pressure measurement, namely patient position, cuff size and the device.

Blood pressure is measured indirectly with a stethoscope and a sphygmomanometer or with electronic devices (see Figure 6.2). The sphygmomanometer consists of the blood pressure cuff, connecting tubes, air pump and manometer. There are two types of manometers: mercury and aneroid. The mercury manometer uses a calibrated column of mercury for blood pressure readings whereas the aneroid manometer is a calibrated dial with a needle that points to the numbers representing the air pressure within the cuff. Various electronic devices for monitoring blood pressure are increasingly being used in the clinical setting to reduce the large variations in measurement due to variability between observers (Cappuccio *et al.*, 2004). However, the accuracy of electronic devices has been questioned (Docherty, 2002;

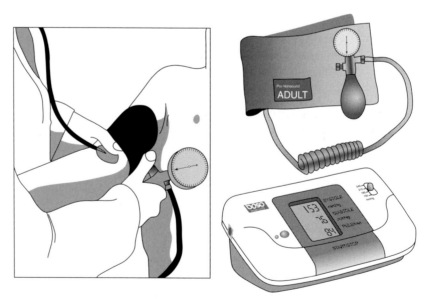

Figure 6.2 Taking the blood pressure and types of equipment that can be used (reproduced with permission from Cox, 2004)

Smith, 2000) and it has been suggested that nurses should maintain their skill in measuring blood pressure manually (Trim, 2005).

Normal blood pressure
Blood pressure varies with age. Typically, normal systolic BP ranges from 100 to 140 mmHg. Normal diastolic BP ranges from 60 to 90 mmHg. The pulse pressure is the difference between the systolic and diastolic pressure readings and gives an indication of stroke volume. A small pulse pressure indicates a low stroke volume (Casey, 2001).

Abnormal blood pressure findings
Hypertension A person is said to have hypertension, or high blood pressure, when the BP readings remain consistently above 140 mmHg systolic and 90 mmHg diastolic on two consecutive visits after initial screening (Estes, 2002).

Hypotension Hypotension, or low blood pressure, is defined as a systolic BP of less than 95 mmHg and a diastolic BP of 60 mmHg or below. Postural or orthostatic hypotension is a drop of both systolic and diastolic BP when a person moves from a supine position to standing position. The systolic BP may fall by more than 30 mmHg and this may cause dizziness, blurring of vision or fainting. When interpreting hypotension, the person's past readings and the clinical state must always be taken into account.

The Joint National Committee on Detection, Evaluation and Treatment of High Blood Pressure (2003) has classified systolic BP of 140–159 mmHg over diastolic BP of 90–99 mmHg as mild hypertension, systolic BP of 160–179 over diastolic BP of 100–109 mmHg as moderate hypertension, and a systolic BP of 180+ mmHg over diastolic BP of 110+ mmHg as severe hypertension.

Section 2: Physical asssessment of the integumentary system

This section will focus on the comprehensive examination of the integumentary system (i.e. skin and its appendages).

Learning objectives

- Describe the assessment of the skin, hair and nails using the techniques of inspection and palpation.
- Identify pathological changes in the skin, hair and nails.
- Relate changes in the skin to abnormal body functions.

A well-lit and comfortably warm room is required for the assessment of the integumentary system. Gloves need to be worn for contact with body fluid or if the client is in isolation.

The skin

Colour (Table 6.4)

Depending on the client's race, the skin has either a uniform whitish pink or dark colour. During the health history, the client will be asked about any changes in skin colour. These can then be validated by inspection. Deviations in skin colour may suggest disorders of oxygenation, circulation or metabolism.

Moisture

Inspection and palpation are used to evaluate moisture. Normally, the skin is relatively dry, with minimal levels of perspiration. Dryness, sweating or oiliness may be abnormal in some cases. There is skin

Table 6.4 Skin colour changes and their significance.

Colour changes	Significance
• Pallor	• Can be generalised or localised. Generalised pallor occurs in anaemia or in shock. In dark-skinned clients, generalised pallor can be detected in the non-pigmented areas such as the sclera, conjunctiva, buccal mucosa, tongue, lips, nail, palms or soles • Localised pallor is observe in marked local arterial insufficiency (e.g. lower extremity when elevated)
• Cyanosis	• Occurs when there is greater than 5 g/dl of deoxygenated haemoglobin in blood. There are two types: central and peripheral. *Central* cyanosis is secondary to marked lung disease, heart disease and congenital heart disease. *Peripheral* cyanosis may be secondary to systemic conditions (e.g. congestive cardiac failure) causing decreased blood flow or vasoconstriction. In dark-skinned clients, the conjunctiva, buccal mucosa, tongue, palms and soles should be examined to detect cyanosis
• Jaundice	• The skin has a yellow-green to orange colouration. This is detected in the sclerae or hard palate in dark-skinned clients. Jaundice suggests liver or haemolytic disease or obstruction of bile duct. High intake of carotene may also give a yellow colour to the skin (carotenaemia)

dryness in hypothyroidism or dehydration. Profuse sweating may occur in shock or hypoglycaemic attack due to sympathetic nervous system activity.

Temperature

The skin is palpated using the dorsal surface of the hand and fingers to determine the temperature. Generalised warmth occurs with fever or pyrexia. Cold and clammy skin is a sign of shock. In local arterial insufficiency, the affected area feels cool on palpation.

Texture

The skin should normally feel smooth in unexposed areas but may feel slightly rough in exposed areas such as elbows, palms and soles. Very rough skin may occur in hypothyroidism, psoriasis and excessive keratinisation.

Mobility and turgor

To assess skin mobility and turgor, a fold of skin on the forearm or sternum is lifted using the thumb and forefinger. The ease with which it is lifted up denotes its mobility and the speed at which it returns into place its turgor. Dehydration as well as the ageing process causes reduced skin turgor.

Oedema

Oedema occurs as a result of excess fluid in the skin. This may be localised or generalised. Localised oedema may be the result of a local trauma or inflammation. Generalised oedema may result from increased capillary hydrostatic pressure (e.g. congestive cardiac failure, renal failure) or decreased capillary osmotic pressure (e.g. plasma protein deficits). Generalised oedema tends to gravitate to the dependent parts of the body. To check for oedema, press down on the skin of the feet or ankle using your thumbs. There will be a skin indentation (pitting oedema) if there is fluid in the tissue.

Skin integrity

Inspection of all pressure point areas (e.g. sacrum, elbows, hips, ankles, heels) is made to determine skin integrity. People who have reduced mobility and are emaciated or elderly are particularly prone to developing pressure ulcers. A reddened area on the skin may be the first sign of skin breakdown. This may progress to ulcer formation of various degrees of severity, ranging from superficial skin loss to full-thickness skin loss. Four stages are assigned to pressure ulcer development (Table 6.5).

Table 6.5 Stages of pressure ulcer development (Potter & Perry, 2001).

Stages	Description
Stage 1	• Erythema of the intact skin, which does not blanch with light palpation
Stage 2	• Superficial loss of skin, involving epidermis or dermis. It may present as a blister, abrasion or erosion
Stage 3	• The damage to the skin involves the epidermis, dermis and subcutaneous tissue. It resembles a crater
Stage 4	• Full-thickness skin loss, involving epidermis, dermis, subcutaneous tissue, muscle, bone and other supporting structures. It resembles a massive crater

Skin lesions

The skin is inspected for the presence of lesions. If a lesion is found, you need to wear gloves if palpation is required. When evaluating a lesion, the following characteristics should be noted:

- colour, texture and appearance
- size: a ruler can be used to measure the lesion
- presence of exudates
- elevation (flat or raised)
- regularity of borders
- distribution: is it localised, regionalised or generalised?

Skin lesions can be the result of carcinoma, infections (viral, bacterial or fungal), infestations, eczema, psoriasis, dermatitis and autoimmune disorders (e.g. systemic lupus erythematosus). When inspecting the skin for lesions, you also need to look for signs of skin discoloration such as those occurring in petechiae, purpura and ecchymosis. These may indicate a blood clotting disorder, microemboli (e.g. subacute bacterial endocarditis), trauma or thrombocytopenia.

Assessment of nails

Colour

Nails appear pink but may have a bluish hue in dark-skinned people. Nail lesions may alter the colour of the nail plate. Bluish discoloration (cyanosis) of the nail bed may result from hypoxia.

Capillary refill time

Depress the nail until blanching occurs. Release the pressure and calculate the time taken for the nail bed to return to its baseline colour. If the capillary refill time is greater than three seconds, this indicates poor tissue perfusion.

Shape and configuration

The nail surface is normally smooth and slightly convex. The angle at the nail base should normally be 160° at the skin–nail interface. If the angle is greater than 180°, it indicates clubbing, which is associated with pulmonary pathology and congenital heart disease. Concave nail plate or spooning is associated with iron deficiency anaemia.

Texture

On palpation, the nails will feel hard and immobile. It is important to note whether the nails are thickened as this may be due to decreased circulation or fungal infection.

Assessment of hair (see Table 6.6)

When assessing hair, the techniques of inspection and palpation are used to note quantity, distribution, infestations and texture.

Table 6.6 Examination of the hair.

Techniques	Possible findings on examination
• Inspection	• *Colour*: scalp, eyebrows, eyelashes become grey with ageing process. Patches of grey hair can be indicative of nerve damage • *Distribution*: males may experience a certain degree of balding due to genetic predisposition and androgen effects. Alopecia (loss of hair) may be secondary to chemotherapy, radiation, infection, lupus and drug reactions. Diminished or absence of pubic hair may occur in endocrine disorders (also see section 10 of this chapter). Hirsutism (excessive body hair) may be secondary to endocrine disorders or side effects of drugs. In females, hirsutism is manifested in excess facial and chest hair • *Infestations*: check the hair for presence of head lice (pediculosis capitis) and nits. Nits can be differentiated from seborrhoea (dandruff) by the fact that dandruff can easily be removed compared to nits. Lice can also be found in body hair, particularly pubic hair
• Palpation	• This is used to note the condition of hair. The hair can be brittle or dull due to malnutrition, hyperthyroidism, certain medications or use of chemicals.

Section 3: Physical assessment of the respiratory system

Learning objectives

- Assess the respiratory system using the techniques of inspection, palpation, percussion and auscultation.
- Identify signs and symptoms relating to respiratory disorders.

Taking a health history

Examination of the respiratory system starts with the general survey and assessment of vital signs. Subjective data from the health history may provide some clues to the likely pulmonary disorders and may help to guide the physical examination. A complete examination of the thorax and lungs will involve the techniques of inspection, palpation, percussion and auscultation in that order. As smoking, pollution, living conditions and certain types of occupation are known risk factors in respiratory disorders, it is relevant to collect data relating to these exposures (Bennett, 2003; Jevon & Ewens, 2001).

Activity Describe how you will assess the following complaints		
Complaints	**Description**	**Examples of questions you could use to elicit the information**
• Dyspnoea	• Also referred to as shortness of breath. Uncomfortable awareness of breathing that is inappropriate to the level of exertion. Sometimes the shortness of breath occurs when lying down (orthopnoea)	
• Cough	• Reflex response to irritation in the larynx, trachea or large bronchi	
• Sputum	• Productive cough. Sputum or blood may be coughed up	
• Wheezing	• Musical respiratory sounds. Suggests partial airway obstruction	
• Chest pain	• Discomfort or unpleasant feelings in the chest	

Physical examination

This is performed in an orderly fashion as follows:

- inspection
- palpation
- percussion
- auscultation.

Depending on the initial findings from the general survey, vital signs and/or patient's complaints, a comprehensive assessment of the respiratory system may be required. Some of the general observations that would have been made in the general survey and vital signs are as follows (Bennett, 2003):

- *Appearance*. General colour, finger clubbing, colour of nails, conscious level and non-verbal expression of pain.
- *Posture*. Erect, slouched or crouched-forward posture, breathlessness when lying down (orthopnoea).
- *Physical symptoms*. Coughing or increased respiratory secretions, unable to complete full sentence, breathlessness only on exertion.
- *Pulse oximetry*. To assess oxygen saturation.
- *Peak expiratory flow rate (PEFR)*. A measurement of the maximum flow rate, in litres per minute, that can be expelled from the lungs during a forced expiration. PEFR measurement gives objective information concerning the severity of airway obstruction.
- *Respiration*. Rate (16 breaths per minute), rhythm (regular) and depth.
- *Cyanosis*. Associated with excessive deoxygenation of haemoglobin and hypoxia (Casey, 2001). *Peripheral* cyanosis is most noticeable in the lips, ear lobes, mouth and finger tips and in the absence of central cyanosis, suggests circulatory problems rather than respiratory disease (Casey, 2001). *Central cyanosis* is best observed in the tongue and is an acute sign of hypoxia (e.g. asphyxia) or a chronic respiratory disease such as chronic obstructive pulmonary disease (Jevon & Ewens, 2001).

The posterior and anterior thorax are systematically examined in turn. The posterior thorax is usually examined while the patient is sitting up and the anterior thorax when the patient is in supine position. The anterior thorax can also be examined in the sitting-up position and the posterior thorax can be examined by turning the patient from side to side. The techniques used and the possible findings on examination are shown in Table 6.7.

Assessment of breathing in an unconscious patient

Where the patient is unconscious, it is important to ascertain the presence or absence of breathing. With the patient lying on his back and

Table 6.7 Examination of posterior and anterior thorax (Figure 6.3).

Techniques	Observations
• Inspection	• *Shape*: note any deformities or asymmetry, abnormal retraction of the interspaces • *Movement*: note impaired chest movement on one or both sides. Respiration rate, depth and regularity
• Palpation	• *Tenderness*: palpate any area where pain has been reported or where there are bruises or other obvious lesions • *Tactile fremitus* or palpable vibrations (the bony part of the palms is used on both sides of the patient's back and ask the patient to repeat fairly loudly the phrase 'ninety-nine'. This will cause a vibration). Fremitus is decreased or absent in COPD, pleural effusion or pneumothorax
• Percussion	• Identify five resonant notes. Normal lungs are *resonant*. *Flat* sounds occur in large pleural effusion, *dullness* in lobar pneumonia, *hyper-resonance* in emphysema or pneumothorax and *tympany* in large pneumothorax
• Auscultation	• Four types of normal breath sounds can be detected. *Tracheal* breath sounds are harsh and high-pitched and are heard over the trachea. *Bronchial* sounds are loud and high-pitched and are heard next to the trachea. *Vesicular* sounds are soft and low-pitched and are heard over most of the lungs. *Bronchovesicular* sounds are heard next to the sternum between the scapula. They are medium in loudness and pitch. Noisy breathing may be heard without use of a stethoscope and is indicative of blocked airway • Abnormal breath sounds are *crackles* (soft, high-pitched and very brief; may indicate abnormalities of the lungs or airways), *wheezes* (high-pitched and have a hissing quality, and suggest narrowed airways due to asthma-induced bronchoconstriction), *rhonchi* (low-pitched and have a snoring quality, and suggest secretions in lung airways). *Grunting* (noise heard on breathing out, usually in infants who have severe breathing problems) may also be present. *Crepitation* may also be audible with stethoscope (Sadik & Elliot, 2002)

with your head facing the patient's trunk, place your cheek close to the patient's mouth and nostrils to listen and feel for expired air, whilst observing the chest for breathing movements. Any noisy and laboured breathing denotes an obstructed airway. This might be accompanied by flaring of the nose, especially in a child (Sadik & Elliot, 2002). A clear airway should be maintained by tilting the head and lifting the chin of the patient. The degree of head tilt for an adult is hyperextension, for

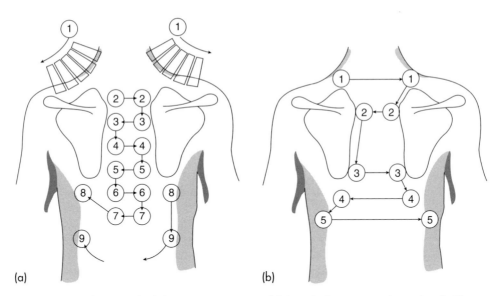

Figure 6.3 (a) Percussion sequence. (b) Auscultation sequence (reproduced with permission from Cox, 2004)

a child is a sniffing position and for infants is a neutral position, as advocated by the Resuscitation Council (2004). Following an incident it is best not to move the casualty, especially where injury to limbs and spinal column might have occurred. Otherwise, the casualty should be placed in a recovery position to help maintain a clear airway (Resuscitation Council, 2004).

Sputum

Where a sputum specimen is produced and collected, it should be observed for its amount and colour (e.g. clear, yellow, green or blood-stained). Sputum should also be assessed for its consistency; that is, whether it is tenacious (sticky and difficult to cough up), frothy, mucoid (like raw egg white), purulent (slimy green/yellowish) or mucopuru-lent (sticky, thick greenish/yellowish in colour) (Law, 2000). A sputum specimen should be sent to the pathological laboratory to be examined for culture and sensitivity.

Section 4: Physical assessment of the cardiovascular system

The cardiovascular system plays an important role in maintaining homeostasis as it transports oxygen and nutrients to the cells and removes waste products. Malfunction of this system will lead to serious repercussions to the body and affect the client's ability to perform activities of daily living. This section will focus on those aspects of cardiovascular assessment not covered in the general survey and vital signs.

Learning objectives

- Collect subjective data specific to cardiovascular functions.
- List the abnormalities that may be detected when performing a cardiovascular assessment using the four techniques of physical examination.
- Differentiate between normal and abnormal findings.
- Identify risk factors associated with coronary heart disease.

Relevant health history

Subjective data are collected in order to identify problems relating to the cardiovascular system. This is followed by a physical examination either to validate these problems and/or to identify other abnormalities. The relevant health history that needs to be taken into account prior to physical examination of the cardiovascular system is outlined in the activity box below.

Activity How will you assess the following symptoms of cardiovascular disorders?

Symptoms	Description	Give examples of questions that you will ask and observations you will make to elicit the information
• Chest pain	• Chest pain may indicate conditions such as angina, myocardial infarction or a dissecting aortic aneurysm	
• Palpitations	• Unpleasant awareness of heart beat. May result from an irregular heart beat or from rapid acceleration or slowing of the heart	

Symptoms	Description	Give examples of questions that you will ask and observations you will make to elicit the information
• Dizziness	• May indicate decreased blood flow to the brain. May be associated with hypotension and hypoxia (diminished oxygen in the tissues)	
• Oedema of ankles; pulmonary oedema	• Oedema results from increased capillary pressure that develops in peripheral circulation (dependent oedema) in congestive cardiac failure and in the pulmonary circulation in left-sided heart failure (pulmonary oedema)	
• Dyspnoea	• Perceived shortness of breath. May be of cardiac or pulmonary origin. It is associated with heart failure or severe anaemia. Exertional dyspnoea is dyspnoea related to an increase in activity. Orthopnoea is shortness of breath when the person is supine	
• Cyanosis/ pallor	• Cyanosis is bluish discolouration of the skin and mucous membranes caused by excess desaturated haemoglobin. May be associated with left ventricular failure, congestive cardiac failure, congenital heart disease and respiratory failure • Pallor is associated with anaemia or shock	
• Cough	• May occur in left ventricular failure. Pink sputum may be produced due to alveolar trauma from pulmonary oedema	

Continued

Symptoms	Description	Give examples of questions that you will ask and observations you will make to elicit the information
• Weakness and fatigue	• Diminished cardiac output from heart failure may lead to tissue hypoxia, resulting in weakness/fatigue. General fatigue increases as activity progresses during the day	
• Weight change	• Collection of fluid in the interstitial spaces will lead to a rapid increase in weight. Generalised oedema occurs in congestive cardiac failure	
• Hypotension/ hypertension	• Hypotension is common in the elderly and occurs particularly when moving from a lying to standing position. It also occurs in shock or heart failure • Hypertension contributes significantly to death from coronary heart disease (CHD) or stroke	
• Pain in legs	• Particularly occurs during activity (intermittent claudication) due to diminished blood supply	
• Peripheral skin changes	• Diminished blood supply to the skin causes the skin to become thin and shiny, affects hair distribution and causes skin ulcers	
• Changes in activities of living	• The symptoms associated with heart disease such as angina, dyspnoea, weakness and fatigue may interfere with activities of living. Limitations of physical activity range from minimal to virtual inability to carry on any physical activity without discomfort	

Risk factors for coronary heart disease

Genetic, lifestyle and socio-economic factors are known to contribute to coronary heart disease (CHD). These are often called risk factors, in that they influence outcomes without necessarily being their sole cause. Identification of risk factors (Table 6.8) is essential in health screening and cardiovascular assessment as their modification may play a key part in the reduction of morbidity and mortality from CHD. The three major risk factors are smoking, hypertension and abnormal cholesterol level (Foxton, 2004). Family history of CHD, diabetes, lack of exercise, abdominal obesity and lack of fruit and vegetables in the diet have also been implicated (Yusuf, 2004).

Table 6.8 Assessment of risk factors.

Risk factors	Description	Assessment
• Smoking	• Cigarette smoking greatly increases the risk of CHD. Carbon monoxide from cigarette smoke may cause microscopic trauma in blood vessel walls, activating the inflammatory response and attraction of lipid material (Timby et al., 1999)	• Do you smoke? How many cigarettes a day? When did you start?
• High fat intake and/or hyperlipidaemia	• The risk of cardiac disease increases as the level of low-density lipoproteins (LDL) rises (Foxton, 2004). LDL has the ability to invade the intimal wall of arteries, triggering the development of atheroma	• Do you take any animal fats and dairy products? How much?
• Exercise pattern	• Diminished exercise is associated with CHD and increase in weight	• Do you exercise? How often?
• Family history	• A genetic predisposition is linked to the development of heart disease	• Is there a history of heart disease, hypertension, high blood cholesterol level or diabetes in your family?

Physical examination

For the physical examination of the cardiovascular system, a stethoscope, sphygmomanometer and a ruler are required. A good light source and a quiet environment are important. In this part, the focus will primarily be on the chest area, using the four techniques of examination. To carry out a methodical assessment of the heart, the clinician will need to be able to identify critical landmarks used in cardiovascular assessment (see Figure 6.4). In Table 6.9, it is shown how the four techniques of examination are applied to cardiovascular assessment.

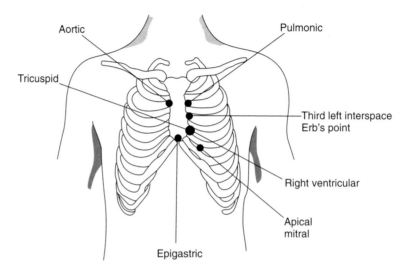

Figure 6.4 Sites for auscultation of the heart (reproduced with permission from Cox, 2004). *Aortic area*: second intercostal space at the right sternal border. *Pulmonic area*: second intercostal space at the left sternal border. *Erb's point*: third intercostal space at the left sternal border. *Mitral (apical) area*: fifth intercostal space near the left mid-clavicular line. *Tricuspid area*: fourth intercostal space at the left lower sternal border

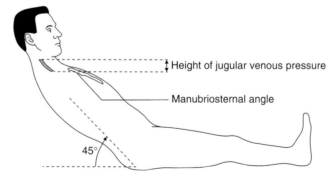

Figure 6.5 Measurement of jugular venous pressure (reproduced with permission from Cox, 2004)

Table 6.9 Cardiovascular assessment.

Techniques	Checklists
• *Inspection*	• *Precordium*: with the client lying supine and the head of the bed elevated at 30–45°, check apical impulse in the fifth intercostal space near the midclavicular line (mitral area). The apical impulse is the result of the ventricle moving outward during systole and is visible in about 50% of adults. Any other pulsations or heaves are abnormal • *Jugular venous pulse (JVP)*: in the position as above, turn the client's head slightly away from you. Then, check JVP in the area of the suprasternal notch. The highest point of pulsations should be no more than 4 cm above the sternal notch. Fully distended jugular veins indicate increased central venous pressure, which may be the result of right ventricular failure, pulmonary hypertension, pulmonary emboli or cardiac tamponade. See Figure 6.5
• *Palpation*	• *Carotid pulse*: palpate carotid arteries alternately – never both at the same time as this may trigger fainting – on the neck medial to the sternocleidomastoid muscle and note any pulse inequality (arterial occlusion or constriction in one artery), weak pulses (decreased cardiac output, shock, hypovolaemia) and thrills. Thrills indicate narrowing of artery
• *Percussion*	• *Cardiac borders*: percussion may be used to locate cardiac borders and note any enlargement. However, a chest X-ray provides more accurate information
• *Auscultation*	• *Heart sounds*: auscultation of the heart sounds can be done with the client lying supine with the head of the bed raised to 30–40°, sitting up or lying on the left side. You need to listen over the precordium, starting at the apex or base and moving in a zig-zag pattern • **Lub**: this is the first heart sound or S_1. It is loudest over the mitral area at the apex of the heart. It is low-pitched and dull and corresponds to the closure of the mitral and tricuspid valves • **Dub**: this is the second heart sound or S_2. It is loudest over the aortic area at the base of the heart. It is high-pitched and corresponds with closure of the aortic and pulmonary semilunar valves • **S_3**: this is a third heart sound and is abnormal, but is normally heard in infants. In adults, it is called ventricular gallop and may be a sign of congestive cardiac failure. It may be due to vibrations caused by ventricular distention and resistance • **S_4**: this is an abnormal sound and is called atrial gallop and may be heard over the tricuspid or mitral areas. It is caused by increased resistance to ventricular filling and may be heard in patients with previous myocardial infarction or elderly patients • **Murmurs**: these are abnormal signs and may be heard during systole or diastole. They may result from stenosis or insufficiency of the aortic, pulmonary, mitral or tricuspid valves • **Pericardial friction rub**: this is a scratchy sound that can be heard in patients with pericarditis. It is best heard using the diaphragm of the stethoscope with the patient sitting upright, leaning forward and exhaling

Section 5: Physical assessment of the nervous system

The patient's chief complaint and the findings on the initial screening will indicate whether or not a full neurological assessment is necessary. This section will focus on the physical assessment of the nervous system.

Learning objectives

- Collect subjective data on neurological function.
- Perform a neurological assessment, using the neurological assessment tool.
- Interpret data and identify abnormal findings.

Relevant health history

Whenever a detailed neurological assessment is conducted, a methodical approach is required. The practitioner will assess the highest level of neurological function (e.g. mental status) and work down to the lowest level (e.g. reflexes). The most common symptoms in neurological disorders and their significance are shown in Box 6.1.

Examination

In a detailed assessment of the nervous system, the examination is focused on five important areas:

- mental status
- cranial nerves
- motor system
- sensory system
- reflexes.

Mental status

Assessment of mental status, particularly level of consciousness (LOC), is aimed at establishing a baseline, detecting changes in the client's medical condition or identifying life-threatening situations requiring immediate medical intervention (Aucken & Crawford, 1998). Assessment of mental status has four components as shown in Table 6.10.

Box 6.1 Symptoms.

• Headache	May be trivial but could indicate serious neurological problems, e.g. brain tumour, subarachnoid haemorrhage or meningitis
• Dizziness	(Feeling light-headed or faint) may be indicative of transient ischaemic attack, stroke, vascular or mass lesions in the central nervous system, or neuromuscular disorders
• Disorientation	May indicate dementia, delirium, toxic confusional states, psychotic disorder and severe anxiety
• Change in mood, attention or speech	Mood change and loss of self-esteem, loss of interest in oneself and the environment may be indicative of depression. Attention and calculation skills are affected in dementia
• Altered or loss of consciousness	This could result from neurological or cardiopulmonary conditions, e.g. stroke, subarachnoid haemorrhage, head injuries, heart attack, suffocation, respiratory arrest
• Weakness or paralysis	May indicate transient ischaemic attack or stroke or lesions of the central nervous system
• Numbness/ altered or loss of sensation	May occur in lesions of the central nervous system or peripheral nerve roots
• Seizures	Caused by excessive electrical discharge in the brain. May occur in organic brain disease or metabolic disorders
• Tremors	Tremors may occur in some types of neurological disorders (e.g. Parkinson's disease)

Glasgow Coma Scale

The Glasgow Coma Scale (GCS), developed by Jennett & Teasdale (1974), is frequently used by doctors and nurses to assess level of consciousness. The GCS is often incorporated in a neurological examination chart, which also includes assessment of intracranial pressure and limb movement, as there could be changes in all three areas in alterations in neurological status. The chart is shown in Figure 6.6.

When using the GCS (Table 6.11) to assess level of consciousness, three activities are examined: eye opening, verbal response which motor response. Each activity is given a score. The total score is 15, which indicates that the client is fully alert. The worst score is three. A score of seven or less indicates deep coma (Aucken & Crawford, 1998; Hickey, 1997).

Table 6.10 Components of assessment of mental status.

Mental status	Observations	Abnormal findings
• Level of consciousness	• Is the patient alert or falling asleep? Can the patient focus his or her attention and maintain it? Do you need to use a stronger stimulus than your voice to get a response? Record what it is and how strong it needs to be to get a response from the patient. Use the Glasgow Coma Scale (Jennett & Teasdale, 1974) if the level of consciousness is altered and there is a high risk of neurological deterioration	• The patient is confused and responds inappropriately to questions • The patient is drowsy Responses to verbal stimuli are delayed • The patient may drift off to sleep during examination • The patient is in coma (Glasgow Coma Scale of 7 or less)
• Appearance and behaviour	• Note dress, personal hygiene, facial expression and action (Potter & Perry, 2001)	• Grooming and hygiene are affected in a number of psychiatric and neurological disorders
• Speech	• Note pace, volume, clarity and spontaneity of the patient's speech; assess comprehension by determining the patient's ability to follow instructions (Springhouse Corporation, 1997)	• Slow speech in depression and fast speech in mania • Defective articulation in stroke, Parkinson's disease or cerebellar disease • Dysphasia in stroke
• Cognitive functions	• Assess level of orientation, concentration, recent memory, remote memory and judgements (Potter & Perry, 2001)	• Cognitive functions are affected in delirium or dementia

Table 6.11 The Glasgow Coma Scale.

Activities	Observations
• Eye opening	• The best response (score 4) is for the client's eyes to open spontaneously, demonstrating that the arousal mechanisms are intact. If clients open their eyes in response to a verbal stimulus, they score 3. Eyes opening to a painful stimulus scores 3. If there is no response to verbal or painful stimuli, the score is 1
• Verbal response	• This assesses whether the client is aware of self and environment. Complete awareness (orientation) of oneself and the environment will score 4. Inappropriate speech scores 3, in comprehensible speech scores 2, and no verbal response to verbal or painful stimuli scores 1
• Motor response	• Obeying commands such as 'Lift up your arm' indicates awareness of environment and is given the maximum score of 6. Ability to localise pain gets a score of 5. Withdrawing from pain scores 4. Abnormal flexion to pain scores 3. Extension of arm in response to pain scores 2, and no response receives a score of 1

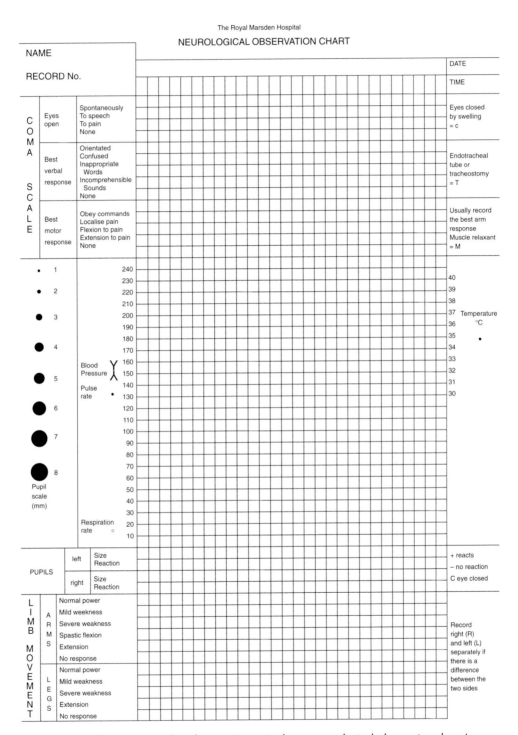

Figure 6.6 The Glasgow Coma Scale – a neurological observation chart (reproduced with permission from Mallet & Dougherty, 2000)

Assessment of pupil reaction and vital signs
Pupillary response
The assessment of pupil size, shape and response to light is vital in the detection of raised intracranial pressure. The oculomotor nerve, which is responsible for pupil constriction, is located in the brainstem; hence any compression of the nuclei of this cranial nerve will affect the pupil response and may cause the pupil to become fixed.

Vital signs
The vital centres such as the respiratory, cardiac and vasomotor centres are located in the brainstem. Damage or compression of the brainstem will lead to ischaemia and affect the control of the vital centres and may cause the blood pressure to rise and pulse to fall. The respiratory centre may become depressed.

Assessment of limb movement
This provides additional information on motor function. A weakness or paralysis of the limbs may indicate increasing intracranial pressure, a stroke or other lesions in the brain. There are 12 cranial nerves, which provide motor and sensory functions for areas from the face to the neck. The assessment of the cranial nerves is shown in Table 6.12.

Motor system

The assessment of the motor system (Table 6.13) includes:

- observation of body position
- inspection of muscle bulk
- testing muscle tone and strength
- assessment of cerebellar function.

Sensory function

When testing for sensory function (Table 6.14), you need to compare the distal with the proximal areas of extremities and symmetric areas on the two sides of the body. You need to scatter the stimuli to cover most of the dermatomes. For all the tests, you need to ask the client to close the eyes and to tell you what they feel and where.

Assessment of reflexes

Two types of reflexes are tested.

Deep tendon reflexes
A reflex hammer is used to strike the tendon briskly, using a head-to-toe and a symmetrical approach. You will test the biceps, triceps, brachioradialis, patellar and Achilles reflexes (Figure 6.7). Reflexes may be diminished or absent in disorders of the relevant spinal segments or peripheral nerves.

Table 6.12 The type, function and assessment of the cranial nerves.

Cranial nerve	Type	Functions	Assessment
• Olfactory (I)	• Sensory	• Smell	• With eyes closed, ask the client to identify a common scent such as coffee or vanilla. Loss of smell may occur in lesions of the olfactory tract or frontal lobe
• Optic (II)	• Sensory	• Responsible for	• Assess near vision by asking the client to sight read a newspaper. Visual fields of each eye are also checked. An ophthalmoscope is used to view the retina and optic disc
• Oculomotor (III)	• Motor	• Responsible for papillary constriction, extraocular movement and elevation of eyelid	• Constriction of pupils in response to light is checked • Extraocular eye movement is also assessed
• Trochlear (IV)	• Motor	• Extraocular movement	• Cranial nerves III, IV and VI all control eye movements. Assess them together by asking the client to follow your finger through six positions of gaze. Abnormalities such as ptosis (drooping of upper lid) may be observed
• Trigeminal (V)	• Mixed	• *Motor*: supplies motor function to the jaw and chewing muscles • *Sensation*: supplies sensation to cornea, nasal and oral mucosa, and facial skin	• *Motor function*: ask the client to clench teeth and palpate the temporal and masseter muscles. Unilateral weakness may indicate lesion of the trigeminal nerve • *Sensory function*: check whether the client can correctly identify sharp and dull stimuli to the forehead, chin and cheeks
• Abducens (VI)	• Motor	• Controls extraocular movement	• Assessed together with cranial nerves III and IV as they all control extraocular movement
• Facial (VII)	• Mixed	• *Motor*: responsible for facial muscle • *Sensory*: taste perception on the anterior part of the tongue	• *Motor function*: ask the client to smile, frown, show teeth, puff out cheeks, purse lips, close eyes and raise eyebrows. Paralysis of facial muscles is seen in Bell's palsy and CVA • *Sensory function*: touch the anterior two-thirds of the tongue with moistened applicator dipped in salt, sugar or lemon juice and ask patient to identify the taste

Continued

Table 6.12 *Continued*

Cranial nerve	Type	Functions	Assessment
• Vestibulo-cochlear (VIII)	• Sensory	• Responsible for hearing and equilibrium	• Whisper words from 1–2 feet away. Vibration sounds using a tuning fork may also be used to assess hearing
• Glosso-pharyngeal (IX)	• Mixed	• *Motor*: responsible for swallowing and salivating • *Sensory*: taste perception on posterior one-third of the tongue	• Cranial nerves IX and X are tested together when assessing swallowing and gag reflex
• Vagus (X)	• Mixed	• Swallowing and gag reflex	• Assessed together with cranial nerve IX
• Accessory (XI)	• Motor	• Controls sternocleidomastoid and upper portion of trapezius muscles	• Ask the client to shrug the shoulders against resistance. Asymmetric contraction or drooping of the shoulder may be seen in paralysis or muscle weakness due to neck injury or torticollis
• Hypoglossal (XII)	• Motor	• Controls tongue movement	• Ask the client to protrude tongue and to move tongue to each side against resistance of a tongue blade

Superficial reflexes

Assessment of superficial reflexes is of two types.

Abdominal reflexes

These are tested by lightly stroking the skin. Briskly stroking both sides of the abdomen and observing contraction of abdominal muscles tests the abdominal reflexes. Absence of abdominal reflexes suggests lower or upper motor neuron lesions.

Plantar reflexes (see Figure 6.7)

The side of the sole of the foot is scratched with a firm implement (e.g. rounded spike of tendon hammer). The normal responses are flexion of all toes. An abnormal response in children and adults will be the extension of the big toe with fanning of the other toes (Babinski response), indicating a lesion of the pyramidal tract.

Table 6.13 The assessment of motor function.

Components	Possible findings on assessment
• Body position at rest and on movement	• Neurological deficits such as paralysis may result in abnormal positions • Involuntary movements such as tremors and tics
• Muscle bulk for contour, size and symmetry	• Muscular atrophy (wasting) to the hands, shoulders and thighs. Atrophy may indicate diseases of the peripheral nervous system or muscles themselves
• Muscle tone and strength	• *Tone*: move the shoulder through a moderate range of motion and check the resistance offered to your movements. Decreased resistance suggests diseases of peripheral nervous system or cerebellum. Increased resistance suggests spasticity • *Strength*: ask the patient to move major muscles or muscle groups against your resistance. Impaired strength is called paresis or weakness. Absence of strength is called plegia
• Cerebellar function	• Assess co-ordination, posture, movements of the legs and general balance by observing the patient walking across the room, turning and walking back. Ataxia or lack of co-ordination occurs in cerebellar disease or intoxication

Table 6.14 Assessment of sensory function.

Sensory function	Assessment and possible findings
• Pain	• Use the blunt and sharp ends of a safety pin or paper clip and ask the patient when the sharp end is felt
• Position	• Grasp the client's big toe and move it up and down, asking the client to tell you when it is up or down. Loss of position sense suggests disease of posterior column or peripheral nerve
• Vibration	• Tap a low-pitched tuning fork on the heel of your hand and place the base firmly on the bony surface of the patient's fingers or big toe. Loss of vibration sense is common in peripheral neuropathy, which is frequently caused by diabetes or alcoholism
• Light touch	• Use a wisp of cotton to lightly touch the client's skin
• Discrimination	• This assesses the ability of the sensory cortex to analyse and interpret sensations. With the client's eyes closed, place a familiar object in the client's hand and ask the client to tell you what it is. Inability to identify familiar objects is called astereognosis. To test for graphesthesia, use a blunt instrument to write a number on the patient's palm. Inability to correctly identify the number suggests a lesion in the sensory cortex

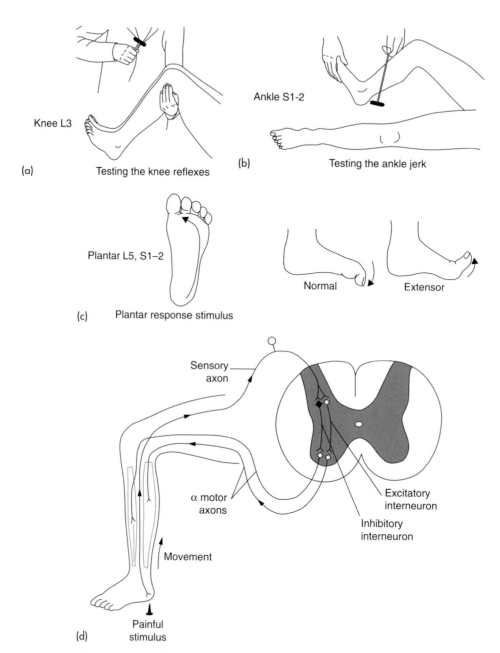

Knee L3

Testing the knee reflexes

(a)

(b)

Ankle S1-2

Testing the ankle jerk

Plantar L5, S1–2

Normal   Extensor

(c)   Plantar response stimulus

Sensory
axon

α motor
axons

Excitatory
interneuron

Inhibitory
interneuron

Movement

Painful
(d)   stimulus

Figure 6.7   (a–d) Normal and abnormal responses on testing reflexes (reproduced with permission from Bray et al., 1999 and Cox, 2004)

Section 6: Physical assessment of the eyes, ears, nose and throat

Learning objectives

- Recognise the normal health of the eyes, ears, nose and throat.
- Perform a physical assessment of the eyes, ears, nose and throat.
- Recognise abnormal findings of the eyes, ears, nose and throat.

The eyes

The incidence of eye disorders and blindness is rising, particularly in older people. As some visual problems occur gradually, it is important to ask the client specific questions about vision. The assessment of the eyes begins by recording subjective data (Table 6.15). This is followed by physical examination using the techniques of inspection and palpation.

Physical examination

The important areas of examination are the external structures of the eyes, visual acuity, extraocular muscles and intraocular structures (Table 6.16).

Visual acuity and visual fields

The Snellen chart is used to test distant visual acuity. It consists of lines of letters that decrease in size from top to bottom with standardised visual acuity numbers at the end of each line of letters. The numbers indicate the degree of visual acuity when the patient is able to read that line at a distance of 20 feet. Normal visual acuity is 20/20. A patient with a visual acuity of 20/70 can read at 20 feet what a person with a visual acuity of 20/20 can read at 70 feet.

For near vision, the clinician will check whether the patient is able to distinguish the letters in a near-vision card placed 14 inches from the eyes. Normal near visual acuity is 14/14. If presbyopia (impaired near vision) is present, the client will move the chart away from the eyes to focus on the letters. Presbyopia is common from middle age onwards.

A visual field is the entire area seen by an eye when it looks at a central point. Four visual field positions are tested: inferior, superior, temporal and nasal. Failure by the patient to see the examiner's moving finger in these positions indicates a reduction in peripheral vision.

Table 6.15 Common eye complaints.

Common complaints	Significance of the complaints
• Changes in vision/ visual acuity	• May be of sudden or gradual onset. Sudden changes may suggest retinal detachment or other acute problems. Gradual changes are related to ageing, diabetes, hypertension or neurological disorders. Difficulty with close work suggests hypermetropia or long-sightedness. Myopia or short-sightedness is difficulty with long distance vision
• Double vision (diplopia)	• May affect one or both eyes; the images may be seen side by side (horizontal) or on top of each other (vertical). Diplopia may arise from a lesion in the brainstem or cerebellum or from paralysis of extraocular muscles (CN III or VI in horizontal diplopia or CN III or IV in vertical diplopia)
• Blind spots	• Complaints of specks in the vision. Moving specks or strands suggest vitreous floaters, vascular spasms or pressure on the optic nerve. Fixed defects (scotomas) may indicate retinal detachment, lesions in the retinas or visual pathways
• Eye pain	• It may indicate a foreign body in the eyes or changes within the eye. Burning pain may indicate allergies or irritation
• Haloes or rings around lights	• Seeing haloes is associated with narrow-angle glaucoma (i.e. raised intraocular pressure due to narrowing of anterior chamber of the eye and outflow impairment when the iris thickens as a result of pupil dilation)
• Difficulty seeing at night	• Night blindness is associated with deficiency of vitamin A, glaucoma or optic atrophy
• Excessive watering or tearing of the eye	• This may occur in blockage of lacrimal apparatus or exposure to irritants or loss of the lipid film
• Eye discharge, redness or swelling	• This is often related to an inflammatory response caused by a bacterial or viral infection or an allergy

Extraocular muscles

The assessment of extraocular muscle function includes the following.

The corneal light reflex

The patient is asked to look straight ahead while you shine a light on the bridge of the nose. The reflection of light should be on the same

Table 6.16 Examination of extraocular structures.

Structures	Possible findings on examination
• Position and alignment of the eyes	• Inward or outward deviation of the eyes. Protrusion of the eyes (occurs in Graves' disease or ocular tumours)
• Eyebrows	• Note quantity and distribution of eyebrows. Sparseness may suggest hypothyroidism
• Eyelids	• Drooping of the lid (ptosis), inflammation (blepharitis) along the lid margin, stye or hordeolum
• Lacrimal apparatus	• Swelling, excessive tearing or dryness
• Conjunctiva and sclera (ask the client to look up while you gently pull the lower eyelid down)	• Nodules or swelling
• Cornea and lens (use penlight to inspect)	• Opacity of lens
• Iris	• The iris should appear flat while the cornea should appear convex. The iris may be pushed forward in glaucoma
• Pupil size, shape and symmetry	• Test for pupillary reactions to light. Neurological damage or raised intracranial pressure may alter the size, shape and response of the pupils

spot on each cornea, indicating parallel alignment. In a condition called strabismus, there is asymmetric position of the light reflex.

Cardinal positions of gaze
The patient follows your finger or pencil while you move it through the six cardinal positions of gaze. You will note any abnormal findings such as nystagmus (where one eye fails to follow the finger or pencil), lid lag and poor convergence.

Intraocular structures
An ophthalmoscope is used for direct observation of the internal structures of the eyes. The examination will focus on the following structures.

Cornea and lens
When the light beam is shone on the pupil, an orange glow (the red reflex) should be seen, indicating a clear lens and cornea. Absence of a red reflex suggests opacity of the lens (cataract) or the vitreous.

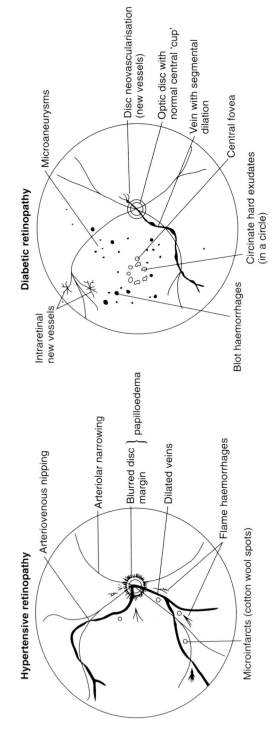

Figure 6.8 Abnormalities in the retina (reproduced with permission from Cox, 2004)

Optic discs and retina
Observation will be made of the sharpness or clarity of the disc, the colour of the disc, scars or pigmentation on the retina, macular degenerations and any tapering of the veins. A swollen optic disc with a blurred disc margin is called papilloedema, signalling raised intracranial pressure (Figure 6.8). Arteriovenous nipping may be seen in hypertension (see Figure 6.8). Shiny yellow patches of lipid in the retina may be noticed in a patient with diabetes mellitus (Figure 6.8).

The ears

The ear has three compartments: external, middle and inner. Each part plays an important role in hearing. The ear is also responsible for balance. The types of ear complaints are shown in Table 6.17.

Physical examination

In the physical examination of the ear, the auricle, canal and tympanic membrane (eardrum) are carefully inspected (Table 6.18). A tuning fork

Table 6.17 Ear complaints and their assessment.

Complaints	Significance
• Hearing loss	• There are two types: conductive (problems in the external or middle ear) and sensorineural (problems in inner ear, cochlear nerve, connections in the brain). People with sensorineural loss tend to have trouble in understanding speech, particularly in noisy environments. People with conductive deafness do not find noisy environment such an hindrance
• Earache	• Inflammation of middle ear (otitis media) or external ear (otitis externa) may cause earache. Could lead to sore throat, cough, upper respiratory tract infection or fever. Discharge from the ear may arise from soft wax, debris from inflammation or rash in external ear or from a perforated eardrum secondary to otitis media
• Tinnitus	• This is a perceived sound (musical ringing) that has no external stimulus. When it is associated with hearing loss, it may suggest Ménière's disease
• Vertigo	• Perception that the environment is rotating. Several questions may need to be asked to clarify what the patient means. Feeling of unsteadiness or being lightheaded may suggest a cardiovascular aetiology whereas a feeling of being pulled to the ground or the room spinning suggests true vertigo, arising from an inner ear problem or a lesion of cranial nerve VIII

Table 6.18 Physical examination of the ear.

Structures	Possible findings on examination
• Auricle	• Deformities, low-set ears, skin lesions, lumps, excessive cerumen, discharge or inflammation. In otitis externa, the auricle is painful if it is moved up and down. Tenderness behind the ear may be present in otitis media
• Ear canal and tympanic membrane (use otoscope – see figure 6.9a)	• To straighten the canal, gently pull the auricle upward, backward and slightly away from the head. Possible findings include discharge, foreign bodies, nodules, redness or swelling in the canal. A red bulging tympanic membrane suggests purulent otitis media
• Auditory acuity	• Test one ear at a time. Occlude one ear and whisper softly towards the unoccluded ear, evaluating the auditory acuity in each ear
• Air and bone conduction	• This is used to distinguish between conductive and sensorineural hearing problems. The Weber's and Rinne's tests are used. In *Weber's test* (*bone conduction*), a vibrating tuning fork is placed firmly on top of the patient's head. In unilateral conductive hearing loss, the sound is heard in the impaired ear. In unilateral hearing loss, sound is heard in the good ear. *Rinne's test* compares air conduction with bone conduction. The vibrating tuning fork is placed on the mastoid bone until the patient can no longer hear the sound. Then the tuning fork is placed close to the ear canal. Normally the sound is heard longer through air than bone conduction. In conductive deafness, sound is heard as long or longer through bone. In sensorineural deafness, sound is heard longer through air

is used to evaluate air and bone conduction. Figure 6.9a also shows an otoscopic examination. Figure 6.9b shows a child's ear being examined.

The mouth, nose, sinuses and throat

Complaints relating to the mouth, nose, sinuses and throat are common. These structures are usually assessed together, not only because of their close proximity to each other but also because some of the disorders in these structures may have shared causes.

Relevant health history

Subjective data are collected from the client to aid in the detection of diseases and abnormalities (Table 6.19).

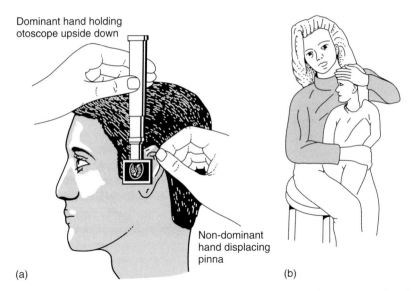

Dominant hand holding
otoscope upside down

Non-dominant
hand displacing
pinna

(a)   (b)

Figure 6.9 (a) Otoscopic examination. (b) Examination of a child's ear (reproduced with permission from Mallet & Dougherty, 2000)

Table 6.19 Subjective assessment of the mouth, nose, sinuses and throat.

Complaints	Significance
• Sore tongue and mouth sores	• Aphthous ulcers (may be associated with stress, extreme fatigue and oral trauma). Smooth red tongue (glossitis) occurs in nutritional deficiency of B12, iron or niacin. Thrush (candidiasis) – curd-like coating of the tongue
• Bleeding from the gums	• Often caused by gingivitis (may be caused by poor oral hygiene, incorrectly fitted dentures, scurvy or stomatitis)
• Rhinorrhoea (nasal discharge)	• May be associated with other symptoms such as tenderness in the face or over the sinuses. Causes of rhinorrhoea include viral infections, allergies and concurrent sinusitis
• Epistaxis (bleeding from the nose)	• May be caused by trauma (nose picking), inflammation, tumours or foreign bodies. Bleeding disorders may also contribute to epistaxis
• Sore throat	• May be due to viral or bacterial infection. A persistent sore throat may be due to a malignant growth
• Hoarseness	• Most common causes are overuse of the voice or upper respiratory infections. Chronic hoarseness may be due to voice abuse, hypothyroidism, malignant growth or tuberculosis
• Tender enlarged lymph nodes	• Enlarged and tender lymph nodes in the neck are normally due to pharyngitis but could be due to a malignant growth of the lymphatic system
• Goitre (enlarged thyroid gland)	• Goitre or enlargement of the thyroid may occur in either hypothyroidism (hyposecretion of thyroid gland) or hyperthyroidism (hypersecretion of thyroid gland)

Physical examination of the mouth, nose, sinuses and throat

The techniques of inspection and palpation are usually employed in the assessment of the mouth, nose, sinuses and throat.

The mouth

You need to wear gloves when examining the mucous membrane. Inspect the following structures.

* *The lips.* Observe for colour, moisture, cracks or ulcers.
* *Oral mucosa.* With the help of a good light and a tongue blade, inspect the oral mucosa for colour, ulcers, nodules and white patches. Curd-like patches over reddened mucosa that scrape off and bleed easily indicate thrush. Leucoplakia are white patches that do not scrape off and are considered precancerous.
* *Gums and teeth.* Note the colour of the gums and whether there are any swellings and ulceration, which occurs in gingivitis. Inspect the teeth and note colour, missing teeth and general state of the teeth.

The throat

With the client's mouth open, ask the patient to say 'ah' and inspect the pharynx, soft palate, uvula and tonsils. Note any ulcers, inflammation, exudates and tonsillar enlargement.

The nose and paranasal sinuses

* *Anterior and inferior surface of the nose.* The application of gentle pressure on the tip of the nose with your thumb will allow you to view each nasal vestibule. Note any asymmetry or deviation of the septum. Note any ulcers or polyps.
* *Nasal obstruction.* To check for obstruction, press on each ala nasi in turn and ask the patient to breathe in.
* *Nasal mucosa.* Note colour, any swelling, bleeding or exudates. In rhinitis the mucosa is reddened and swollen.
* *Paranasal sinuses.* Palpate the frontal sinuses from under the bony eyebrow and then the maxillary sinuses in the lower part of the cheek. Tenderness suggests sinusitis.

The throat

Inspect the neck, particularly noting its symmetry. Note any enlargement of the thyroid gland, visible lymph nodes or scars.

Examination of the lymph nodes (see Figure 6.10)
Using the pads of the index and middle fingers, palpate the lymph nodes and note size, shape, mobility, consistency and any tenderness. Tender nodes suggest inflammation. Hard or fixed nodes suggest malignancy.

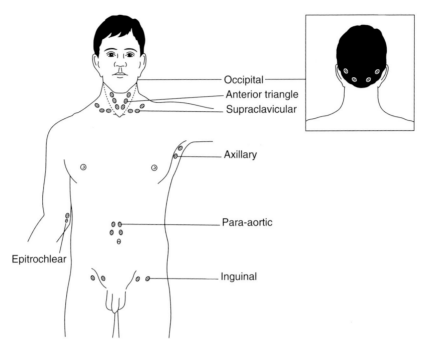

Figure 6.10 Examination of lymph nodes

Section 7: Physical assessment of the digestive system

> ## Learning objectives
>
> - Obtain a health history of the digestive system.
> - Undertake a physical assessment of the anus and rectum.
> - Differentiate between normal and abnormal findings.

The digestive system consists of the gastrointestinal tract and the accessory organs of digestion – liver, gall bladder and pancreas (see Chapter 1). Before you go any further, please give an outline of the functions of the gastrointestinal tract and its accessory organs in the activity box on the following page.

Activity	
Structure/Organ	**Function**
• Teeth /tongue	
• Oesophagus	
• Stomach	
• Small intestines	
• Large intestines	
• Liver	
• Gall bladder	
• Pancreas	

Relevant health history

Assessment of the digestive system initially involves obtaining a health history. Here the nurse should collect subjective data relating to the following areas:

- usual dietary intake
- ability to chew food and swallow
- presence of indigestion, nausea, vomiting
- anorexia or recent weight loss
- presence of pain or discomfort such as indigestion or with defaecation
- normal bowel pattern and any recent changes
- frequency of elimination
- colour and consistency of the faeces
- use of laxatives and any recent increase in frequency or dosage
- past medical and family history of problems or surgery associated with the digestive system.

Risk factors

Certain risk factors also need to be taken into account:

- Age of patient (increased risk of bowel cancer for people over age 50 years).
- Any exposure to hepatitis B virus (e.g. sexual contact with a carrier, intravenous drug user).

Physical assessment

Physical assessment of the digestive system employs the techniques of inspection, palpation and auscultation. These techniques are all used during the abdominal assessment and are largely performed by the medical team and are therefore outside the scope of this text. The nurse will, however, be involved in the preparation and support of the patient and doctor during this time.

The nurse will be required to inspect and report on materials such as vomit and faeces (Table 6.20) and to undertake auscultation of the abdomen to ascertain the presence or absence of bowel sounds (see Table 6.21) with a view to reintroducing oral fluids after abdominal surgery or if the patient complains of nausea.

It is also important to observe the amount, odour, frequency and time of any vomit or faecal matter collected. The presence or absence of any foreign substances in the specimen collected should also be noted.

Procedure for auscultation of the abdomen

This procedure should be performed before palpating the abdomen to ensure bowel sounds, if present, are not altered. The nurse should ensure patient comfort by warming the diaphragm of the stethoscope before use.

Ascultation of the abdomen (see Table 6.21) should be performed systematically by placing the diaphragm in each quadrant, starting with the right upper quadrant and proceeding in a clockwise direction. Apply light pressure. Due to the nature of bowel sounds, the nurse should spend about five minutes undertaking the procedure, spending an equal amount of time within each quadrant.

Assessment of the anus and rectum (perianal region; Table 6.22)

Inspection and palpation of the anus and rectum are skills the nurse also needs to develop. These procedures are both uncomfortable and embarrassing for the patient. The nurse must therefore ensure privacy is maintained throughout the assessment and that the patient is allowed to express their concerns.

The most commonly used position for this assessment is the left lateral position. The patient should be asked to lie on their left side with their buttocks as close to the edge of the table as possible. They should then be asked to bend their right leg at the hip and knee. The patient should be covered to maintain comfort and dignity throughout the procedure. Some of the possible findings on examination of the anus and rectum are outlined in Table 6.22.

Table 6.20 Inspection of vomit and faeces.

Physical/chemical characteristics	Normal – observation and analysis	Deviations and possible causes
Vomit • Quantity, frequency, presence of blood	• Absent	• *Haematemesis*: vomiting or regurgitation of blood arising from bleeding in the upper GIT. Bright red – recent bleeding. Brown or 'coffee grounds' – bleeding is old and has mixed with stomach acid leading to alteration of the haemoglobin. Possible causes – oesophageal varices, oesophagitis, erosion of gastric or duodenal ulcer, Mallory-Weiss tear (tear in the mucous membrane at the junction of the oesophagus and stomach that results in massive bleeding. Usually caused by protracted vomiting and is often seen in alcoholics and people where the pylorus is obstructed
Faeces • Colour	• Brown to dark brown	• *Melaena*: black, tarry, foul-smelling stool. Possible cause – upper GIT bleeding • *Fresh blood loss*: this may be mixed in with the faeces or located on the outside. Mucus may or may not be present. Possible causes – cancer of the colon, inflammatory bowel disorders such as ulcerative colitis and Crohn's disease, anal fissures, haemorrhoids and diverticular disease • *Pale, putty-coloured stool*: results from the absence of bile pigments. Possible causes – obstructive jaundice due to gallstone, carcinoma of head of pancreas, cholangiocarcinoma (cancer of the biliary ducts)
• Consistency	• Formed but soft	• *Diarrhoea*: passage of 3 or more unformed or watery stools per day. Possible causes – infection, e.g. *Salmonella*, inflammatory bowel disorders

Continued

Table 6.20 *Continued*

Physical/chemical characteristics	Normal – observation and analysis	Deviations and possible causes
		• *Constipation*: infrequent passage of hard stools. Possible causes – dehydration, embarrassment, difficulty in accessing toilet facilities, neurogenic disorders such as Hirschsprung's disease, painful anal lesions such as a fistula, drugs such as opiates and antacids (aluminium hydroxide) and systemic disorders such as hypothyroidism and diabetic neuropathy • *Steatorrhoea*: stool with high fat content. It tends to be bulky, greasy in appearance and has an offensive odour and may result in diarrhoea. Possible causes – malabsorption syndromes (failure of the intestinal mucosa to absorb digested nutrients), e.g. deficiency of the enzyme lactase which is responsible for the digestion of lactose (milk sugar) to the monosaccharide sugars glucose and galactose

Table 6.21 Possible finding on auscultation of the abdomen.

Assessment	Normal findings	Deviations/abnormalities
• Auscultation for bowel sounds. Note intensity, pitch, frequency	• High-pitched irregular gurgles in all 4 quadrants. Occur between 5–30 times per minute • May be hyperactive (loud and prolonged gurgles known as borborgymi)	• *Absent*: possibly due to intestinal obstruction, peritonitis, abdominal surgery following handling of the gut • *Underactive*: following abdominal surgery, late stage of bowel obstruction, constipation • *Hyperactive*: might occur in early stage of bowel obstruction, diarrhoea, gastroenteritis

Table 6.22 Possible findings on assessment of the perianal region.

Assessment	Normal findings	Deviations/abnormalities
• **Perianal region** Inspect by separating the buttocks with gloved hands. Note colour, presence of swelling, lumps, fissures or discharge, infection	• The anal opening is hairless, moist and tightly closed	• *Swelling or lump*: may be due to cancer, haemorrhoids, perianal haematoma, sexually transmitted disease (e.g. anal warts) or rectal prolapse • *Pain and redness*: possible causes include thrombosed haemorrhoid, perianal abscess, fissure and fistula • *Pruritus +/– redness*: might be caused by fungi or worm infestation • *Ulceration*: may indicate Crohn's disease • *Discharge*: Faecal soiling – possible causes include tumour, incontinence amd haemorrhoids; mucus may be due to inflammatory change in rectal or anal mucosa, or haemorrhoids; pus – possible causes include abscess, fissure in ano and infection
• **Sacrococcygeal region** Note colour, presence of hair	• Smooth and free from hair. No redness	• *Pilonidal disease*: lesion located in the midline of the natal cleft with one or more openings; may be covered by a small tuft of hair. Redness, pain and possibly pus

Further investigations

Further investigations of the digestive system involve blood analysis, imaging techniques such as barium studies and ultrasound and direct visualisation via an endoscope. Endoscopies are now being undertaken by nurses who have completed extended training.

Section 8: Physical assessment of the urinary tract system

The urinary system consists of two kidneys and ureters, one bladder and one urethra. A further structure closely associated with the male urethra is the prostate gland which is a component of the male reproductive system.

The kidneys perform the main functions of the urinary system, while the remaining structures are involved in transport and storage of urine prior to its evacuation from the body. The primary function of the kidneys is to regulate the volume and composition of blood and in so doing maintain homeostatic balance. The product of this activity is urine. Urine is composed of approximately 95% water, with the remaining 5% consisting of products from cell metabolism and external sources such as drugs.

Several factors influence renal function including age and various disease processes. The latter may be acute or chronic in nature and they may also reflect pathology within another body system.

The prostate gland is located at the base of the bladder where it encircles the urethra. The gland enlarges with age and in so doing may lead to symptoms of benign prostatic hyperplasia (frequency, hesitancy, urgency, nocturia) in men and may result in either acute or chronic urinary retention.

Prostate cancer is the second most common cancer in men in Britain, accounting for about 4% of all deaths annually in England and Wales (DoH, 2000). It primarily affects men over the age of 50 and with the global trend toward an ageing population, it is predicted that the number of individuals dying from the disease will rise substantially within the next two decades (Kirby *et al.*, 2001). In the United Kingdom 19 000 new cases are diagnosed annually. In addition, 10 000 men die which accounts for 3% of those diagnosed with the disorder (Brewster, 2001).

The clinical features arising are similar to those for benign enlargement. Due to the adverse effects the gland may exert on both micturition and renal function, it will be discussed under assessment of the urinary system.

Learning objectives

- Perform a physical assessment of the urinary system.
- Recognise abnormalities associated with the urinary system.

Assessment of the urinary system

The main assessment of the urinary system performed by the nurse involves collection and analysis of urine along with enquiry into micturition and associated symptoms, such as pain, low back pain, burning sensation on micturition, hesitancy or frequency. Where there is prolonged retention of urine, the patient should be examined for lower abdominal distension.

Other investigations, such as urodynamic studies or imaging by X-rays or ultrasound, are ordered and performed by other health professionals, although this is an area that has opened up to the specialist nurse.

Whilst collecting a specimen of urine is a common nursing activity, this may not be the case for the patient. It is important therefore that the nurse ensures the patient understands the type of specimen required and maintains privacy and dignity.

Types of urine sample

Mainstream specimen

First and final flows are passed into a toilet with approximately 30 ml of the mainstream being passed into a clean receptacle. This type of specimen is used for routine urinalysis using a reagent strip. This is then read at the stated times to identify the presence or absence of various substances (see Table 6.23 for normal characteristics of urine).

Midstream specimen (MSU)

Involves collection of a urine sample into a sterile container. The patient or nurse should carefully clean the labia or glans with soap and water. An antiseptic should not be used as it may affect the urinalysis (Mallett & Dougherty, 2000). The first part of the urine flow should be discarded and the remainder collected in a sterile container. An MSU is collected for laboratory examination.

Early morning specimen (EMU)

First urine excreted in the morning. Undertaken for pregnancy and tuberculosis tests.

Catheter specimen of urine (CSU)

Involves removal of a specimen via an indwelling catheter. The specimen is taken via either a rubber cuff situated on the tubing or an access point located on the drainage bag. If no urine is present in the tubing a clamp should be applied below the rubber cuff until sufficient urine has collected. Following hand cleansing, the portal is swabbed using 70% isopropyl alcohol and the required amount of urine aspirated using a sterile syringe and needle (if required). A CSU is collected for laboratory examination.

Twenty four-hour urine specimen

Involves collection of a patient's urine over a 24-hour period. The first sample at 08.00 hours is discarded. The remainder is then passed into a clean receptacle and transferred to a large container. The investigation is required when a substance which is being investigated does not have an even excretion rate over a 24-hour period. Examples include hormones, such as cortisol, or hormonal metabolites.

Table 6.23 Normal and abnormal characteristics of urine.

Physical/chemical characteristics	Normal – observation and analysis	Deviations and significance
• Volume	• 1.5–2 litres daily (1 ml/kg per hr – Sadik & Elliot, 2002). Variable due to a variety of influencing factors	• *Oliguria*: impaired renal function, dehydration • *Polyuria*: impaired renal function, high intake
• Colour	• Yellow or amber	• Varies with concentration, diet and presence of abnormal substances
• Turbidity	• Transparent when fresh	• Becomes cloudy on standing or if abnormal substances present
• Odour	• Faint aromatic odour when fresh	• Develops an ammonia-like odour on standing • Fishy odour indicates infection
• PH	• Ranges between 4.6 and 8.0; average about 6	• Affected by diet – high protein intake increases acidity (low pH) • Inability to regulate urinary pH – Infection, prolonged vomiting
• Specific Gravity (solute concentration of urine)	• Ranges between 1.001 and 1.035	• Inability to concentrate or dilute urine • Renal failure, presence of abnormal constituents, e.g. glucose
• Haemoglobin – haemoglobinuria	• Negative	• Transfusion reaction, haemolytic anaemia, severe burns
• Erythrocytes – haematuria	• Negative	• Bleeding into urinary tract due to trauma, renal calculi and infection • Menstruation
• Glucose – glycosuria	• Negative	• May be present during pregnancy. Uncontrolled diabetes mellitus (diabetic ketoacidosis)
• Ketones – ketonuria	• Negative	• Uncontrolled diabetes mellitus, prolonged vomiting, dieting, starvation
• Leucocytes	• 0–4	• Infection
• Protein – proteinuria	• Negative	• Infection, glomerular or tubule damage

Assessment of the prostate gland

Assessment of the prostate gland involves a variety of techniques and investigations that collectively contribute to the final diagnosis. The methods used include palpation, imaging and blood analysis. Imaging involves ultrasound via a rectal transducer (transrectal ultrasound – TRUS).

Blood investigations are mainly concerned with the detection of prostatic cancer through the presence of a substance called prostate-specific antigen (PSA). Normal value is <4ng/ml but this increases with age and it is also higher in black than white males. Levels are also elevated with benign enlargement and infection. For these reasons, it is considered to be insufficiently specific or sensitive to be used alone for screening (Brooker & Nicol, 2003).

Palpation of the prostate gland involves digital examination via the rectum. Such an examination may be embarrassing and therefore the nurse should be sensitive to the patient's body language (muscle tensing) and ensure all aspects of the procedure are explained and understood before proceeding.

The patient should be placed in the left lateral position with the buttocks as close to the edge of the examining table as possible. The knees should be bent upward toward the chest with the upper knee higher than the lower. This position ensures the colon lies in its natural anatomical position and thus assists access into the rectum. The patient's privacy and dignity must be maintained throughout the examination by careful draping and ensuring entry to the room is controlled.

Table 6.24 Palpation of the prostate gland.

Assessment	Normal	Deviations/abnormalities
Place index finger into the rectum and rotate it in an anticlockwise fashion until its inner surface faces the patient's umbilicus. Rub the pad of the index finger over the prostate gland and try to identify the sulcus between the two lateral lobes (Weber & Kelley, 2003). Identify the *size, shape* and *texture* of the gland. Note the presence of any lumps and tenderness	• The prostate gland is approximately the size of a walnut, weighing about 20 g • Enlargement occurs in most men over 50 years • Texture is smooth and rubbery	• *Infection* • *Prostatitis*: tender, swollen gland. Patient may complain of low back pain and symptoms of a urinary tract infection (dysuria, frequency, urgency) • *Benign prostatic Hyperplasia*: enlarged but smooth rubbery gland • *Cancer*: hard area or presence of hard fixed nodules within the gland

The nurse should use a gloved finger that has been well lubricated prior to insertion into the rectum. The normal findings and any possible deviation from these that might be noted on palpation of the prostate gland are shown in Table 6.24.

Section 9: Physical assessment of the musculoskeletal system

Learning objectives

- Undertake a physical assessment of the musculoskeletal system.
- Differentiate between normal and abnormal findings.

The musculoskeletal system (also see Chapter 1)

The musculoskeletal system comprises the following structures.

Skeleton
Composed of 206 bones (Courtnay, 2002) divided into two divisions: the axial (80 bones) and appendicular (126 bones) skeletons. The former makes up the skull, vertebral column and the thorax and the appendicular skeleton makes up the upper and lower extremities and the pectoral (shoulder) and pelvic girdles.

Skeletal muscles
Composed of more than 350 voluntary muscles, which occur mainly in pairs. Skeletal muscles show a great deal of variation in size and shape. Each muscle is made up of millions of indivdual fibres arranged in bundles held together by connective tissue. Each muscle is attached to the skeleton by fibrous cords (tendons).

Joints/articulations
Site where two or more bones meet. The primary function of joints is to provide stability and movement to the skeleton. Joints are classified according to structure or the degree of movement allowed:

- *Fibrous joints* are joined together by fibroconnective tissue allowing little or no movement, e.g. sutures of the skull.
- *Cartilaginous joints* are united by a pad or disc of fibrocartilage allowing slight movement, e.g. intervertebral joints.

- *Synovial joints* are the most movable and complex joints in the body. Each possesses a joint cavity containing synovial fluid, the function of which is to promote sliding movement where the bone surfaces articulate. The bones are held together by ligaments, e.g. hip, shoulder.

Assessment

Assessment of the musculoskeletal system involves the collection of both subjective and objective data. Prior to a physical examination, using observation and palpation, the nurse needs to identify the patient's concerns and views. This will include questions concerning the following:

- presence and location of pain
- past medical history relating to previous injuries or treatment
- level of exercise and activity
- past and present occupation.

Also the nurse needs to consider *potential risk factors*, such as:

- alcohol intake
- smoking
- osteoporosis and the fact that muscle strength and tone are usually greatest on the patient's dominant side.

During the physical assessment, the patient (if able) will need to assume standing, sitting and lying positions. The nurse needs to inform the patient that the examination may be quite lengthy and that frequent changes of position will be required. Clear and simple explanation of the various tasks the patient needs to perform should be given and, where appropriate, the nurse should precede these by demonstration.

Patient comfort, dignity and privacy must be maintained by only exposing the area of the body requiring assessment at a given time.

Assessment should start with observation of the patient's gait. This can be best achieved when the patient enters the room and walks around prior to taking a seat. Weight should be evenly distributed with the ability to bear this on both heels and toes. The toes should point directly ahead. Posture should be erect and movements should be co-ordinated.

Guidelines for assessing joints and muscles

The assessment should be performed in a systematic manner. This can be best achieved by commencing at the head and moving down to the toes. For each part of the examination, the patient should, if possible, assume the neutral position (Figure 6.11) and the nurse should use

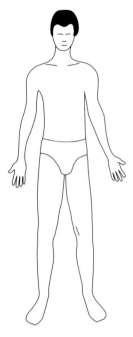

Figure 6.11 The neutral position (reproduced with permission from Cox, 2004)

Box 6.2 Assessment of the joints.

- **Observe** for colour, shape and size. Note any abnormalities. Since most joints are present in pairs, a bilateral comparison should be undertaken.
- **Palpate** for heat, oedema, tenderness, crepitus or nodules.
- **Test range of movement (ROM).** It is important for the nurse to be familiar with the normal ROM of a joint in order to ensure force is not applied. The patient should be asked to copy the nurse's demonstration of each movement. If this is not possible the nurse should support the area with his/her non-dominant hand and slowly move the joint through its ROM with the other. A comparison between sides should be made. It may be sufficient to estimate the ROM but if greater accuracy is required a goniometer should be used (instrument that measures movement in degrees).

---

anterior, posterior and lateral views. During the general inspection the nurse should observe for the presence of extra digits (polydactyly) or webbing between either the fingers or toes.

Assessment of the joints

Conditions that may lead to deformation of joints include osteoarthritis and rheumatoid arthritis. The former is a degenerative condition that affects the articulating surfaces of a joint, whereas rheumatoid arthritis is an inflammatory disorder affecting many joints and although its exact pathology remains unknown, it is considered to have an autoimmune component.

Assessment of the muscles

Muscle strength is tested by asking the patient to move each limb through its ROM against resistance offered by the nurse. Each finding should be compared to a rating scale as described by Weber & Kelley (2003). In their scale, a full range of movement against full resistance is rated 5; a range of movement against some resistance is rated 4 and an active movement against gravity is rated 3. Webber & Kelley (2003) also rate any movement without gravity as 2, slight muscle contraction as 1 and absence of muscular contraction as zero. A bilateral comparison should also be made.

Following a general inspection, the nurse will undertake an examination of various regions relating to specific areas of the musculoskeletal system. An in-depth discussion of this is outside the remit of this book but specific points relating to the spine will be included as the student may experience these in various care areas.

Assessment of the spine

Each area of the vertebral column should be inspected and palpated, starting from the cervical spine and working downward. Each spinous process should be palpated using the thumbs. The nurse is aiming to ensure presence and continuity for each vertebra. This is particularly important for the newborn infant where the condition of spina bifida may be present. Degeneration of the vertebrae may also be seen in the elderly or nutritionally compromised patient where bone resorption has occurred. The patient should then be observed as they move their head through a ROM:

- *Bending*: shrug each shoulder separately upward towards the ear.
- *Extension*: raise head from chest back to neutral position.
- *Flexion*: chin to chest.
- *Hyperextension*: bend head backwards.
- *Rotation*: turn head form side to side.

Following palpation of the spinous processes of the thoracic and lumbar vertebrae, the nurse should observe for any abnormal curvatures of the spine. The healthy spine has three curves, two being concave (cervical and lumbar) and one convex (thoracic). To achieve this observation the patient should be asked to stand with their feet approximately 15cm apart and to then bend forward as if trying to touch their toes. In order to prevent injury the patient should be told not to go beyond their maximum ROM and to stop if they experience discomfort or pain. Abnormal curvatures (Figure 6.12) may include the following:

- *Gibbus*: convex curvature of the spine, that has a sharply defined edge (Cox, 2004). May result following collapse of a vertebra, fracture or tuberculosis (TB).
- *Kyphosis*: convex curvature of the thoracic spine when viewed from the side, commonly termed 'dowager's hump'. The condition may result from rickets or TB. It also is seen in individuals with osteoporosis.
- *Lordosis*: exaggeration of the normal curvature of the lumbar spine.
- *Scoliosis*: lateral curvature of the spine, commonly seen in childhood where it may result from several conditions including

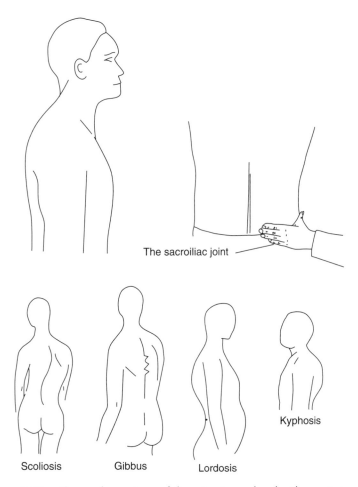

The sacroiliac joint

Kyphosis

Scoliosis   Gibbus   Lordosis

Figure 6.12 Abnormal curvatures of the spine (reproduced with permission from Cox, 2004)

congenital malformations of the spine and unequal limb length (Cox, 2004).

Section 10: Physical assessment of the female and male reproductive systems

In this section, information related to the physical assessment of the breast and the reproductive systems will be provided. This requires good knowledge of the anatomy and physiology of the breast, and of the female and male reproductive systems. Refer to the information given on this in Chapter 1 and in other anatomy and physiology books.

Learning objectives

- Determine deviations from normal during physical assessment of the breast.
- Distinguish between normal and abnormal findings during physical examination of the female external and internal genitalia.
- Differentiate between normal and abnormal findings during physical examination of the male reproductive system.

Examination of the breast

According to national statistics (ONS, 2003), the mortality rate for breast cancer is about 30 per 100 000 women in England and Wales. It is estimated that 1 in 9 women will develop breast cancer at some point in their lives. Physical examination of the breast is important for early detection and treatment of breast cancer, particularly in women. Breast screening is also offered to women aged between 50 and 64 and to those 65 years of age and over on request (ONS, 2003).

Risk factors associated with breast cancer include the following:

- age, e.g. cancer is more common in the menopausal years
- personal or family history of breast cancer
- early onset of menarche and late onset of menopause
- nulliparous (never borne a child)
- having first child after the age of 30 years
- use of oral contraceptives (ONS, 2003)
- use of Hormone replacement therapy (Chambers *et al.*, 2004; Million Women Study Collaborators, 2003).

History relevant to the physical examination must therefore take into account the following:

- age
- age of patient at onset of menarche
- first day (date) of last menstrual period
- age when menopause occurred if relevant
- family history
- child-bearing history
- personal history, e.g. any nipple discharge, if so onset, colour, frequency, consistency, amount, any associated pain and odour
- any lumps felt or noticed.

Physical examination of the breast

The pre-pregnant/non-nursing state

The main techniques necessary for physical assessment of the breast are inspection and palpation. Such examination may be carried out by a nurse, midwife and/or the client. Table 6.25 outlines the possible findings during inspection of the breast and nipple.

Following inspection, the breast should be palpated with the patient sitting or standing upright. Further palpation should be carried out with the flat of the hand in a circular motion. Ensure that each quadrant is examined (Figure 6.13: Cox, 2004), as shown by the arrows in Figure 6.14 but with the woman lying down on a small pillow, with the arm that is being examined placed over the head.

Table 6.25 Inspection of the breast and nipple.

Structure	Normal features	Deviations from normal
• *Breast and nipple* for size, symmetry, shape and contour of breast	• Variable but relatively equal in size • Roundish and firm or roundish and pendulous	• Increase in size of one breast or part of the breast; oedema • Surface appears irregular: lumpy, dimpled or retracted
• *Nipple*: colour	• Roundish/everted (some have inverted nipples) • Pinkish/dark brown in white race. Dark brown or black in people with dark skin	• Dimpled or retracted
• *Discharge*, if any, for amount, consistency, smell and frequency	• None	• Spontaneous discharge, thick or thin in consistency

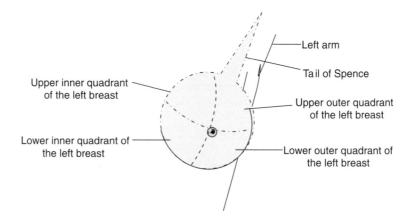

Figure 6.13 Quadrants of the breast

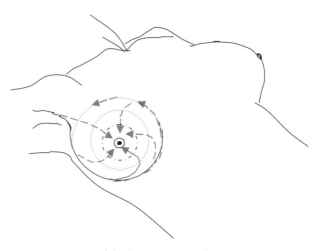

Figure 6.14 Examination of the breast. Arrows show direction and areas for palpation (adapted with permission from Cox, 2004)

Self-examination of the breast (Figure 6.14) and report of deviation from the norm should be taught and encouraged to help early detection and treatment. Self-examination of the breast may be carried out with the person standing upright and in front of a mirror, with the arm on the side of the breast being examined placed over the head (Carcio, 1999; Cox, 2004).

Mammography and ultrasound breast scan may also be carried out to confirm any deviation from the norm. These may be followed

Table 6.26 Palpation of the breast and nipple.

Structure	Normal findings	Deviations from normal
• Type • Lumps	• Erectile nipple tissues • None	• Inverted, flat, bifid • Lumpy, nodular. The upper outer quadrant (Figure 6.13) is a common place for malignant tumours
• Texture and mobility • Pain/tenderness	• Smooth, elastic • Not painful, slightly full and tender about a week before menstruation	• Irregular • Painful (but be aware that not all malignant lesions are painful)
• Temperature • Discharge	• Warm • Nil	• Might be hot if inflamed • Discharge on palpation

---

Box 6.3 Changes that occur in (physiology of) the breast during pregnancy.

- 3 weeks: slightly enlarged, tender and tingling.
- 6 weeks: soft tissues of breast become nodular. Enlargement of breast due to growth of breast tissue and oedema becomes obvious. Feels full. Subcutaneous blood vessels become visible as blood supply to breast increases.
- 12 weeks: pigmentation of areola around breast nipple deepens. Sebaceous glands enlarge and become known as Montgomery tubercles. There is an increase in sebum from these glands, which lubricates the nipple.
- 16 weeks: colostrum (clear fluid) is secreted and can be expressed from the nipple. Mottled area surrounding the areola darkens and is known as secondary areola.

---

by biopsy and pathological examination and analysis of the breast tissue.

Breast examination during pregnancy and following childbirth

During pregnancy and following childbirth, the breasts undergo certain physiological changes in response to high oestrogen and progesterone levels, which are regarded as normal. Physical examination to ascertain normality and to detect any deviations from the norm during such periods is therefore important. On inspection and palpation the normal physiological changes outlined in Boxes 6.3 and 6.4 should be detected.

Box 6.4 Noticeable changes in the breast after delivery of the baby, placenta and membranes.

- Milk: breast milk is produced under the influence of hormones. This can be expressed.
- Maintenance of milk: stimulation and emptying of breast through breast feeding encourages more milk production, hence its maintenance.
- Tenderness: there is some tenderness, especially by the third day after delivery as the breast fills with newly produced milk.
- Size: enlarged and feels very full due to milk production.

Examination of the female genitalia

A good knowledge of the basic anatomy of the genitalia is important for you to be able to make an accurate assessment of it. Please label Figures 6.15 and 6.16. The answers are at the end of the chapter.

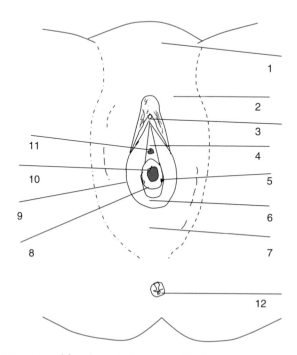

Figure 6.15   External female genitalia (please label)

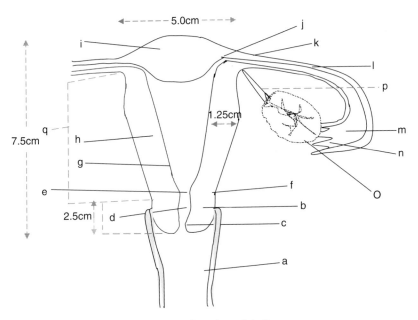

Figure 6.16 Internal female genitalia (please label)

Activity	
Structure	**Please give an outline of the functions**
• Vagina	
• Cervix	
• Uterus	
• Ovaries	

History relevant to the physical examination must also take into account the risk factors for development of any deviations from the norm. These include the following:

- age
- age of patient at onset of menarche
- age when menopause occurred where relevant
- family history
- child-bearing, medical and surgical history
- first day (date) of last menstrual period
- if pregnant, how many weeks? Any changes in the body noted? Foetal movements felt? Any foetal parts palpable? Foetal heart audible on auscultation?

Other information that will be useful during assessment includes the following:

- *Menstruation history*: regularity, frequency and nature of menstrual periods, e.g. associated with or without pain.
- *Head-to-toe examination*: to include examination of body systems.
- *Personal history*: general hygiene, any discharge per vaginam, if so onset, colour, frequency, consistency, amount, any associated pain and odour.
- *Any observable or palpable lesions/lumps.*
- *If patient is taking any medication*: contraceptive pills, any hormone replacement therapy, etc.

Assessment of the female external genitalia

Prior to assessment of the genitalia, the patient should be asked to empty her bladder.

The assessment should be carried out with the patient's informed consent and with sensitivity. The patient should be asked to lie in the supine recumbent position (on her back with the knees bent and thighs externally rotated). *Inspection* and *palpation* (sterile gloves should be worn as necessary) of the external genitalia should elicit the information in Table 6.27 and in Figure 6.17 below.

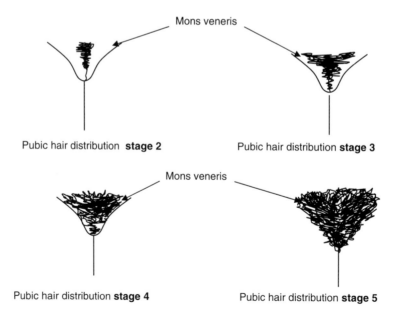

Figure 6.17 Tanner staging. Pubic hair distribution stages 2–5 which assists in rating sexual maturity (Tanner, 1966)

Table 6.27 Possible findings on assessment of the external genitalia.

External genitalia	Normal findings	Deviation from normal
• General hygiene	• Clean	• Dirty, scaly plaques due to psoriasis. Pus from infected spots
• Pubic hair growth	• Growth of pubic hair starts from about age 8–14 years. Coarse hair over mons veneris in an inverse triangle (Tanner staging (Tanner, 1966): Figure 6.17). The growth of hair occurs in stages which demonstrate sexual maturity and normal pituitary ovarian axis function. The stages are described below	• Sparse distribution, hirsutism, dirty-looking hair shafts, inflammation at root of hair, psoriasis
Tanner stage 1	• Fine body hair similar to that on abdomen but no pubic hair	• As above. Also lack of hair growth may indicate malfunction of the pituitary ovarian axis
Tanner stage 2	• Slightly pigmented, straight or slightly curled long downy hair grows sparsely along the labia. Hair is tightly curled, black and shorter in black people	• As above
Tanner stage 3	• Hair is curlier, darker and coarser. It grows thinly over the mons veneris	• As above
Tanner stage 4	• Coarse curly hair covering most of the mons veneris	• As above
Tanner stage 5	• Hair growth spread over medial surfaces of the thigh	• As above
• Vulva	• Labia should be equal in size. Clitoris should be present. Glistening mucosal surfaces	• Mutilation of genitals: bruises might be indicative of sexual assault; mutilation/ circumcision of clitoris
Lesions	• Nil	• Boils, spots, inflamed areas, warts, cysts, ulceration, chancre, swelling, genital herpes, varicosity
Colour	• Pink	• Discolouration, blue, shiny lesions
Skin texture	• Soft, smooth, loose skin	

Continued

Table 6.27 *Continued*

External genitalia	Normal findings	Deviation from normal
• Vaginal orifice *Colour*	• Pink in colour	• Bluish (but normal in pregnancy)
Discharge	• Clear/whitish discharge in small amount during pregnancy or blood-stained menstrual flow in non-pregnancy state monthly	• Thick, white, cheese-like, irritating discharge may be due to thrush; purulent; offensive; very rarely, greenish discharge may denote gonorrhoea while yellowish discharge indicates syphilis; yellow-green irritating discharge nay denote trichomonas. Thick, white/creamy discharge may denote lactobacillosis (Carcio, 1999)
Observe for		• Any vaginal tissue or cervix bulging through the orifice, indicating uterine prolapse
• Urethral orifice *Colour*	• Pink in colour	• Bruised/bluish
Discharge	• Nil	• Urine incontinence: irritating whitish discharge may be due to thrush. Any purulent discharge. Blood-stained or offensive urine
Observe for		• Caruncle (small red protrusion via the orifice) more common in older women due to oestrogen deficiency • Oedematous red ring around the urethral opening
• Bartholin's and Skene's glands	• Not palpable, no discharge and no tenderness	• Any tenderness, swelling or discharge

Assessment of the female internal genitalia

The internal genitalia include the vagina, cervix and the uterus. Any vaginal examination should be carried out carefully and with great sensitivity. A vaginal examination involves the use of two fingers for palpation and/or a vaginal speculum, with the patient in the supine recumbent or lithotomy position. The patient may also be asked to bear down during inspection of the vaginal walls for bulging of the anterior and/or posterior vaginal walls, for cystocele and rectocele respectively. Information that may be gathered during a vaginal examination is outlined in Table 6.28.

Other investigations that may be carried out include the following.

Swab for culture

When any abnormal discharge is noted or reported, a swab should be taken for culture and sensitivity. The discharge should be observed for amount, colour and odour.

Vaginal microscopy

When a patient presents with any vaginal symptoms, a vaginal smear test is taken; the smear is taken from the vaginal sidewall, pool or both but never from the cervix.

Papanicolaou smear (cervical smear)

A cervical smear test is carried out to screen for uterine cancer once every 1–3 years in women aged 18–40 years and yearly for women over 40 years (Kozier *et al.*, 2003). It helps to prevent 70% of potential uterine cancers (Carcio, 1999). Early detection and treatment of cervical cancer are also possible. Either the central long bristles of the *cytobrush* or the tip of the long end of the *spatula* may be used for taking the smear from the external cervical os (Figure 6.18). The cytobrush should not be used on pregnant women (Carcio, 1999). The spatula or the brush is then rotated 3–5 times to the left and right, before being withdrawn. The sample is then transferred on to a slide.

If a patient is found to be at high risk of developing uterine cancer, an endometrial tissue sample may be taken for closer examination under the microscope.

Table 6.28 Assessment of internal genitalia.

Structure/ Assessment	Normal findings	Pregnancy	Deviations from normal
• Vagina (inspect colour)	Pink	Lilac discolouration (Jacquemier's sign)	Discolouration not associated with pregnancy
• Vaginal wall (inspect and palpate)	Smooth, in folds warm, moist	Softening of tissues; warm; moist; increased vascularity; pulsation of uterine arteries felt through lateral fornices, called Osiander's sign	Thin, atrophic, varicosity; oedema; dryness; foreign bodies, e.g. forgotten tampons; lesions; masses; tenderness; warts; polyps. Prolapsed cervix or uterus may be felt or seen in between vaginal wall
(Patient to cough/strain)			Bulging of anterior and/or posterior wall indicative of cystocele or rectocele respectively
Discharge (inspect)	Menstrual flow or small, clear, thin, odourless mucous	No menstrual flow, increased amount of clear, thin discharge	White, thick and curdy discharge (monilial/yeast infections). Grey, offensive (bacterial infections); watery, profuse, frothy, greenish and offensive (trichomonal infections – Kozier et al., 2003)
• Uterine cervix Colour (inspect)	Intact Pink	Softens and elongates. Lilac in colour due to increase in blood supply	Discolouration due to erosion and or ectropion
Lesions (palpate) (smear test)*	No lesions or tenderness		Polyps; cysts; wart-like excoriation indicative of advanced cervical/uterine cancer*
Secretion (inspect)	Mucus in canal thins out during ovulation.	Operculum in canal. Show during labour	Discharge post coital or inter-menstrual bleeding
• Uterus (abdominal and vaginal exam)	In pelvis; size of a fist anteverted and anteflexed; Wt = 60g No lesion Menstruation	Palpable abdominally from 12 wks (fig 6.19) No menstruation; Wt = 1000 g by term; foetal heart audible from 14 wks with sonicaid; foetal parts felt and palpable from about 16–18 wks	Retroverted; retroflexed; double uterus; bicornuate; subseptate; polyps, cysts, cancer; fibroids; endometriosis; ectopic pregnancy; incarceration of gravid uterus; amenorrhoea during childbearing years. Pain, tenderness, bleeding during pregnancy; uterus too large for periods of gestation and no foetal parts felt; sub/infertility

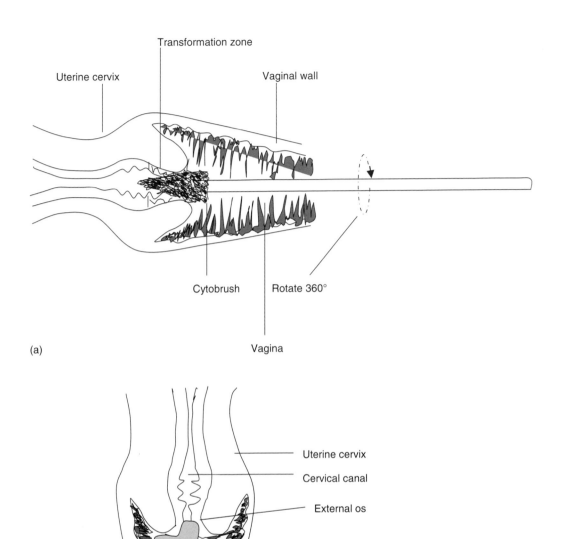

(a)

(b)

Figure 6.18 Cervical smear. (a) Cytobrush in cervical canal. (b) Cervical smear with spatula

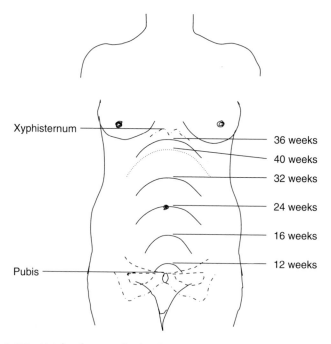

Figure 6.19 Height of uterine fundus during pregnancy

Activity

Changes that occur in the reproductive system during pregnancy have been highlighted. It is also important to have knowledge of the changes that occur in the other body systems.

- List some of the main changes that occur in the following systems during pregnancy: endocrine, cardiovascular, renal, nervous, respiratory, integumentary (skin and nails), musculoskeletal.
- Now refer to a current midwifery textbook and/or the following website: www.nice.org.uk to find out about the examination/screening tests available for pregnant women. (Also see NICE, 2003.)

Infertility: postcoital test

The postcoital test is usually performed to evaluate fertility. Infertility has been defined as a failure to conceive, in the absence of any reproductive pathology, after two years of unprotected sexual intercourse (NICE, 2004). McCance & Heuther (2002) have identified that up to 50% of infertility cases have a male contribution. The examination of both the woman and her partner is therefore important. The timing of this test is also important.

Important information to be gathered during interview includes the following:

- genetic history
- health history – complete physical examination of all body systems
- psychosocial examination
- family history/congenital anomalies
- medical and surgical history
- menstrual history
- sexual history.

Preparation
- Recommend use of ovulation predictor or luteinising hormone surge kits to determine day of ovulation, as these tend to be more accurate than the basal body temperature chart (Carcio, 1999). Education of the woman regarding these is important to ensure accuracy.
- No lubricant should be used during intercourse.
- The postcoital test needs to be carried out at least three hours but no longer than 12 hours after intercourse so the woman and her partner should be made aware of this but sensitively.
- The woman should be advised not to have a bath after intercourse. A shower is fine.

Other information necessary on the day of the test includes the following:

- first day of last menstruation
- hours since sexual intercourse took place (ensure that no lubricant is used)
- days of abstinence before intercourse
- method by which ovulation is determined (the use of ovulation predictor kits should be encouraged)
- records of ovulation.

Procedure for the postcoital test
An endometrial biopsy pipelle is inserted 2–3 mm into the cervix via a vaginal speculum to withdraw a drop of cervical mucus 3–12 hours after sexual intercourse. The sample is placed on a slide and immediately covered with a cover slip, and examined under a microscope to evaluate the number of sperm.

The residual mucus on the pipelle tip should then be spread evenly across a second slide. This is left to dry while the first slide is being examined. The second slide sample is also viewed under the microscope. Ferning is evaluated and graded on the second sample.

Other tests that may be carried to evaluate fertility include:

- physical examination of the thyroid (female)
- abdominal/pelvic examination – may include endometrial biopsy
- blood tests for HIV and rubella, for both partners; hormonal assays.

Assessment of the male reproductive system

The male reproductive system is composed of two divisions: internal and external genitalia. The former includes the testes and various ducts and glands. The scrotum and penis make up the external genitalia. It is also important for the nurse to be familiar with the inguinal region and the reproductive structures (spermatic cord) that run through the inguinal canal, due to the frequent occurrence of hernias within this area. Knowledge of the functions of the different structures is also important (Table 6.29).

Conditions affecting the male genitalia range from life-threatening to painful disorders. It is important therefore that abnormalities are detected early. During the assessment the nurse should take the opportunity to check the patient's knowledge and performance of testicular self-assessment and to teach if a deficit is identified (Figure 6.20).

Prior to performing a physical assessment, the nurse needs to obtain a nursing history relating to the following areas (Weber & Kelley, 2003):

Table 6.29 Functions of the male reproductive system.

Structure	Function
• Testes (2)	• Formation of spermatozoa and hormone testosterone
• Ducts: Epididymis (2) Vas deferens (2) Ejaculatory ducts (2) Urethra (1)	• Site of sperm maturation and motility • Transportation of sperm • Urethra is also responsible for passage of urine
• Accessory glands: Seminal vesicles (2) Bulbourethral glands (2) Prostate (1)	• Secrete various fluids into ducts forming semen (sperm plus fluid)
• Scrotum	• Contains testes and accessory structures. External location of the scrotum provides temperature necessary for sperm survival (3°C below core body temperature)
• Penis	• Male organ of copulation; passage for ejaculated semen into vagina. Also passage for elimination of urine

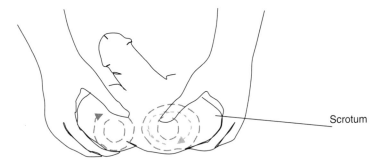

Figure 6.20 Self-examination of the testes. Each testis should be gently grasped between the thumb and fingers and rolled to ensure all surfaces are palpated, as shown by the arrows

- biographical data, i.e. name, date of birth, age, weight, height, occupation
- current symptoms
- past individual and family history, e.g. mumps, undescended testicles, tumours, sexually transmitted infections, e.g. syphilis, herpes, chlamydia, gonorrhoea
- lifestyle and sexual practices, e.g. caffeine, smoking, alcohol intake daily/weekly, any medication
- sexual history – include difficulty achieving or maintaining erection
- surgical history, e.g. hernia repair, vasectomy, pelvic surgery.

Physical assessment

Assessment of the male reproductive system involves the skills of observation and palpation. Due to the sensitive nature of the assessment, it is important that the nurse creates a relaxed and private environment where the patient feels able to express his concerns and ask questions. To promote comfort further, the patient should be asked to empty his bladder prior to the assessment. He also needs to be aware that the assessment is mainly performed standing (if able). Table 6.30 shows possible findings on physical assessment of the male reproductive system.

Semen analysis

Semen analysis may be carried to investigate infertility. Analysis involves identifying the quality of the seminal fluid along with an ability of sperm to survive in and move through cervical mucus and to penetrate and fertilise an ovum. This involves determination of the number, motility and structure of the spermatozoa (Box 6.5).

Table 6.30 Assessment of the male reproductive system.

Structure/Assessment	Normal findings	Deviation from normal
• Penis (*observation*)	• No infestation, lesion or tenderness	• *Infestation*: presence of lice or nits at base of penis or in pubic hair due to pediculosis pubis – 'crabs' • *Redness and lesions/lumps*: may indicate the presence of a sexually transmitted infection (STI) or cancer, e.g. syphilitic chancre, genital herpes/warts. The former is a single painless lesion that regresses spontaneously
• Glans of penis (*observation*) Shape and size	• The glans varies in shape and size from round to pointed	
• Urinary meatus Note its location	• Urinary meatus is usually located in the middle of the glans	• May be on the ventral (underneath – known as *hypospadias*) or dorsal (on top – known as *epispadias*) surface of the penis. Both are congenital defects requiring surgical correction
Note presence of any discharge, inflammation, etc. Gently squeeze the urethral opening to identify the presence of any discharge	• No discharge • Smegma (presence of whitish material that accumulates under the foreskin)	• *Discharge*: indicative of a STI, e.g. gonorrhoea (yellowish green in colour) • Accumulation may be associated with phimosis or poor hygiene
Presence/absence of the foreskin (prepuce). Gently retract the foreskin or ask the patient to do so	• If present, the foreskin should retract and return easily. (Absence may be due to circumcision)	• *Balanitis*: inflammation of the glans – associated with poor hygiene and phimosis • *Phimosis*: tight foreskin which cannot be retracted back over the glans
• Penile shaft (*palpation*)	• In non-erect state, the pens is soft and non-tender	• *Paraphimosis*: following retraction, the foreskin cannot be returned to cover the glans (both conditions may lead to penile pathology • *Hardness*: may indicate cancer. Tenderness may be due to infection • *Peyronie's disease* (McCance & Huether, 2002): there is dense fibrous plaque on dorsal surface of shaft. Lateral curvature on erection

Continued

Table 6.30 *Continued*

Structure/Assessment	Normal findings	Deviation from normal
• Scrotum (*observation*)	• Scrotal skin is thrown into a series of folds (rugae)	• Pain, tenderness, feeling of heaviness
Size and shape of scrotum and the skin surface for colour and form	• Size and shape vary. Left side of the scrotum is normally lower than the right. Slightly darker in colour than penis. Scant hair	• Increase in size and shape may result from presence of: fluid – hydrocele; blood – haematocele; bowel – hernia; cancer
Ask the patient to hold his penis away from the examination field. Ensure all surfaces of the scrotum are inspected and that rugae are smoothed out	• Sebaceous cysts (benign, yellow lesions) may be present	• Redness, swelling and pain may indicate infection or torsion • *Orchitis*: inflammation of testes • *Epididymitis*: inflammation of the epididymis • *Torsion* of the spermatic cord requires urgent surgical intervention to prevent loss of a testis
Transillumination: in presence of an abnormal swelling or growth, transillumination should be performed. Darken room and shine a light through the scrotal wall from the back	• Normal structures do not transilluminate	• Swellings such as hydrocele or spermatocele, which contain serous fluid, produce a red glow • Masses that are solid do not, e.g. cancer, hernia
• Scrotum (testes) (*palpation*) Located within the scrotal sac are the testes. The sac should initially be examined to confirm the presence of both testes	• Testes descend through the inguinal canal into scrotum during seventh month of gestation	• *Cryptorchidism*: (undescended testis) • *Absence of testis* from scrotal sac arises in about 3% of full-term babies and about 30% of premature infants (Henry & Thompson, 2001)
Each testis with its accompanying epididymis should then be palpated for size, shape, texture, lumps and tenderness. Each testis should be gently grasped between the thumb and fingers and	• Testes are oval organs measuring 3.7–5 cm in length and about 2.5 cm in width and depth • The epididymis is slightly softer and non-tender, less than 3.5 cm in length	• *Atrophy*: may result after orchitis or from cirrhosis, oestrogen therapy or a prolonged illness

Continued

Table 6.30 *Continued*

Structure/Assessment	Normal findings	Deviation from normal
rolled to ensure all surfaces are palpated (Figure 6.20). Too much pressure during this procedure will cause pain	• Smooth, soft, firm and rubbery in texture. Tender to pressure	• *Enlarged or nodular testis* may indicate cancer, particularly if painless • *Spermatocele*: small, mobile but non-tender cystic lesion • *Pain or swelling*: may indicate infection, torsion, varicocele (dilation of veins in spermatic cord) or strangulated hernia. In the latter situation urgent surgical referral is required to preserve bowel function

Box 6.5 Semen analysis – normal values.

- Volume
- pH
- Sperm concentration (number)
- Total sperm number
- Motility

- Morphology
- Viscosity

- WBC
- Antisperm antibodies

- 3 ml (range 2–6 ml)
- 7.2 or more
- 20 million spermatozoa per ml
- 100–600 million per ejaculate
- 50% or more motile, or 25% or more with progressive motility, within 60 minutes of ejaculation
- 15–30% normal structure and shape
- Liquefaction of ejaculate within 60 minutes
- Less than 1 million per ml
- No sperm agglutinins present

A second investigation involves the detection of antisperm antibodies in seminal fluid; 3–7% of infertile males have antisperm antibodies. NICE (2004) does not recommend screening since there is no evidence of an effective treatment to improve fertility in such cases.

In the event of the first analysis being abnormal, a second confirmatory test should be offered. Analysis should be done three months after the initial analysis to allow for the cycle of spermatozoa formation to be completed but where the spermatozoa deficiency is severe, the analysis should be repeated as soon as possible (NICE, 2004).

Record keeping

The subjective and objective data collected help health professionals to make a diagnosis. It is important to ensure that written records of any information gathered during health assessment are kept. Such records must be signed and dated by the one who carries out the assessment and must be in accordance with the Nursing and Midwifery Council (2004b) requirements for record keeping.

Summary

In this chapter, we have identified and outlined some of the main symptoms (the relevant health history) that need to be considered prior to physical examination of each of the body systems. Some of the main possible deviations from the norm, during physical assessment of the patient, have also been explored. The need to keep appropriate records has also been highlighted.

Activity

- Describe the observations you will make in the general survey of a client and the assessment of vital signs.
- Explain how the health history and general survey would help you to prioritise and organise the physical assessment.
- Describe the four techniques of physical examination.
- Describe how you will use the four techniques of physical examination to assess each system of the body.
- Discuss the advantages of using a systematic approach in the physical assessment of the client.

Answers

Figure 6.15

1. Mons veneris
2. Labia majora
3. Clitoris
4. Vestibule
5. Duct of Bartholin's gland
6. Fourchette
7. Perineum
8. Hymen
9. Labia minora
10. Vaginal orifice
11. Urethral meatus
12. Anus

Figure 6.16

a. vagina	b. cervix	c. external os	d. cervical canal
e. internal os	f. isthmus	g. endometrium	h. myometrium
i. fundus	j. cornua	k. interstitial portion	l. fallopian tube
m. ampula	n. fimbria	o. ovary	p. ovarian
q. body of			ligament
uterus			

References

Ahern, J & Philpot, P (2002) Assessing acutely ill patients on general wards. *Nursing Standard* 16 (47): 57–64.

Alcock, K, Clancy, M & Crouch, R (2002) Physiological observations of patients admitted from A&E. *Nursing Standard* 16 (34): 33–7.

Aucken, S & Crawford, B (1998) Neurologiocal assessment. In: Guerrero D (ed.) *Neuro-Oncology for Nurses*. Whurr, London.

Bennett, C (2003) Nursing the breathless patient. *Nursing Standard* 17 (17): 45–53.

Bernando, L (1999) Temperature measurement in pediatric trauma patients: a comparison of thermometry and measurement routes. *Journal of Emergency Nursing* 25 (4): 327–9.

Bickley, L S & Szilagyi, P G (2003) *Bates' Guide to Physical Examination and History Taking*, 8th edition. Lippincott, Philadelphia.

Bray, J, Cragg, P, Macknight, A & Mills, R (1999) *Human Physiology*, 4th edition. Blackwell Science, Oxford.

Brewster (2001).

Brooker, C & Nicol, M (eds) (2003) *Nursing Adults: the practice of caring*. Mosby, Edinburgh.

Cappuccio, F P, Kerry, S M, Forbes, L & Donald, A (2004) Blood pressure control by home monitoring: meta-analysis of randomised trials. www.bmj.com.

Carcio, H (1999) *Advanced Health Assessment of Women: clinical skills and procedures*. Lippincott, Philadelphia.

Carroll, M (2000) An evaluation of temperature measurement. *Nursing Standard* 14 (44): 39–43.

Carroll, L (2004) Clinical skills for nurses in medical assessment units. *Nursing Standard* 18 (42): 33–40.

Casey, G (2001) Oxygen transport and the use of pulse oximetry. *Nursing Standard* 15 (47): 46–53.

Chambers, R, Wakley, G & Jenkins, J (2004) *Demonstrating Your Competence 2: women's health*. Radcliffe Medical Press, Oxford.

Chestnutt, M & Prendergast, T (2004) *Current Medical Diagnosis and Treatment*. McGraw-Hill, Columbus, Ohio.

Childs, C, Harrison, R & Hodkinson, C (1999) Tympanic membrane temperature as a measure of core temperature. *Archives of Disease in Childhood* 80: 262–6.

Courtnay, M (2002) Movement and mobility. In: Hogston, R & Simpson, P M (eds) *Foundations of Nursing Practice: making the difference.* Palgrave Macmillan, Basingstoke.

Cox, C (2004) *Physical Assessment for Nurses.* Blackwell Publishing, Oxford.

Department of Health (2000) *The NHS Plan: a plan for investment, a plan for reform.* DoH, London.

Department of Health (2001) *Comprehensive Critical Care: a strategic programme of action.* Stationery Office, London.

Docherty, B (2002) Cardio-respiratory physical assessment for the acutely ill: 1. *British Journal of Nursing* 11 (11): 750–8.

Dougherty, L & Lister, S (2004*) Manual of Clinical Nursing Procedures,* 6th edition. Blackwell Publishing, Oxford.

Estes, M E Z (2002*) Health Assessment and Physical Examination,* 2nd edition. Delmar, USA.

Foxton, J (2004) Coronary heart disease: risk factor management. *Nursing Standard* 19 (13): 47–56.

Gordon, M (2000) *Manual of Nursing Diagnosis,* 9th edition. Mosby, St Louis.

Hamric, A (2000) *Advanced Nursing Practice: an integrative approach.* W B Saunders, Philadelphia.

Henry, M M & Thompson, J N (eds) (2001) *Clinical Surgery.* W B Saunders, Edinburgh.

Hickey, J V (1997) Intracranial pressure: theory and management of intracranial pressure. In: *The Clinical Practice of Neurological and Neurosurgical Nursing,* 4th edition. Lippincott, Philadelphia.

Holland, K, Jenkins, J, Solomon, J & Whittam, S (2003) *Applying the Roper Logan Tierney Model in Practice.* Churchill, Livingstone, Edinburgh.

Jamieson, E M, McCall, J M & Whyte, L A (2002) *Clinical Nursing Practices,* 4th edition. Churchill Livingstone, Edinburgh.

Jennett, B & Teasdale, G (1974) Assessment of coma and impaired consciousness. *Lancet* 2: 81–4.

Jevon, P & Ewens, B (2001) Assessment of breathless patient. *Nursing Standard* 15 (16): 48–53.

Joint National Committee on Prevention, Detection, Evaluation and Treatment of High Blood Pressure and the National High Blood Pressure Education Coordinating Committee (2003) *The Seventh Report of the Joint National Committee on Prevention, Detection, Evaluation and Treatment of High Blood Pressure.* Ovid MEDLINE (R): http://gateway.ut.ovid.com/gw2/ovidweb.cgi.

Kirby, R S, Anderson, M, Gratzke, P, Dahistrand, C & Hoye, K (2001) A combined analysis of double/blind trials of the efficacy and tolerability of doxanzosin-gastrointestinal therapeutic system, doxazosin standard and placebo in patients with benign prostatic hyperplasia. *BJU International* 87 (3): 162–200.

Knies, R (2003) Temperature measurement in acute care. www.enw.org/research-thermometry.htm.

Kozier, B, Erb, G, Blais, K & Wilkinson, J (2003) *Fundamentals of Nursing.* Addison-Wesley Longman, New York.

Law, C (2000) A guide to assessing sputum. *Nursing Times* 96 (24): 7–10.

Mallet, J & Dougherty, L (2000) *Manual of Clinical Nursing Procedures*, 5th edition. Blackwell Science, Oxford.

McAlister, F & Straus, S (2001) Measurement of blood pressure: an evidence-based review. *BMJ* 322: 908–11.

McCance, K L & Huether, S E (2002) *Pathophysiolog: the biologic basis for disease in adults and children*, 4th edition. Mosby, Edinburgh.

Million Women Study Collaborators (2003) Breast cancer and hormone replacement therapy in the Million Women Study. *Lancet* 362: 419–27.

National Institute for Clinical Excellence (2003) *Clinical Guidelines – Antenatal Care. Routine care for the healthy pregnant woman.* NICE, London.

National Institute for Clinical Excellence (2004) *Fertility: assessment and treatment of people with fertility problems. Clinical Guideline 11.* NICE, London.

Norman, J & Cook, A (2000) Medical emergencies. In: Shepherd, M & Wright, M (eds) *Principles and Practice of High Dependency Nursing.* Baillière Tindall, London.

Nursing and Midwifery Council (2004a) *Code of Professional Conduct. Standard for conduct, performance and ethics.* NMC, London.

Nursing and Midwifery Council (2004b) *Guidelines for Records and Record Keeping.* NMC, London.

Office for National Statistics (2003) *Breast Cancer. Incidence rate rises while death rate falls.* National Statistics Online: www.statistics.gov.uk.

O'Neil, D & Legrove, A (2003) Monitoring critically ill patients in accident and emergency. *Nursing Times* 99 (45): 32–5.

Ostrowsky, B, Ober, J, Wenzel, R & Edward, M (2003) The case of the cold thermometers. *American Journal of Infection Control* 31 (1): 57–9.

Potter, P A & Perry, A G (2001) *Fundamentals of Nursing*, 5th edition. Mosby, St Louis.

Pritchard, A P & Mallett, J (2001) *The Royal Marsden Hospital Manual of Clinical Nursing Procedures.* Blackwell, Oxford.

Resuscitation Council (2004) *Basic Life Support. Resuscitation guidelines.* Resuscitation Council, London. www.resus.org.uk.

Rolfe, G & Fulbrook, P (1998) *Advanced Nursing Practice.* Butterworth-Heinmann, Oxford.

Royal College of Nursing (1997) *Nurse Practitioners.* RCN, London.

Sadik, R & Elliot, D (2002) Respiration and circulation. In: Hogston, R & Simpson, P (eds) *Foundations of Nursing Practice: making the difference.* Palgrave Macmillan, Basingstoke.

Singh, M, Pai, M & Kalantri, S P (2003) Accuracy of perception and touch for detecting fever in adults: a hospital-based study from a rural, tertiary hospital in central India. *Tropical Medicine and International Health* 8 (5): 408–14.

Smith, G (2000) *ALERT: acute life-threatening events recognition and treatment.* University of Portsmouth, Portsmouth.

Springhouse Corporation (1997) *Assessment Made Incredibly Easy.* Springhouse, Pennsylvania.

Stevenson, T (2004) Achieving best practice in routine observation of hospital patients. *Nursing Times* 100 (30): 34–5.

Tanner, J M (1966) *Growth at Adolescence*, 2nd edition. Blackwell Scientific Publications, Oxford.

Timby, B K, Scherer, J C & Smith, N E (1999) *Introductory Medical-Surgical Nursing*, 7th edition. Lippincott, Philadelphia.

Trim, J (2005) Performing comprehensive physiological assessment. *Nursing Times* 100 (50): 38–42.

Weber, J & Kelley, J (2003) *Health Assessment in Nursing*, 2nd edition. Lippincott, Williams and Wilkins, Philadelphia.

Woodrow, P (2004). Arterial blood gas analysis. *Nursing Standard* 18 (21): 54–5.

Yusuf, S (2004) Effect of potentially modifiable risk factors associated with myocardial infarction in 52 countries (the INTERHEART study). Case control study. *Lancet* 364 (9438): 937–52.

Assessment of nutritional status

M. Ingham and J. O'Reilly

Learning objectives

- State the reasons for the assessment of clients' nutritional status.
- Describe the components of a normal nutrition.
- Discuss some of the factors that influence food choice.
- Describe the constituent of a balanced diet.
- Discuss the nutritional requirement for different age groups.
- Identify and discuss how a patient's/client's nutritional status might be assessed.

Introduction

Human nutrition is the process of obtaining food for energy, growth and repair. A complete definition of human nutrition also needs to embody the social factors influencing food choice. According to Carpenito-Moyet (2004), nutrition is the sum of the processes involved in taking in food then assimilating it for body functioning and the overall maintenance of health.

The foods that are habitually eaten can be described as forming part of a diet. Diets are often described in an infinite number of ways. We hear about diets of developing countries as being high in dietary fibre and low in fat, which is in contrast with the diets of many industrialised nations which are often high in fat, salt and sugar and low in fruit and vegetables. It is noteworthy that there is no such thing as good or bad foods but a diet may be described as healthy or unhealthy. A healthy diet is normally balanced with respect to macronutrient and micronutrient composition.

It is now established that diet is one major environmental influence in the aetiology of degenerative conditions such as cardiovascular disease, cancer and dental caries. The aim of this chapter is therefore to give a better understanding of nutrition to help facilitate an assessment of the nutritional status of patients.

Purpose of nutritional assessment

Nutritional assessment determines the factors that affect or reflect nutritional health and can be used to evaluate the status of individuals or populations (Lee & Nieman, 2003). Assessment of nutritional status provides the information required to determine the degree to which an individual's nutrient requirements are being met and as such, it needs to consider environmental as well as homeostatic changes (Fuller & Schaller-Ayres, 2000). Initial screening forms a key part of the process of nutritional assessment, where specific data can offer an indication of under- or overnutrition which may in turn prompt further investigations and subsequent actions. This first requires us to remind ourselves of the various components of food.

Components of food

Nutrients can be described as substances which the body digests and absorbs from food. There are two main types, namely macronutrients and micronutrients. Macronutrients are those that make up the bulk of the food we eat and include carbohydrate, fat, and protein. These nutrients can all be utilised by the body to provide energy. The micronutrients, collectively includes a wide range of vitamins and minerals.

Macronutrients

Carbohydrate and sugars

Carbohydrates provide energy of around 3.8 kcal per gram. Carbohydrates can be classified as monosaccharides, disaccharides or polysaccharides. Monosaccharides are simple sugars such as fructose found in most fruits. Glucose, a minor sugar in foods (mainly fruits), is also a monosaccharide and is central to human energy metabolism. Hence glucose is sometimes referred to as blood sugar.

Disaccharides

As their name suggests, these are formed from the chemical bonding of two simple sugars. Sucrose (table sugar) is a disaccharide formed from glucose and fructose. Lactose is the disaccharide responsible for the sweetness of milk and is formed from the monosaccharides glucose and galactose. A significant proportion of adults, especially within Eastern populations, are lactose intolerant. Consumption of significant quantities of milk by lactase-deficient adults results in diarrhoea (Smeltzer & Bare, 2000).

Polysaccharides

These are long chain polymers formed from simple sugars. The principal polysaccharide in most plant foods is starch, which is composed of chains of glucose units. Rich sources of starch include potatoes, bread and rice. In the UK carbohydrates are the main source of energy in the diet, typically contributing 45–50% of total energy intake (Barker, 2002). Wholegrain foods also contain indigestible carbohydrates that are often collectively referred to as dietary fibre. There is evidence that increasing the proportion of wholegrain products may lower the risk of premature heart disease and colorectal cancer (British Nutrition Foundation, 2003).

Fat and cholesterol

Fats

Fats impart considerable palatability to foods and facilitate the absorption of fat-soluble vitamins. Fats consist of triacylglycerol (triglyceride) molecules, which are composed of three fatty acid units joined to a single glycerol component (Figure 7.1). The fatty acids are described as either saturated, monounsaturated or polyunsaturated, reflecting the presence or absence of a double bond within the chain. The type of fatty acid determines whether triglycerides are liquid or solid at room temperature – hence the terms fats and oils. Animal fats tend to be rich in saturated fatty acids whereas fats from plant sources are rich in monounsaturated and polyunsaturated fatty acids (Eastwood, 2003).

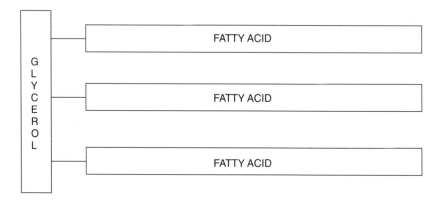

Figure 7.1   Triacylglycerol

There is currently much interest in fish oils as they contain long-chain omega 3 polyunsaturated fatty acids which may have a anti-inflammatory effect in the body. Fish oils are thought to alleviate the inflammation associated with conditions such as arthritis and psoriasis. Consumption of fish oils may also help reduce the risk of heart disease and healthy eating policy in the UK advocates that people regularly consume oily fish such as mackerel (HEA, 1997).

Some types of saturated fatty acids raise the concentration of cholesterol in the blood. Hence displacing saturated fatty acids from the diet with monounsaturated and polyunsaturated fatty acids will lead to a lowering of blood cholesterol. Regardless of fatty acid composition, fats add considerably to the calorie content of food. Fats contain more than 9 kcal per gram, more than double that of carbohydrates.

The rapid rise of obesity in the UK, including abnormal or excessive fat accumulation among children, has led to a focus on diet as a contributing factor. Currently the prevalence of overweight adults in the UK is 63% of men and 54% of women.

Perhaps more worrying are the corresponding statistics in relation to clinical obesity, with 19% of men and 21% of women falling into this category (British Nutrition Foundation, 2003). Many processed foods have a high fat content, contributing significantly to high energy content. Potato crisps and milk chocolate are high in calories mainly because of their high fat content. Adding fats to food increases the energy density of the average UK diet. At present, fat contributes around 40% of energy intake. It is widely thought that lowering fat content of the UK diet and increasing the proportion of carbohydrates would have significant health benefits.

Cholesterol
This fat-like substance is found in most animal foods but not foods of plant origin. Rich sources of cholesterol are liver and eggs. Cholesterol has a number of key roles in the human body. It is a component of biological membranes and required for the synthesis of steroid hormones, including vitamin D. It is not an essential nutrient as the body can synthesise cholesterol, mainly in the liver. Cholesterol is transported in the blood within lipoproteins. These are spherical structures composed of protein and lipid including triacylglycerol and cholesterol. Low-density lipoprotein (LDL) causes heart disease (Smeltzer & Bare, 2000). In the past, it was considered that dietary cholesterol affected blood cholesterol levels by increasing the concentration of LDL. For most people, lowering cholesterol intake has no marked effect on blood cholesterol levels as the liver synthesises cholesterol to make up for the deficit. However, most dietary sources of cholesterol are also rich in saturated fatty acids. Intake of saturated fatty acids has the more significant effect on LDL concentration compared with cholesterol.

Protein

Average protein requirements for men and women in the UK are estimated to be 56 g and 45 g per day respectively (Bender, 2002). Typical UK diets contain protein well in excess of minimal requirements and even in excess of the incremental increase associated with pregnancy and lactation. An average lean beefsteak or chicken breast contains around 30 g of protein. Excess nitrogen in the diet, mainly as a result of protein intake, is excreted in the urine as urea.

Individual protein molecules consist of one or more chains of amino acids (polypeptides). There are 20 different kinds of amino acids. The specific sequence or order of individual amino acids in a protein molecule determines the function of a particular protein. Proteins have a diverse array of functions (Table 7.1). Many proteins are enzymes, which are protein catalysts (facilitate chemical reactions) that drive and regulate metabolic reactions in the body. Enzymes are also key to breaking down large molecules during digestion. Some hormones are proteins, which bind to specific receptors expressed by target cells. These receptors are also proteins.

The strong acidic environment in the stomach facilitates digestion of dietary protein. Specific enzymes (proteinases) released into the small intestine break up proteins into their constituent amino acids. These are subsequently absorbed into the blood, providing the building blocks for the synthesis of new protein molecules. However, the body utilises excess amino acids as a source of energy.

Amino acids are described as essential and non-essential. Non-essential amino acids can be synthesised in the body whereas the essential amino acids need to be provided in the diet from protein. Animal foods such as meat and eggs contain proteins which have the full spectrum of essential amino acids. This is not the case with most plant proteins, which may be lacking in one or more of the essential amino acids (Mann & Trusswell, 2002). However, consuming plant proteins from different sources allows complementation to occur in that one protein source makes up for the deficit in the other protein source and vice versa.

Table 7.1 Examples of proteins in humans.

Examples	Function
• Amylase	Starch to glucose
• Insulin	Hormone
• Collagen	Structural role in tissues
• Haemoglobin	Transports oxygen
• Ferritin	Iron storage

Alcohol

Alcohol (ethanol) is a macronutrient because it can be broken down to yield energy. There is some evidence that consuming alcohol (Guinness) may help prevent heart attacks in middle-aged men. The popular perception regarding the health benefits of alcohol is a concern to many health professionals. This reflects the adverse acute effects of binge drinking among young people and the chronic effects of excess consumption with respect to liver disease. Alcohol may also contribute to obesity in some individuals as a single gram of alcohol contains 7 kcal. Alcoholics also tend to displace food from their diet in exchange for alcoholic beverages that are invariably low in most vitamins and minerals. Alcoholics are thus considered to be at risk of nutrient deficiency.

Water

Water, although a large constituent of the diet, is not a macronutrient because it does not provide energy. However, humans cannot survive for more than a week or so without water. Water is the medium in which biochemical reactions take place. The minimum requirement for water is given as around 1 ml for every calorie of energy expended. Thus average men and women require 2500 and 2000 ml of water per day respectively. Much of this water is supplied from food and beverages consumed but additional water may be required, especially in hot humid conditions and/or during exercise, which leads to loss of water as sweat. Furthermore, alcohol and caffeine have a diuretic effect, promoting the net loss of water in urine. Drinking plenty of water is advised by many health experts to avoid dehydration. Lethargy, thirst and low urinary output are initial symptoms of dehydration. Excess intake of water is a requirement for proper functioning of the kidney since the majority of toxic metabolites such as urea are excreted in urine. Higher intakes of water lead to formation of larger volumes of more "dilute" urine, which may help reduce the risk of kidney disease.

Micronutrients

Vitamins

Vitamins are essential micronutrients. Insufficient intake has adverse effects on health. Vitamins A, D, E and K are fat-soluble vitamins as opposed to vitamin B and the C vitamins, which are water soluble. Most vitamins are sensitive to heat and considerable losses can occur on heating. Vitamin C is perhaps the most heat sensitive of the vitamins and prolonged cooking of food followed by storage in heated containers, as used in many catering establishments, leads to considerable losses of this and other vitamins. However, certain cooking methods, such as stir-frying, minimise losses of heat-labile vitamins. A summary of the vitamins is provided below.

Fat-soluble vitamins
Vitamin A
- Rich sources include eggs, liver, oily fish and margarine.
- Can be synthesised in the body from beta-carotene, the orange pigment present in carrots.
- Required for the synthesis of 11-*cis* retinol (constituent of visual pigments) and maintenance of epithelial tissues.
- Deficiency symptoms: night blindness, xerophthalmia (can lead to permanent blindness). Marginal deficiency impairs the immune system.

Vitamin D
- Rich sources include eggs, liver and oily fish.
- Can be synthesised in the body utilising UV radiation from sunlight.
- Required for the regulation of calcium metabolism.
- Deficiency symptoms: muscle weakness and skeletal abnormalities including rickets and oesteomalacia (adult rickets). Low exposure to sunlight is a risk factor for deficiency.

Vitamin E
- Rich sources include wheatgerm, vegetable oils and wholegrain cereals.
- Functions as an antioxidant – protects lipids from oxidation.
- Deficiency results in neurological degeneration but very rarely occurs.

Vitamin K
- Rich sources include green leafy vegetables but widely distributed in many foods.
- Required for the effective clotting of blood.
- Deficiency results in excessive bleeding but normally confined to premature infants, in whom it can result in fatal brain haemorrhage.

Water-soluble vitamins
Vitamin B1 (thiamin)
- Rich sources are wholegrain cereals, pulses and nuts.
- Required as a co-factor in energy metabolism.
- Deficiency leads to beri-beri and Wernicke-Korsakoff encephalopathy, a neurological disorder occurring among alcoholics.

Vitamin B2 (riboflavin)
- Rich sources are liver and dairy products but widely distributed in many foods.

- Required for the function of several enzymes.
- Deficiency is characterised by reddening of the lips.

Niacin
- Rich sources are liver and dairy products but widely distributed in many foods.
- Can be synthesised by the body from the essential amino acid tryptophan.
- Required in synthesis of nicotinamide adenine dinucleotide, which is required as a co-factor in many biochemical reactions.
- Deficiency leads to pellagra, a condition characterised by diarrhoea, dermatitis and dementia.

Vitamin B6
- Widely distributed in food.
- Required in amino acid metabolism.
- Deficiency is very rare.
- High dose supplements have been used to treat carpal tunnel syndrome and alleviate symptoms associated with premenstrual syndrome. However, there is some evidence that high doses may cause neurological damage.

Folate
- Rich sources are liver, green leafy vegetables and fortified breakfast cereals.
- Interacts with vitamin B12 in the synthesis of DNA and hence plays a fundamental role in cell division.
- Deficiency causes megaloblastic anaemia. Deficiency during early pregnancy increases the risk of giving birth to a child with a neural tube defect.
- UK women are advised to take folate supplements if they are considering pregnancy although a significant number of pregnancies are unplanned.

Vitamin B12
- Almost exclusive to animal foods, meat, milk and eggs being rich sources.
- Interacts with folate in the synthesis of DNA.
- Deficiency causes megaloblastic anaemia followed by neurological degeneration, which can lead to permanent paralysis.
- Following a vegan diet greatly limits intake of this vitamin but the substantial storage of the vitamin in the liver and availability in fortified foods prevent overt deficiency.

Vitamin C (ascorbic acid)
- Rich sources include fruit, fruit juices and green leafy vegetables. In the UK, potatoes make an important contribution to vitamin C

intake, especially among individuals with a limited intake of fruit and vegetables.

- Required for the synthesis of collagen (protein constituent of bone and skin), serves as an antioxidant by scavenging free radicals and promotes absorption of iron from the gut.
- Marginal deficiency can cause fatigue, as opposed to prolonged deficiency, which leads to scurvy, a condition characterised by bleeding gums and skin lesions which fail to heal.

Minerals

Minerals can be categorised as major minerals, such as sodium and potassium, or trace elements, such as copper, zinc, magnesium, iron, iodine and selenium. Dietary intake of trace elements is much lower than that of the major minerals. Some minerals are required in very small amounts, such as chromium. Unlike vitamins, minerals cannot be destroyed by heating or other food-processing techniques. However, they can be physically lost during cooking as they may leach out of food during heating in water.

Sodium, potassium and chloride
- Major electrolytes in the body fluids, regulating the distribution and movement of water.
- Considerable quantities of sodium are added to food in the form of salt (sodium chloride) during food processing. Sodium is particularly high in meat products such as bacon. In the UK around 80% of sodium intake is from processed foods.
- Excess sodium intake may raise blood pressure in some individuals. Salt should be restricted in young infants as they excrete excess sodium in relatively large volumes of urine, leading to dehydration.
- Fruit and fruit juices have a high proportion of potassium compared with their sodium content. It is thought that increasing the ratio of potassium to sodium in the diet may help attenuate the tendency for sodium to raise blood pressure.

Calcium, phosphorus and magnesium
- Minerals found in bone which function to give rigidity to the skeleton but these minerals also have many other important biochemical functions in the body.
- Rich sources of calcium and phosphorus are dairy products including milk and cheese. Magnesium is widely distributed in most food.
- Insufficient bone mineralisation causes skeletal abnormalities, rickets in children and osteomalacia in adults.
- Calcium is deposited into bone for the first 30 years or so of life. A peak bone mass is attained, after which there is decline of bone mineral. It is thought that high intakes of calcium in adolescence

may allow the attainment of higher bone density, which may lower the risk of osteoporosis in later life.

Iron
- Iron is a constituent of haemoglobin, providing the means by which oxygen can be transported to the tissues. There are also a number of enzymes that contain iron.
- Meat, especially red meat, is the best source of iron since iron in plant foods is less well absorbed. Most breakfast cereals in the UK are now fortified with iron.
- Insufficient intake of iron leads to iron deficiency anaemia, which is characterised by a low red blood cell count and low haemoglobin concentration, resulting in fatigue and poor cold tolerance. Many women of menstruating age, although not anaemic, have low liver iron stores. This can be problematic during pregnancy as the liver serves to provide extra iron for the developing foetus.
- Iron absorption from plant sources can be greatly affected by other components of the diet. Dietary fibre-rich foods and milk inhibit absorption whereas vitamin C enhances uptake.

Selenium
- Functions as a key constituent of a number of enzymes.
- There are significantly low levels of selenium in the soil in the UK so wheat flour and cattle fed on wheat hay may not be good accumulators of selenium in the diet.
- Changes in dietary patterns, with lower consumption of red meats and bread products, may reduce selenium intake and, in turn, protection against heart disease.
- Seafood and organic meat are good sources with some nuts, notably Brazil nuts, being the richest source.
- Deficiency leads to heart abnormalities and low selenium may increase the risk of some forms of cancer.

Iodine
- Functions as a constituent of thyroid hormones, which regulate metabolic rate.
- Fish and shellfish are rich sources. Milk provides around one-third of the intake in the UK but the iodine content of cow's milk is variable depending on the use of fortified feed.
- Deficiency of iodine leads to swelling of the thyroid gland in the neck and subsequent lethargy. Goitre is reversible but iodine deficiency during pregnancy can lead to children with cretinism, which is irreversible brain damage.
- Goitre and cretinism, although now absent in the UK, are still prevalent in some less economically developed countries due to

low iodine content of the surrounding soils which subsequently compromises the iodine content of the food supply.

Copper and zinc
- Function as constituents of a broad range of enzymes, influencing all areas of metabolism.
- Copper is present in many foods, although milk is notably a poor source. Meat, fish and dairy products are major sources, whereas fruit and vegetables are relatively poor sources.
- Copper deficiency can lead to anaemia and neurological abnormalities and affects the formation of connective tissue. Likewise, zinc deficiency can have several adverse effects on the body, including retarded growth, impaired sexual development, delayed wound healing and even impaired taste sensitivity. Marginal deficiency may also compromise immune function.

Other components present in the diet

Food and drink are complex mixtures of many components in addition to the nutrients discussed above. Many herbs and spices contain compounds which provide flavour and aroma. Many foods contain naturally occurring toxins but eating a varied diet protects against possible adverse effects. Some toxins occur in food as contaminants or accumulate in the food chain. Additives are frequently added to food during processing as colourants, flavours or preservatives. In the UK there is tight control over the use of additives but consumers often express concern about the salt, fat and sugar content of foods.

Caffeine

Caffeine occurs in some beverages such as tea and coffee and is added in some soft drinks. Small amounts of caffeine also occur naturally in chocolate. An average cup of black tea contains between 30 and 50 mg of caffeine whereas around 60 mg is typical of instant coffee. However, a cup of filter coffee may contain 120 mg of caffeine. Caffeine influences the central nervous system and has a stimulant-like effect in promoting alertness. Caffeine also has other metabolic effects on the body such as promoting the release of the hormone adrenaline. The safety of consuming coffee has been debated for many years but at present there is little evidence to suggest any adverse effects. However, some individuals have an intolerance of caffeine, which may lead to headaches, elevation of blood pressure and cardiac arrhythmia.

Flavonoids

Tea, red wine and fruits and vegetables are significant sources of flavonoids in the diet. Flavonoids have attracted much interest in recent years since some population studies suggest that diets rich in flavonoids protect against heart disease. Red wine which is rich in flavonoids may in part explain the so-called 'French paradox'; the French population have lower than expected rates of heart disease given the high prevalence of cigarette smoking and high intake of saturated fatty acids. Numerous laboratory studies demonstrate that flavonoids are potent antioxidants and have the capacity to inhibit aggregation of platelets, effects which are consistent with preventing heart disease. However, it remains unclear whether these compounds are sufficiently absorbed, at least to levels high enough to exert biological effects within the body.

Carotenoids

Carotenoids are compounds present in plant foods. They impart characteristic colour to fruit and vegetables. Carotenoids have attracted much interest in recent years as an active constituent of fruit and vegetables. It is thought that carotenoid intake may help prevent heart disease and some forms of cancer. However, large well-controlled supplementation trials in humans have yet to provide sufficient support for recommending increased intake.

Nutritional requirements

Since the identification of the vitamins and minerals required by humans, there has been much focus on determining the actual amounts needed in the diet. Early studies tended to consider the amounts of nutrients required to prevent overt deficiency. For example, daily intake of 10 mg of vitamin C was shown in early studies to be sufficient to prevent scurvy. However, later studies showed that 20 mg/day was needed for normal wound healing and an intake of 30 mg/day reduced the risk of gum disease (gingivitis). Recently it has been suggested that higher intakes may be protective against developing cancer and heart disease.

Optimum daily intakes of some nutrients may be considerably higher than the amount needed to prevent deficiency symptoms. Iron deficiency may result from inadequate intake resulting in low storage in the liver but intake may remain sufficient to prevent iron deficiency anaemia. Dietary reference values (DRV) refer to a set of estimates of the nutritional requirements of populations. In the UK, reference nutrient intake (RNI), estimated average requirement (EAR) and safe intake (SI) are used (DoH, 1991). The EAR is an estimate of the amount of a nutrient needed to prevent deficiency and maintain normal biochemical and physiological function. For example, the EAR for vitamin C for healthy men and women is 30 mg/day.

Some nutrient requirements vary significantly depending on age and gender. For example, the iron requirement of premenopausal females is markedly higher compared with men and postmenopausal women in order to compensate for losses of iron during menstruation. There is also variation in the nutrient requirements of individuals of the same sex and age. It follows that some individuals have a requirement for a specific nutrient that is above the EAR. The RNI accommodates this variation and is a higher value compared with the EAR. In the case of vitamin C, the RNI is 40 mg/day and this is considered sufficient to meet the requirement of almost all the adult population. Recommended daily allowance (RDA) values are used for the purposes of UK food labelling and represent a level sufficient to meet the needs of all members of the population, whatever age, sex or stage of the life cycle. The RDA for vitamin C is at present 60 mg/day.

Dietary guidelines

The primary focus of recent dietary guidelines has been on minimising the risk of diet-related diseases, namely obesity, cardiovascular disease, cancer and dental caries. In the interests of reducing the risk of obesity, the UK DRVs for total fat and carbohydrate intake are 35% and 50% of total food energy respectively. It is thought unlikely that individuals would overeat, because fat provides more energy per gram compared with carbohydrate and so it follows that replacing fat with carbohydrate-rich foods increases the bulkiness and hence satiety of the diet. Diets high in saturated fatty acids are associated with heart disease. Saturated fatty acids should constitute no more than 10% of total food energy.

Other DRVs have focused on salt intake, dietary fibre, sugars and alcohol. Dietary guidelines have been devised to translate these numerical data of DRVs into foods, providing a means by which individuals can make informed choices. Food pyramids or a tilted plate are used to pictorially show the relative proportions of different food groups that constitute a balanced diet (Figure 7.2 and Table 7.2).

Eating five portions of fruit and vegetables daily, increasing consumption of wholegrain cereals, replacing fatty meat products with leaner cuts of meat and fish are examples of practical dietary guidelines aimed at complying with current DRVs.

Assessing nutritional status

There is a wealth of literature which plots the problems associated with malnutrition and hospitalisation, a key element of which appears to be lack of awareness of nutritional risk (ACHC, 1997; Lennard-Jones, 1992). McWhirter & Pennington (1994), in a study of 500 adult hospital patients, identified that 40% were undernourished on admission

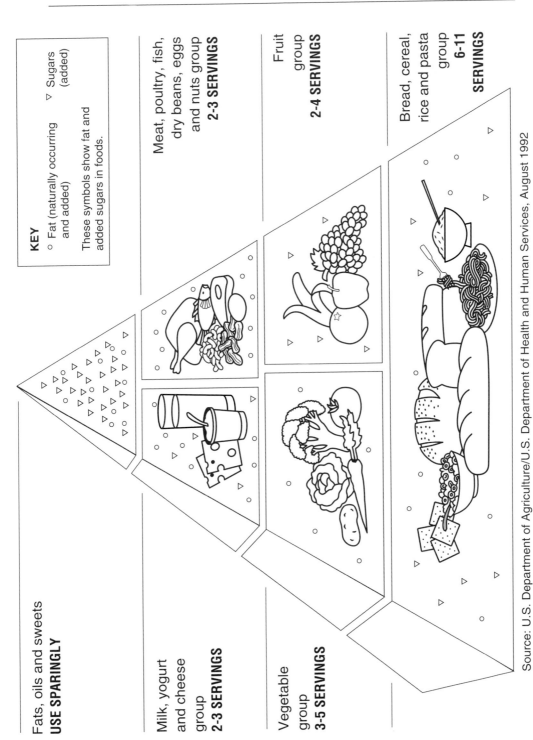

Fats, oils and sweets
USE SPARINGLY

KEY
○ Fat (naturally occurring and added)   ▽ Sugars (added)

These symbols show fat and added sugars in foods.

Milk, yogurt and cheese group
2-3 SERVINGS

Meat, poultry, fish, dry beans, eggs and nuts group
2-3 SERVINGS

Vegetable group
3-5 SERVINGS

Fruit group
2-4 SERVINGS

Bread, cereal, rice and pasta group
6-11 SERVINGS

Source: U.S. Department of Agriculture/U.S. Department of Health and Human Services, August 1992

Figure 7.2   The US Department of Agriculture food guide pyramid (www.usda.gov)

Table 7.2 Serving sizes for the food groups in the Food Guide Pyramid.

Food group	Serving size
Grain	1 slice bread $\frac{1}{2}$ cup cooked cereal, rice, other grain or pasta
Vegetables	1 cup raw leafy vegetables $\frac{1}{2}$ cup other vegetables, cooked or chopped raw
Fruits	1 medium apple, banana or orange $\frac{1}{2}$ cup chopped, cooked or canned fruit $\frac{3}{4}$ cup fruit juice
Dairy	1 cup milk or yoghurt $1\frac{1}{2}$oz natural cheese 2oz processed cheese
Protein	2–3oz cooked lean meat, poultry or fish $\frac{1}{2}$ cup cooked dry beans* 1 egg* 2 tablespoons peanut butter*

*Count as 1 ounce of meat.
Reprinted with permission of the US Department of Agriculture (USDA) and the US Department of Health and Human Services (DHHS) 1996; www.usda.gov.

and that this got worse during the hospital stay for 74% of patients where nutritional support failed to be instigated. This is despite indications in Lennard-Jones' influential King's Fund report *A Positive Approach to Nutrition as Treatment*, which clearly pointed out the cost-effectiveness of appropriate nutritional support. There are serious consequences associated with undernutrition, namely poor wound healing, immune dysfunction, sepsis, hypothermia, increased incidence of fractures, delayed recovery from illness and delayed drug elimination, problems which are particularly obvious in the elderly (Jordan *et al.*, 2003). Problems associated with malnutrition cost the NHS £70 million per annum (Holmes, 2004).

A number of nutritional assessment tools have been developed (Cotton *et al.*, 1996; Guigoz *et al.*, 1996; Scanlan *et al.*, 1994). Some are fairly generic, others target specific client groups, but all are designed to improve awareness of nutritional status and give indications of the need for dietary interventions. However, there has been considerable criticism of the lack of evidence base for these (Lyne & Prowse, 1999), their reliability and validity have come into question and Arrowsmith (1999) suggests the need to retest for specificity and sensitivity. Ferguson *et al.* (1999) emphasises the limitations of many of the previous tools as not being cost-effective, too complicated and time-consuming, advocating a much simpler tool. The result was a subjective global assessment, concentrating on medical history, examination and lifestyle but anthropometric, biochemical and body mass index measurement was excluded.

A thorough nutritional assessment needs to be undertaken to determine a plan of action for improving a person's nutritional status. A number of techniques can be used depending on the particular individual and situation. However, there is currently no single "gold standard" method by which nutritional status can be determined (Ledsham & Gough, 2000). Reilly (1996) supports a dual approach which assesses status, i.e. the degree of over- or undernutrition, and also assesses intake to see if nutrition is adequate for needs. In principle, then, the following methods are used in determining nutritional status and in combination may provide a more reliable assessment:

- sociological evaluation
- clinical evaluation
- anthropometry
- biochemical evaluation.

Use of sociological evaluation in assessing nutritional status

Use of variables that are non-nutrient related can provide valuable insights to nutritional status. These data, sometimes referred to as historical (retrospective) information, can be obtained by formal or informal interviewing or by the use of structured questionnaires using open-ended and closed questions. The approach used needs to take into account the individual involved. It may include details of previous illness, bereavement or other traumatic experience, type of accommodation and financial support (Edwards, 1998). Historical information can be categorised as to whether the data are personal and socio-economic, health related or diet related. Groups at risk of nutrient deficiency can be identified from such information and examples are discussed below.

Historical information can be gained from questionnaires and/or interviews. Interviews can be used to determine a number of factors that influence the individual choice of foods which make up a person's usual diet.

Activity

- Reflect on the kind of food you choose to eat.
- Give reasons why you prefer certain foods over others.
- Can you outline other factors that influence food choices?

You will note that the factors that influence food choice include:

- values and beliefs
- flavour and appearance of food
- religious issues, familiarity and cultural background
- health influences
- availability and cost
- personal preferences
- convenience
- social influences
- emotional influences
- environmental concerns (Leeds, 1998).

By understanding the various factors that influence food choices, we can more easily change them when necessary. What we choose to eat affects our nutritional status.

Validated questionnaires are often used to ensure the accuracy and reliability of data obtained. However, undertaking successful interviews reflects the skill of the interviewer. Subjects may be unco-operative or unwilling to discuss past experiences, medical problems, eating habits or economic circumstances. In order to obtain personal data, assessors need to establish trust and rapport with subjects, thus enabling them to communicate freely and honestly. The following simple techniques are used to help subjects feel at ease:

- selecting a time for the interview that is convenient for the subject
- explaining the purpose of the interview, allowing the subject to understand what is expected
- assuring subjects that all information will be treated with confidentiality
- ensuring that the subject is seated comfortably
- offering refreshment
- allowing sufficient time for the interview.

Age and gender

Age has a significant effect on food choice and nutritional requirements. Young children are dependent on their parents or guardians for food choice, which may not always be appropriate. In the UK there have been reports in recent years of parents providing young children with low-fat diets, which may actually provide insufficient energy to support normal growth. Older children and teenagers increasingly make their own food choices and are especially influenced by peer pressure and food marketing. Much of the advertising and marketing of food focuses on products containing high fat and sugar levels. This continues to generate controversy with respect to ethical standards and the rapid rise in the prevalence of obesity in the UK. In contrast, a significant number of young females abstain from eating meat, which (especially red meat) is an important source of iron in the UK diet. Iron deficiency anaemia is prevalent in the UK, especially among adolescent females who, after the onset of menstruation, have high iron requirements. Furthermore, young females may limit food intake in attempts to conform to the ideal "slim" body image portrayed in advertising. Fad diets and restricting food intake may increase the risk of eating disorders such as anorexia nervosa and bulimia.

The frail elderly represent a group vulnerable to poor nutrient intake, as they are less able to physically obtain and prepare food. In addition, they may also suffer from poor dentition, so limiting food choice and reducing appetite. Elderly residents of nursing and residential homes may be subjected to limited food choice and/or availability. Unlike younger adults in the UK, older people have a requirement for dietary vitamin D to prevent deficiency. This is because the elderly (as a group) have limited exposure to sunlight by which vitamin D can be synthesised.

Religion and ethnicity
Religion and ethnicity are strong determinants of lifestyle and food choice (Leeds, 1998). Recently, bone abnormalities have re-emerged in the UK among Asian women in parts of northern England. This has been attributed to low vitamin D status due to insufficient sunlight exposure and a diet containing significant amounts of unleavened bread products such as chappiti. Unleavened bread is rich in phytate, a compound that binds calcium and prevents absorption of this major bone mineral. Recent immigrants arriving in the UK may be unfamiliar with the available food and thus depend on a very limited range of products. Any factor reducing variety of food in the diet increases the risk of nutritional inadequacy.

Poverty
Limited food choice and restricted facilities for the preparation of food have been identified as affecting the nutritional status of those with insufficient income. Information regarding employment, education, financial status, family circumstances, housing and other environmental factors can provide an insight as to the likely meal pattern and food choices made.

Health information
The health of an individual may significantly influence nutritional status. As discussed above, the frail elderly can be identified as at risk as they often have limited capability to prepare food, which may be further exacerbated by conditions such as arthritis. Illness is often accompanied by loss of appetite. This is of particular concern in hospitals where a significant number of patients are malnourished. Many patients, for example cancer and postoperative patients,

normally require nutritional support in terms of specialised feeds to prevent them becoming malnourished. It is also noteworthy that a side effect of some medications is a loss of appetite.

Diet history

Information on diet history can be obtained from a general health questionnaire, which can ask questions relating to alcohol intake, food avoidance, etc. It should comprise questions which determine likes and dislikes of certain foods, changes in the quantity and texture of foods taken due to illness and the ability to obtain and prepare food (Edwards, 1998). There are a number of more specific methods by which diet history can be obtained. A simple 24-hour recall requests that subjects simply list all the food and drink consumed in the last 24 hours. Subjects can forget some foods but may recall greater detail when questioned as part of a structured interview in which the assessor can help the subject recall past events. The use of food frequency questionnaires allows more information to be obtained about diet over the longer term compared with a 24-hour recall. The questionnaire can gain information about specific food groups such as fruit and vegetables.

Clinical evaluation

Clinical examination or assessments can be used to determine characteristic symptoms of nutrient deficiency or toxicity. Simple observations include whether clothing is ill-fitting, examination of the oral cavity, whether dentures fit properly, evidence of sore mouth or any difficulty chewing and swallowing. As discussed previously, vitamin C deficiency is characterised by specific physical symptoms. Scurvy was historically common in sailors where a chronic low intake of vitamin C was found to be responsible for the condition. In industrialised nations, overt deficiency is now relatively uncommon among free-living subjects. However, iron deficiency anaemia affects a significant proportion of premenopausal females in industrialised nations. The clinical deficiency symptoms associated with other nutrients may also be present within some groups such as the frail elderly, the homeless, alcoholics and hospitalised patients. Clinical symptoms arising from specific nutrient deficits as well as protein energy malnutrition are also widely observed in many less economically developed nations. There are some classic physical signs of poor nutrition which healthcare professionals need to be alert to when making a health assessment of a patient (Box 7.1).

Clinical indicators are absent during suboptimal intake of nutrients which may impair physiological functions or increase the risk of disease, as discussed previously for iron and vitamin C. Clinical symptoms are therefore of limited use as they represent an extreme mani-

Box 7.1 Physical signs of poor nutrition (Smeltzer & Bare, 2000; Weber, 2001; Kozier et al., 2003).

General appearance	• Listless, appears acutely or chronically ill
Hair	• Dull and dry, brittle, easily plucked, thin, sparse
Face	• Skin dark over cheeks and under eyes, skin flaky, face swollen or hollow/sunken cheeks
Eyes	• Eye membranes pale, dry, increased vascularity, cornea soft
Lips	• Swollen, puffy, angular lesions at the corners of the mouth
Tongue	• Smooth appearance, swollen, beefy red, sores, atrophic papillae
Teeth	• Dental caries, malpositioned
Gums	• Spongy, bleed easily, marginal redness
Glands	• Thyroid enlargement
Skin	• Rough, flaky, dry, swollen, pale, pigmented, lack of fat under skin
Nails	• Spoon-shaped, ridged, brittle
Skeleton	• Poor posture, beading of ribs, bowed legs, knock knees
Muscles	• Flaccid, poor tone, wasted, underdeveloped
Extremities	• Weak and tender, oedematous
Abdomen	• Swollen
Nervous system	• Ankle and knee reflexes absent or decreased
Weight	• Overweight or underweight

festation of nutrient deficiency. Therefore most clinical indicators are regarded as insensitive and merely warn of the need for preventive measures. Another limitation of clinical evaluation is that symptoms are often non-specific, reflecting a spectrum of deficiencies in addition to conditions unrelated to nutrition.

Anthropometrical evaluation

The scientific study of physical measurement of the human body is known as anthropometry. Anthropometry can be used to determine body composition, which can significantly reflect nutritional status. Excess food intake can lead to accumulation of body fat (adiposity) and subsequent weight gain. Levels of obesity have risen markedly in recent years in many industrialised nations including the UK. In contrast, in many developing countries, insufficient food intake (malnutrition) leads to loss of body weight. Much of this weight loss is predominantly adipose tissue but increasingly lean body tissue is lost.

Box 7.2 Body mass index.

Under 20 kg m	Underweight
20–24.9 kg m	Ideal
25–29.9 kg/m²	Overweight
30–34.9 kg/m²	Obese class I
35–39.9 kg/m²	Obese class II
>40 kg/m²	Obese class III

Body mass index

Use of height and weight measurement allows calculation of the body mass index (BMI) in adults, which is an indicator of body composition. Similar calculations for children and adolescents can be made using percentile charts. BMI is defined as the weight of an individual in kilograms divided by the square of their height in metres:

$$BMI = \frac{body\ weight\ (kg)}{height\ (m)^2}$$

BMI is quantitative and simple to determine, accounting for its use by the World Health Organisation. Difference in BMI between individuals is assumed to be due to variation in the ratio of adipose (fat) tissue to lean (muscle) tissue. It follows that low BMI is associated with being "lean" whereas high BMI is associated with being 'fat'. UK adults are classified as follows.

Being underweight or overweight increases the risk of mortality or morbidity. Ideal BMI (20–25 kg/m²) is the range in which individuals are at the lowest risk of mortality compared with those with a BMI outside this range. The correlation between adiposity and BMI is strong but BMI is not a direct measure of body composition and may not be able to differentiate between fat loss and muscle loss, particularly in older people.

There are a number of situations (discussed below) in which classifying subjects based on BMI does not reflect adiposity and is therefore inaccurate:

- *Oedemic and dehydrated subjects.* Rapid changes in weight are associated with fluid balance, not changes in fat or muscle stores (Reilly, 1996). Gaining or losing body fluid may lead to significant changes in body weight with no change in adiposity. Athletes who need to "make weight" may induce loss of body fluid (dehydration) using sweating techniques (e.g. saunas) and diuretics. Oedema (accumulation of excess body fluid) occurs as a symptom of a number of conditions, including malnutrition. Poor nutritional status may be masked using BMI in subjects with oedema.

- *Ethnic variation.* Studies now indicate that the relationship between BMI and percentage body fat varies with ethnicity. For example, it has been demonstrated that some Asian populations have up to 5% more body fat compared with Caucasians matched for age and gender. This variation may reflect differences in build and/or frame size. It follows that an individual with a "heavier build" may have an identical BMI but significantly lower percentage body fat compared with an individual of smaller build.
- *Athletes.* Some strength athletes, especially body builders, and sprinters have a highly developed musculature. This substantially increases body weight so that such individuals have a high BMI yet their body fat (adiposity) is low.
- *Older people.* As people age there is a gradual increase in the ratio of adipose to lean tissue. In older people, the mass of lean tissue and bone may be significantly less than in younger adults. It follows that an elderly subject may have a BMI in the ideal range but actually have high levels of body fat.

BMI determination requires accurate measurement of height. Many elderly and disabled subjects are unable to stand upright so that height measurements are difficult to obtain. An alternative to height as a measure of skeletal size is the demi-span measurement. This is defined as the distance from the web of the middle and right finger and the sternal notch when the arm of the subject is held out horizontally. BMI can be determined from the demi-span measurement as follows:

Height for men = (1.2 × demi-span) + 71
Height for women = (1.2 × demi-span) + 67

Skinfold thickness

The thickness of a skinfold is dependent on the amount of subcutaneous adipose tissue (Kozier *et al.*, 2003). Measurement of skinfold thickness allows total fat to be determined since subcutaneous fat stores are positively associated with total adipose tissue (the sum of the subcutaneous and internal fat stores). The use of skinfold callipers allows the thickness of skinfolds to be measured quantitatively. Skinfold thickness is normally measured at four specific sites:

- upper arm biceps
- upper arm triceps
- under the scapula (subscapular)
- above the iliac crest (suprailiac).

These four measurements are added together and translated into an estimate of percentage total body fat using a conversion table, which allows an assessor to simply read off the value. Separate tables are used for males and females and children.

The method seems simple but it requires considerable experience to take accurate skinfold readings. Particular difficulties can occur in taking accurate measurements in severely obese subjects or subjects with oedema in whom it is easy to make overestimates. Other factors also need to be considered. First, subjects need to partly undress, which adds time to the procedure and the need for male and female investigators. Second, there is much between-subject variation in the distribution of body fat. For example, older people subjects have increased proportion of internal adipose tissue compared with younger adults. Similarly, patients with human immunodeficiency virus (HIV) lipodystrophy lose subcutaneous adipose tissue in favour of an increased proportion of abdominal fat. Finally, the conversion of skinfold measurement to percentage body fat relies on tables derived from measurements of body density. Therefore, the errors in determining body density become errors in the use of skinfold measurements.

Waist-to-hip circumference ratio

This is the circumference of the body at the waist divided by the circumference at the hips. Unlike BMI or bio-electrical impedance, this simple measurement provides information on the distribution of body fat. Some individuals can be described as ovoid or "apple shaped" in contrast to others who can be described as gynoid or "pear shaped". The female body shape is typically gynoid and is influenced by the female sex hormones, especially oestrogen. A low waist-to-hip ratio is of the gynoid body shape. Men and postmenopausal women have a body shape that is more ovoid so they have a higher waist-to-hip ratio. The significance of waist-to-hip ratio measurements is that body fat distribution may have profound health implications. Several lifestyle factors, including smoking, lack of physical activity and excess alcohol intake, promote a high waist-to-hip ratio. In addition, ageing usually (but not inevitably) leads to a rise in waist-to-hip ratio, predisposing to "middle age spread". Adipose tissue accumulating internally around the abdomen (visceral fat) appears to increase the risk of diabetes and heart disease. The WHO has suggested that waist-to-hip circumference ratio should not exceed 1.00 and 0.85 for men and women respectively.

Bio-electrical impedance

Water is distributed within cells (intracellular) and between cells (intercellular) and contains dissolved electrolytes. Solutions of electrolytes are good conductors of electric current. Measurement of bio-electrical impedance involves placing electrodes in contact with hands or feet and applying an alternating electric current that passes from one electrode to the other. It is assumed that the impedance to the flow of electric current is proportional to the percentage body fat. This is due to the low water content of adipose tissue which makes it a relatively poor conductor of electricity compared with the non-fat mass of the body. Impedance analysers can be calibrated by inputting an individual's age, height, weight and sex. Subjects are able to get an instant reading of percentage body fat. The availability of inexpensive analysers providing an electronic reading has led to the widespread personal use of the method. However, the accuracy and/or validity of the technique remain controversial. The method is also considered inappropriate for subjects with disturbances in fluid balance. For example, inaccurate readings are likely in dialysis patients or those with oedema or dehydration.

Biochemical measurements

The use of sensitive biochemical assays or tests provides a quantitative and objective evaluation of nutritional status. The most common are serum albumin, serum transferrin and serum haemoglobin (Edwards, 1998). Specific nutrients can be estimated in body fluids or samples of tissue to obtain a direct measurement, which can be compared with normal ranges. For example, the best method to evaluate folate status is to measure the concentration of the vitamin in plasma/serum or within red blood cells. Serum folate and red blood cell concentrations below 7 nmol/l and 320 nmol/l suggest a depletion of folate reserves. For some nutrients it is more appropriate to measure some function of the nutrient in the body, i.e. a functional biomarker. For example, selenium status can be determined from measuring the activity of the enzyme glutathione peroxidase in tissues. Selenium is a constituent of the enzyme so if a subject has a low selenium status, the activity of the enzyme will be compromised. Similarly, iron status can be ascertained from red blood cell count and serum ferritin, both of which are affected by low iron status. There are biochemical tests for most nutrients but some tests may be invasive or reflect the previous meal only. It must also be considered that several nutrients are extensively stored in the body, providing reserves lasting over a year in the case of vitamin B12 (stored in the liver).

Dietary assessment

A dietary assessment of an individual can be obtained from a food record which is a detailed log of all food and drink consumed over a given time. Food records are obtained prospectively and therefore do not rely on recall of past events. In hospitals or nursing homes, the patient's food intake can be recorded in diet dairies by medical staff. Food intake by free-living subjects is also recorded in carefully designed diaries containing clear instructions. The amount of food and drink consumed can be estimated in a number of ways. The most accurate method is to weigh all food and drink consumed. Alternatively, estimates of the amount of each food consumed can be gained using a food atlas. Food atlases contain photographic images of a spectrum of foods of differing portion size.

However, use of weighing scales or food atlases may not always be convenient, particularly over several days. Alternatively, food can be described in household measures such as a tablespoon, cup, bowl, etc. What is of particular importance is that subjects need to be carefully instructed to give precise descriptions of food. 'A glass of milk' does not describe whether the milk was skimmed or full fat. As with obtaining a diet history, diet records aim to provide an estimate of habitual intake. Hence food records need to be recorded over at least 3–7 days. Longer periods may not increase accuracy as subject compliance may decline.

Mean daily intake of energy and nutrients in addition to some non-nutrients such as cholesterol can be obtained using food composition tables. These normally extensive databases provide information on the nutrient composition of foods. Diet analysis software greatly facilitates processing the data of food records. Mean intake of nutrients can be compared with appropriate dietary reference values. In the UK, the extent of any excesses or shortfalls is usually expressed relative to the reference nutrient intake. Food records can also provide information on eating patterns as the diet diaries indicate the time of day when food is consumed.

Dietary assessment using food records and food tables has a number of disadvantages. Food records can be inaccurate, especially in free-living subjects who may not comply fully with the procedure. Some subjects may subtly alter their diet when recording their intake by avoiding certain foods with an unhealthy image, such as cream cakes, and eating more fruit and vegetables. Heavy drinkers of alcohol frequently may report consuming only a fraction of their actual intake. Recording dietary intake requires a degree of numeracy and is therefore not suitable for some subgroups such as individuals with learning difficulties. Low compliance is likely to make the method unsuitable for determining the nutrient status of the homeless.

Food composition tables may not be available for some foods such as those of ethnic origin or entirely new products. There may also be considerable variation in the nutritional content of similar food products. For example, the content of the mineral selenium in fruit and vegetables reflects the soil content from which the crop was harvested. Hence determination of selenium intake using food composition tables is not considered accurate. Low-fat or low-salt alternatives and the fortification of foods with vitamins and minerals augment variation and constitute a source of error.

Duplicate analysis is a method of recording food intake by the provision of exact duplicate samples of what an individual has consumed.

The duplicate sample is analysed for energy and nutrient content. Thus, the method avoids the use of food composition tables. However, the method is relatively expensive and subjects inevitably require compensating for expense incurred in collecting duplicate samples. This may induce subjects to adjust their habitual diet to one containing more expensive and luxurious foods. In addition, it can be difficult to obtain duplicate samples such as food consumed in a social setting.

Nutritional interventions

Alongside all the above means of assessment, the health professional needs to exercise clinical judgement (Arrowsmith, 1999). Nurses are well placed to not only make initial assessment of status and intake but also to continue to monitor the nutritional requirements of patients (Kowanko *et al.*, 2001), although Palmer (1998) identified that patients' nutritional status was not always reviewed despite comprehensive initial assessment. If a multidisciplinary approach is taken to nutritional responsibilities then nurses can work with medical staff and the scarce resource of dieticians to ensure that patients' dietary needs are met. Some hospitals are still without specialist nutrition teams (Perry, 1997) but where they exist, there is better interprofessional communication and improved staff morale. A most effective contribution would be in assuming responsibility for feeding patients (Pedder, 1998). There is clearly a need to ensure that meals are within reach, the patient is in an upright position and that patients are helped to choose and eat their meal. Attention must be paid to the amount and presentation of food and that mealtimes are protected time without investigations, cleaning or doctors' rounds going on at the same time. Feeding patients has always been a nursing role but it is increasingly delegated to unqualified and unskilled workers. Weight loss in hospital patients has been directly attributed to a lack of nursing interventions at mealtimes (ACHC, 1997).

Summary

Overall better understanding of nutrition, gaining skills in assessment and interventions to make dietary intake a priority will eventually pay dividends in better outcomes for patients, their families and the service at large. Positive change in poor practice may be driven by initiatives such as the 'red tray' system (Bradley & Rees, 2003) and the fundamental approach to food and nutrition established by *Essence of Care* (DoH, 2001). This gives hope not just for nutritional assessment as a nursing priority but the advent of a holistic nutritional care process.

Activity

1. Using the following list of food components, complete the sentences below.

vitamin C	sodium
calcium	vitamin A
protein	flavonoids
sucrose	glycerol
omega 3 fatty acids	beta-carotene
lysine	sodium chloride
dietary fibre	saturated fatty acids
potassium	starch
iron	glucose
vitamin D	iodine
niacin	vitamin E
lycopene	vitamin K

- The major fat-soluble antioxidant in humans is _____.
- Short chain peptides and _____ are formed from the digestion of protein.
- Table salt is the chemical compound called _____.
- Some types of _____ raise blood cholesterol levels.
- Major bone minerals include _____ and phosphorus.
- Starch is a polysaccharide that is digested to _____.
- Fat molecules are composed of _____ and three fatty acid units.
- _____ are compounds responsible for the colour of red wine.
- The trace element involved in binding oxygen is _____.
- Deficiency of _____ leads to goitre.
- _____ can be made in the body utilising sunlight.
- _____ is poorly digested: it promotes the health of the intestine and facilitates weight control.
- _____ is a micronutrient that promotes blood clotting.

2. Using the following list of foods, complete the sentences below.

orange juice	potato crisps
cow's milk	fresh oysters
sardines	milk chocolate
mineral water	chicken breast
margarine	egg
soya milk	porridge
tea	kiwi fruit
fried liver	grilled beef steak
breakfast cereals	digestive biscuits
tomato ketchup	bacon
instant coffee	stir-fried broccoli

- A major source of cholesterol in the UK diet is _____.
- _____ contains no macronutrients.
- Consuming _____ with meals increases absorption of iron whereas consuming _____ may impair iron absorption from the gut.
- One rich source of polyunsaturated fatty acids would be _____.
- Cured products such as _____ contain high amounts of sodium.
- Some foods such as _____ are said to contain hidden fats whereas some foods such as _____ are said to contain hidden sugars.
- Pregnant women are advised to avoid foods such as _____ because they contain large quantities of vitamin A which may increase the risk of birth defects and miscarriage.
- Many foods such as _____ and _____ are fortified with extra vitamins and/or minerals.
- _____ contains lycopene, a type of carotenoid which may help reduce the risk of cancer.
- Some meats such as _____ and _____ are typically less than 4% fat by weight.
- _____ and _____ are sources of caffeine.
- Rich sources of vitamin C include _____ and _____.
- Women considering pregnancy are advised to consume foods such as _____ which are rich in folic acid.
- Foods such as _____ are associated with "soluble fibre".
- Many adults are intolerant of _____ because of the presence of lactose.

References

Arrowsmith, H (1999) A critical evaluation of the use of nutritional scoring tools by nurses. *British Journal of Nursing* 8 (22): 1483–90.

Association of Community Health Councils (ACHC) (1997) *Hungry in Hospital.* Association of Community Health Councils in England and Wales, London.

Barker, H M (2002) *Nutrition and Dietetics for Health Care*, 10th edition. Churchill Livingstone, Edinburgh.

Bender, D A (2002) *Introduction to Nutrition and Metabolism*, 3rd edition. UCL Press, London.

Bradley, L & Rees, C (2003) Reducing nutritional risk in hospital: the red tray. *Nursing Standard* 17 (26): 33–7.

British Nutrition Foundation (2003) *BNF Information.* www.nutrition.org.uk/information/dietandhealth.

Carpenito-Moyet, L J (2004) *Nursing Diagnoses: application to clinical practice.* Mosby, Philadelphia.

Cotton, E, Zinober, B & Jessop, J (1996) A nutritional assessment tool for older patients. *Professional Nurse* 11: 609–12.

Department of Health (1991) *Dietary Reference Values for Food Energy and Nutrients for the United Kingdom: Report of the Panel on Dietary Reference Values of the Committee on Medical Aspects of Food Policy.* HMSO, London.

Department of Health (2001) *Essence of Care.* HMSO, London.

Eastwood, M (2003) *Principles of Human Nutrition*, 2nd edition. Blackwell Science, Oxford.

Edwards, S L (1998) Malnutrition in hospital patients: where does it come from? *British Journal of Nursing* 7 (16): 954–8 & 971–4.

Ferguson, M, Capra, S, Bauer, J & Banks, M (1999) Development of a valid and reliable malnutrition screening tool for adult acute hospital patients. *Nutrition* 15 (6): 458–64.

Fuller, J & Schaller-Ayres, J (2000) *Health Assessment: a nursing approach.* Lippincott, Philadelphia.

Guigoz, Y, Vellaz, B & Garry, B J (1996) Assessing the nutritional status of the elderly: the Mini Nutritional Assessment as part of geriatric evaluation. *Nutrition Reviews* 11: 559–65.

Health Education Authority in association with the Ministry for Agriculture, Fisheries and Food and the Department of Health (1997) *Guidelines for Nutrition Educators.* HEA, London.

Holmes, S (2004) Malnutrition in hospital: an indictment of the quality of care? *British Journal of Healthcare Management* 10 (3): 82–5.

Jordan, S, Snow, D, Hayes, C & Williams, A (2003) Introducing a nutrition screening tool: an exploratory study in a district general hospital. *Journal of Advanced Nursing* 44 (1): 12–23.

Kowanko, I, Simon, S & Wood, J (2001) Nutritional care of the patient: a nurse's knowledge and attitude in an acute setting. *Journal of Clinical Nursing* 8 (2): 217–24.

Kozier, B, Erb, G & Berman, A D (eds) (2003) *Fundamentals of Nursing*, 6th edition. Addison Wesley Longman, New York.

Ledsham, J & Gough, A (2000) Screening and monitoring patients for malnutrition. *Professional Nurse* 15 (11): 695–8.

Lee, R D & Nieman, D C (2003) *Nutritional Assessment*, 3rd edition. Mosby, Philadelphia.

Leeds, M (1998) *Nutrition for Healthy Living.* McGraw Hill, New York.

Lennard-Jones, J E (1992) *A Positive Approach to Nutrition as Treatment.* King's Fund Centre, London.

Lyne, P A & Prowse, M (1999) Methodological issues in the development and use of instruments to assess patient nutritional status or the level of risk of nutritional compromise. *Journal of Advanced Nursing* 30 (4): 835–42.

Mann, J & Trusswell, A S (2002) *Essentials of Human Nutrition*, 2nd edition. Oxford University Press, Oxford.

McWhirter, J & Pennington, C (1994) Incidence and recognition of malnutrition in hospital. *BMJ* 308 (6943): 945–8.

Palmer, D (1998) The persisting problem of malnutrition in healthcare. *Journal of Advanced Nursing* 28 (5): 931–2.

Pedder, L (1998) Nursing's nutritional responsibilities. *Nursing Standard* 13 (9): 49–55.

Perry, L (1997) Nutrition: a hard nut to crack. An exploration of attitudes and activities of qualified nurses in relation to nutritional nursing care. *Journal of Clinical Nursing* 6 (4): 315–24.

Reilly, H (1996) Nutritional assessment. *British Journal of Nursing* 5 (1): 18–24.

Scanlan, F, Dunne, J & Toyne, K (1994) No more cause for neglect: introducing a nutritional assessment tool and action plan. *Professional Nurse* 9 (6): 382–5.

Smeltzer, S C & Bare, B G (2000) *Medical and Surgical Nursing*. Lippincott, Philadelphia.

Weber, J R (2001) *Nurses' Handbook of Health Assessment*, 4th edition. Lippincott, Philadelphia.

Further reading

Ashwell, M (1997) *British Nutrition Foundation: diet and heart disease*. Chapman and Hall, London.

British Nutrition Foundation Task Force (1995) *Iron: nutritional and physiological significance*. Chapman and Hall, London.

Cardiovascular Review Group (1994) *Committee on Medical Aspects of Food and Nutrition Policy: nutritional aspects of cardiovascular disease*. Report on Health and Social Subjects, 46. HMSO, London.

Department of Health (1998) *Working Group on Diet and Cancer of the Committee on Medical Aspects of Food and Nutrition Policy*. Report on Health and Social Subjects, 48. Nutritional Aspects of Diet and Cancer. HMSO, London.

International Task Force for the Prevention of Coronary Heart Disease. *Coronary Heart Disease: reducing the risk*. www.chd-taskforce.com/guidelines.

McClaren, D S (1992) *Colour Atlas and Text of Diet-Related Disorders*. Wolfe Medical Press, London.

Webb, G P (2002) *Nutrition: a health promotion approach*, 2nd edition. Arnold, London.

World Cancer Research Fund in association with the American Institute of Cancer Research (1997) *Food Nutrition and the Prevention of Cancer: a global perspective*. Washington, DC: American Institute for Cancer Research.

Social assessment in healthcare

S. O'Brien

Learning objectives
• Outline the purpose of social assessment in nursing.
• Outline the integral relationship between nursing models, social influences and assessment.
• Discuss the place of interprofessional frameworks for social assessment.
• Outline a framework for social assessment and analysis, which examines various levels and dimensions of social assessment.

Introduction

The social aspects of health assessment cannot be divorced from the other aspects explored in the health assessment process as applied to an individual or group of individuals. Therefore the issues discussed in this chapter interrelate with the other aspects of assessment discussed in other chapters. It is generally accepted within the healthcare professions that any form of healthcare assessment should embrace the philosophy of humanism and as such, attention should be paid to all facets of the human experience. Within this chapter the social dimensions of health assessment will thus be explored.

The purpose of social assessment

All healthcare and nursing commentators agree that in order to complete a holistic assessment of patient need, you have to examine the biological, psychological and social dimensions of the patient. This point is taken up in the many assessment tools utilised by a wide range of health- and social care professionals. It is known that ill health does not occur by chance. Apart from genetic, biological, psychological, cultural and spiritual factors, social factors such as environmental and lifestyle factors tend to affect health. All of these factors need to be captured in the overall assessment of health and nursing need.

Environment, housing and health

The environment within which people live or work could affect health. Evidence, for example, suggests that people who are exposed to X-rays over a long period of time and those living close to chemical or nuclear plants are more likely to develop certain types of blood disorder (Busby & Scott Cato, 1997). Pollutants such as sulphur dioxide (an acid gas) can affect human health as it could damage the lining of the nose, throat and lungs, especially of patients with asthma and chronic lung disease (National Statistics, 2004). Poor housing conditions such as dampness, lack of toilet and/or bathing facilities and overcrowding have also been linked to high rates of respiratory disorders, stress and infection (Townsend *et al.*, 1990). High-density housing and the lack of adequate play amenities are also associated with higher accident rates in children (Naidoo & Wills, 2000). However, poor housing conditions and the type of house one chooses to live in tend to be influenced by a range of other important factors such as low income, family ties, social support networks and cultural identity. The points made above highlight the need for careful collection of biographical data from patients during the health assessment process.

Lifestyle and health

Lifestyle or health behaviours are usually given as explanations for certain health problems. It needs to be highlighted, however, that these are influenced by certain social factors. Those with low income, for instance, tend to eat food that is high in fat and sugar and less fruit and vegetables. This means low income can affect the amount as well as the quality of resources that can be purchased. This is a recognised determinant of standard of living (National Statistics, 2004). A disease such as atherosclerosis (hardening of the blood vessel walls) is, in turn, linked to cigarette smoking, stress, high blood sugar, a high-fat diet and increased pressure from hypertension (Philippe & Whittaker, 2004). Atherosclerosis predisposes to coronary heart disease. The actual determinant of health in the previous examples could be described as low income. During a comprehensive health assessment, however, questions related to lifestyle and health behaviour are important as they help to plan and facilitate appropriate health promotion activity (Naidoo & Wills, 2000). In the example above, it is likely that if the person has had a low income for some time they would be unable to buy more healthy but expensive foodstuffs.

Health policy: assessing social needs

From a policy perspective, however, the assessment of need in a social context has been contentious. The 1989 White Paper *Working for Patients* (DoH, 1989) and the 1990 NHS and Community Care Act (DoH, 1990) created a cascade of change in which a contract culture was introduced into healthcare (Leathard, 2000). Local authorities were given the overall responsibility for the assessment of individual needs where these needs went beyond health and encompassed a more explicit social dimension. This was to be completed in collaboration with health authority staff. As Leathard suggested, in order for this to work the agencies involved would all need to work together to provide a 'seamless service' Vernon *et al.* (2000), in their examination of politics and practice in primary care, suggest that in 1993 local authority social service departments became the lead agencies for assessing the social care needs of vulnerable groups, including older people. They suggested that need is a nebulous term but 'needs-led' assessment would appear to imply that the aim is to meet the needs identified by the patient.

The DoH *Practitioner's Guide* (1991) states that it is essential that all care agencies and practitioners share a common understanding of the term 'need'. Local authorities are advised to publicise their definition of needs, stating clearly those they are required by law to meet and those where they have the discretion to act. Ultimately, however, having weighed the views of all parties, including their own observations, the assessing practitioner is responsible for defining the patient's needs (DoH, 1991). This would seem to indicate that a 'needs-led' assessment is different from a patient-led approach and that ultimately the assessor will define need (Meredith, 1993). Indeed, Ford & McCormack (1999) identify the assessment of individuals' need for health and/or social care as being a constant theme within the continuing care debates.

It is increasingly difficult to define the difference between health- and social care and as a result, the value of the nursing contribution in continuing care has often been under-recognised or even questioned. Nurses working with individuals who need continuing care will recognise that they have interrelated health- and social care needs. When the links between health and social needs are ignored, the care of people and in particular the most vulnerable is in danger of being broken down into a series of tasks and becoming fragmented. This undermines the holistic nature of professional nursing care.

Nursing models, social influences and assessment

A number of recognised nursing theorists acknowledge within their work the significance of the social dimension of health assessment. The vast majority of nursing models are built upon the four metaparadigms of nursing, the person, the environment and health. The relationship between the person and the environment has a strong social element, which is often explicitly captured in the theorist's work. The most popular nursing model with arguably the greatest influence on practical assessment in the United Kingdom is that developed by Roper, Logan and Tierney (2000). Within their model they accept that assessment of the activities of living will be influenced by sociocultural, environmental and socio-economic factors. For example, Roper *et al.* outline the need to examine social aspects as part of the overall assessment. Against the activity of maintaining a safe environment, it would be important to review societal differences across and within societies, appreciate the influence of social disorder, which appears to be a common feature of modern-day living, and finally appraise the spiritual influences. The spiritual influences may be religious, cultural or other forms of belief. Similarly, when examining this activity, Roper *et al.* suggest that one would need to be aware of environmental aspects such as pollution, accident, infection and fire.

Outlined below are the key social assessment factors within a number of well-recognised conceptual models for nursing. All of these nursing theorists have developed their work embracing the concept of individuality but although it is recognised that the individual is important, one must not neglect the collective/social dimensions within the assessment process. Nurses may find it difficult to attend to social needs in their assessment as the concept of individuality has been so emphasised over the past few years within the recognised nursing assessment frameworks. The emphasis on the individual can provide a tension with the broader complexities of social need.

- *Rogers (1989).* Embraced the social dimensions of health assessment within her framework as the ongoing relationship between the person and their environment.
- *Neuman (1995).* Defined the person as a dynamic composite, which would include sociocultural variables. In addition, she outlines the importance of external social stressors. Social assessment would

need to include a review of the person's ability to adapt to environmental change, which she refers to as accommodation.

- *Roper, Logan and Tierney (2000).* Identified activities of daily living as a framework for assessment. Factors influencing the activities include sociocultural, environmental and politico-economic factors, all of which should be considered as part of the social assessment.
- *Orem (2001).* Emphasised the assessment of how individuals maintain a balance between activity, rest, solitude and social interaction. Additionally, development of the individual within social groups needs to be considered.
- *Roy (2005).* Suggested that nurses should explore the following social-based concepts within assessment: self-concept and group identity, role function and the concept of interdependence.

Nursing and interprofessional approaches to social assessment

The importance of assessing social status has been made clear in the community care legislation and the requirements of the GP Contract to carry out health checks on people over 75 years of age. Increasingly there is recognition of the need to develop tools that can be shared across agencies (Lewis & Glennerster, 1996). However, there is virtually no consensus on how this should be done. There is tremendous variation in assessment schemes being developed in local authorities, from checklists to open-ended client-led questionnaires, from home-grown to well-established and validated assessment tools.

Lewis & Glennerster (1996) noted the beliefs that underpin development of a common assessment:

- User benefit from a seamless service; seamless service is achievable when there is established interagency working.
- Identifying and working on a common task (such as a joint assessment) to achieve good interagency working.
- Developing a common assessment form as a good beginning to joint working.

A nursing assessment cannot be divorced from other professional assessments, especially given the contemporary relevance of interagency/interprofessional working. Lewis & Glennerster (1996) suggested that a common assessment tool was a good start to such 'joined-up' working. Joint assessment as a common task could achieve good interagency working. The differing agency perspectives of assessment can enhance the nature of assessment and add to the social elements that nursing has a tendency to neglect. Lockwood & Marshall (1999) explored the use of a standardised needs assessment tool in the care of people with severe mental health disorders. They suggested that improvements that bordered on the significant were noted for aspects such as social functioning. In this study, a nurse specialist in the field undertook assessment of social need.

The development of interprofessional assessment tools is problematic on a number of counts. Miller *et al.* (2001), examining patterns of team working, outlined a range of factors that suggest that multiagency and multidisciplinary team working is difficult to realise. The working practices examined included the process of assessment and care planning. They proposed that multiprofessional working could be observed in three typologies.

Integrated working

A high degree of collaborative assessment is demonstrated. Organisational stability and predictability are evident with professionals planning their work together, developing an in-depth understanding of each other's roles, contributions and patient needs. Miller *et al.* (2001) identify clear benefits for patients in this style of working, including:

- consistency within the assessment approach
- reducing ambiguity in assessment
- appropriate and timely referral
- holistically based action planning and decision making
- problem solving.

Fragmented working

This is seen where individual teams may wish to work together but are essentially dissimilar. The organisational context may lack stability or be subject to change. As individual teams, they see that their specific assessment is effective but have little recognition of the benefits that could be achieved for the client if a more collaborative assessment style were adopted.

Core and periphery working

Here a combination of integrated and fragmented assessment approaches is used. A core team established as part of the service development and with a history of integrated working attempts to collaborate with another element of the service provision working essentially at the periphery of the core team despite being located in the same geographical area.

Activity

- Examine the extent to which the social assessment scheme used in your current placement is interprofessional in nature. Discuss your findings with your mentor.

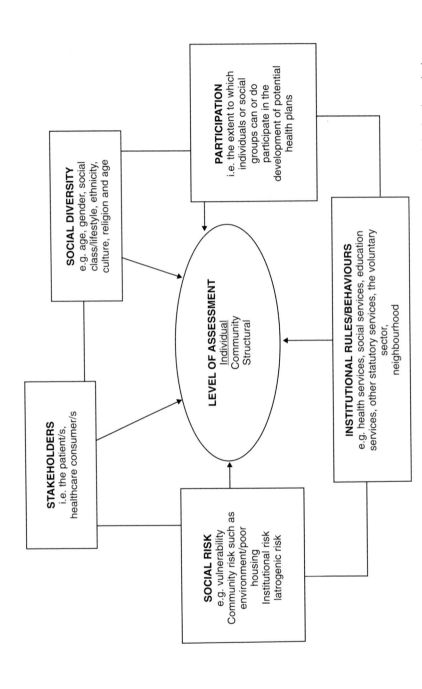

Figure 8.1 Overview of the social assessment/analysis framework. Entry points and dimensions of enquiry and the level at which assessment may be carried out at each entry point. Developed from the work of the World Bank (2002) and Stimson et al. (2003)

The social assessment/analysis framework

The framework outlined and discussed in this section has been developed by the author based upon work originally published by the World Bank (2002), within a social analysis sourcebook. This sourcebook provides a conceptual framework for the systematic analysis of social situations. The original framework offers five entry points or 'dimensions of enquiry' to facilitate a better understanding of social complexity. These dimensions of enquiry can be broken down into a number of key elements. Furthermore, if the nurse applies the series of questions generated by the level of assessment criteria to these elements then a comprehensive social assessment of health and nursing need can be facilitated. An overview of the proposed social assessment/analysis framework is set out in Figure 8.1.

Entry points/dimensions of enquiry

The entry points/dimensions of enquiry for social assessment are:

- the stakeholder(s)
- social diversity
- participation
- institutional rules/behaviours
- social risk.

These entry points offer a starting point for the construction of a comprehensive social assessment. Each entry point can be examined in turn by asking a series of questions at the three distinct levels indicated in Figure 8.1. Not all questions for all levels will be relevant in each situation. However, it would be good practice to try to apply the questions when encountering a patient for the first time. This will ensure that all the required questions are asked and that something which could be crucial is not overlooked.

Set out below are some of the initial questions that could be explored for the entry point of the stakeholder related to the patient profile of Morag below. The stakeholder would be Morag primarily but could also include all the people named in the scenario.

Patient profile

Morag (39 years) telling her story to her GP

I have been happily married to David (42 years of age) for the past 18 years. About four months ago we all moved down from Aberdeen as David was promoted within his company. This was a difficult decision for us all as we loved living in Aberdeen. I have two children, William aged 14 and Margaret aged 8. They are still settling into their new schools. I feel that the move has affected William more than Margaret.

I am having a few problems settling myself. I think this is mainly because my parents, who still live in Aberdeen, are having problems. My father is unwell and has suffered from coronary heart disease for some time. He recently had an angiogram suggesting that he needs a bypass operation. He is currently waiting to see the cardiac surgeon. I can't help feeling a little guilty about 'not being there' for them at this time.

Our new house is wonderful and the neighbours have been very welcoming, especially Derek and Joan. David wouldn't agree as he thinks Joan is overly friendly. He has said that he feels she is always there when he gets home from work and this has caused a bit of tension between us. I mean, when all is said and done Joan has only just come out of hospital following a hip replacement and probably welcomes the company. The other bone of contention at the moment is David's brother Clive. He has been in touch recently, which I am not at all happy about. Clive's a bit of a waster really and he only ever gets in touch when he is in trouble or needs something. Reading between the lines, it looks like he has lost his job. No doubt this was drink related.

So what with one thing and another, this golden opportunity is becoming a bit tarnished. I haven't been sleeping well and I saw you last week when you suggested I go onto antidepressants. I don't think that the pills have made any difference; if anything, I feel worse. I think I need something stronger.

Individual-level assessment
- Could Morag become stigmatised as a result of her presenting problems?
- Are Morag's health problems affecting her social and economic role in society?
- Does she require additional social support at this time?

Community-level assessment
- Has Morag's situation been influenced by her community setting, housing, etc.?
- What are the social consequences for Morag, her husband and her children?

Structural-level assessment
- Are we aware of any national policies that could influence Morag's care?
- Would public attitudes have an impact on Morag, her feelings and willingness to seek help?

Clearly this is only a starting point and is certainly not an exhaustive assessment; however, this example could be extrapolated to the other entry points such as her ability to participate in the assessment process and other factors such as social risk.

Having outlined briefly how the framework could be used, each of the entry points will now be examined, throughout which a series of assessment-related issues will be outlined and discussed based upon the levels mentioned on the previous page and expanded on page 284. Examples of assessment influences will be described and potential assessment tools will be outlined that could be used in a real practical sense.

The stakeholders

Stakeholders are essentially the individual or groups of individuals within society who are subject to the process of health assessment. Any social assessment would need to embrace both the positive and negative influences that individuals and groups have on one another.

Social assessment is fundamentally 'people assessment'. People will have opinions, viewpoints and perspectives either as individuals or held collectively as part of organisations (formal and informal). They have something personally at stake as indeed does the community within which they live and work. The World Bank (2002: p24) recognises that some stakeholders are 'vocal, demanding, well-organised and influential'. Others are less visible and fail to be heard, perhaps because the powers-that-be fails to recognise that the processes of social exclusion have disempowered some organisations or social groups. Some stakeholders may also be vulnerable to manipulation by political parties or other powerful interest groups. In addition, the experiences of the stakeholders need to be recognised across the whole social spectrum, as this will certainly have a bearing upon current and future health behaviours.

It is recognised that the stakeholder commands a pivotal position within the framework. The notions of health ownership and health behaviour empowerment are crucial factors in relation to the social dimension of health assessment and future health outcomes. The effective engagement of stakeholders in the processes of social assessment demands an understanding of the patient's scope of interests and their individual degree of influence.

One way of capturing the social perspective of the stakeholder would be collecting a personal biography as often our health behaviours are programmed by our environmental backgrounds, i.e. who we are, how we see ourselves, where we come from and how this has influenced our lives. The expectations and aspirations of the individual can also be captured as these can often have a bearing on prognosis.

Sociogram

The relationship between the individual and their social circle/contacts (a personal social network) can be mapped out using a spidergram. The

spidergram (sociogram) can include relationships within social institutions such as family, friends, work, other social groupings and other
social networks (see Figure 8.2).

Activity

• Refer to the profile of Morag on pages 271–72 and develop a sociogram for
  Morag and her family.

A broader type of sociogram, a community health profile, can also be
developed which embraces a wider profile of the social community
within which the patient lives. The community health profile, sometimes referred to as a neighbourhood profile or study, can be mapped
against the individual sociogram and is often viewed as an extension
of the individual sociogram to include a wider community context.
This could indicate aspects of social exclusion, social deprivation
including poverty indices, housing issues, employment, education
resources, crime, social stability, the cultural/ethnicity profile and
social mobility/migration in any given community, for example
asylum seekers.

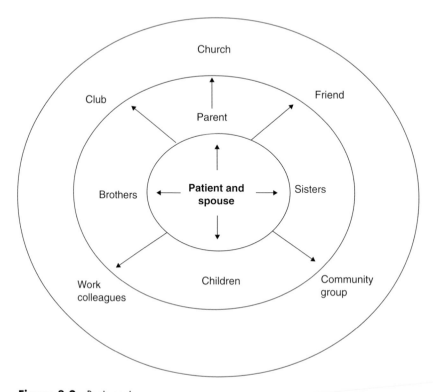

Figure 8.2 Basic sociogram

Social diversity

All societies comprise a range of socially diverse groupings that may be identified on the basis of gender, social class, ethnicity, religion, age, culture and social role as well as 'spatial' (geographical) and economic characteristics. These social categories are important to the health assessment investigator and the patient for the simple reason that they are a means of defining themselves and their neighbours. The social categories can form the basis for identification of personal/vested interests, provoke a set of health-related actions or provide restraints to action, and determine access to opportunity. The health status of individuals and groups can be directly linked to a number of these factors.

Gender

There is evidence that gender differences play a part in the perception and interpretation of symptoms (Edelmann, 2000). This may be affected by the process of gender socialisation, perceptions of gender roles and the interpretation of those roles by healthcare professionals.

Social class

The link between social class and health status has been established for many years. The Black Report (Townsend *et al.*, 1989) identified that there was a clear correlation between an individual's social circumstances and social group and their health status. Social class is also associated with financial income and spending power. For example, earlier in the chapter we looked at the relation between low income and lifestyle and how this may affect the health of individuals. The drive to address inequalities is at the heart of the current government's reforms of healthcare and the new modern and dependable NHS (DoH, 1997). The media have coined the term 'postcode lottery' related to inequalities in healthcare provision based upon geographical differences in levels of resource and funding.

Ethnicity, culture and religion

An understanding of transcultural issues can aid a social assessment by helping the assessor to appreciate culturally sensitive elements for any given patient. It has to be remembered, however, that there is an inherent danger of cultural or ethnic stereotyping when these types of issues are taken into account.

Age

The diversity in the age of any given population will certainly have an influence upon the services provided and the approaches taken by healthcare professionals in the assessment of social need. The demographic changes within the United Kingdom's population demonstrate, for example, that the elderly population is rising and will continue to rise over the next ten years (DoH, 2000a). This is high-lighted in the recently published National Service Framework (NSF) for the older person, which reflects a growing concern about the care and treatment of the elderly. Similarly the NSF for children emphasises the diversity in the population and related specific health issues with a clear attempt to provide standards based upon a number of key principles around:

- respect for the individual
- the need for intermediate care
- the provision of evidence-based specialist care
- the promotion of active living.

Returning to the social categories mentioned previously, people have no choice about some of them, such as gender, age, ethnicity, language, race and religion. If, for example, you are a 44-year-old woman of African origin, this is not a matter of choice. However, social diversity also includes achieved categories, such as those based on occupation, other social roles or membership in social movements. So if the 44-year-old woman of African origin is a nationally known journalist, working for a daily newspaper, and is married with two children she has a number of achieved social categories explicit within her personal biography (wife, mother, journalist). Collecting biographical data such as this is important and has been addressed earlier in this chapter related to environmental and housing issues. Table 8.1 presents a checklist of social categories that could be used to assist a social assessment in terms of diversity.

Activity

- With reference to Table 8.1, identify the ascribed, mixed and achieved categories for a patient you are currently nursing. What are the health/nursing implications associated with these roles and categories?

Table 8.1 Checklist of social diversity categories (adapted from World Bank, 2002).

Ascribed	Mixed	Achieved
• Age • Ethnicity or race • Tribe • Gender • Sexual orientation	• Language • Native/immigrant • Religion • Spatial and geographical location • Disability	• Citizen/migrant • Education • Ideology • Land ownership • Occupation/livelihood • Political affiliation • Urban/rural

Callista Roy (2005) examined the weight of the socially diverse roles of individuals within her conceptual model for nursing and suggested that changes in health status had the potential to alter the role concepts held by the individual. Additionally, the perception of these social categories held by the healthcare professional conducting the assessment can be challenging. Furthermore, how individuals and groups perceive themselves and their relationship with others does not always match how they are perceived by others. It is therefore important for the assessor to keep an open mind about social categorisation. There is no doubt that social categorisation helps the assessor to identify a range of commonly held healthcare perceptions about that category; however, they must avoid adopting a stereotypical view of the category. For example, not all Muslims behave in exactly the same way. Indeed, there can be as much social diversity within groups as there is between groups.

In reality, individuals, and occasionally groups, 'cross over' from one social category to another and the degree of social mobility can be a good indicator of social development. With increasing interethnic marriages, even the notion of ethnicity has become fluid in many societies and occasionally the gender barrier is also crossed. Furthermore, the phenomenon of social ethnicity is not static within a community; we may see quite distinct differences between the behaviours of the same community across the age ranges. For example, in the UK there is a difference between the social and health behaviours of first-and second-generation immigrants from the Caribbean. What makes social diversity complex and important in social assessment is that all these forms of identity can be reinforced or weakened by other elements in society, such as institutions or technology.

Participation

When using participation as a dimension of social assessment, we need to examine the extent to which individuals or social groups can and do participate in the development of potential health plans constructed in collaboration with healthcare professionals. We also need to appreciate the potential levels of engagement/participation and the strategies we may ultimately utilise to improve the effectiveness of that participation.

Participation is viewed as problematic for a number of reasons. First, the recent emphasis on patient participation in the nursing process has challenged nurses to consider how this can be achieved. Some have attempted to include the patient in the decision-making processes about care provision. However, a criticism of this emphasis is centred upon approaches adopted by nurses as being tantamount to coercion. Waterworth & Luker (1996) describe patients as reluctant collaborators, with some patients preferring nurses to actively exclude them from participation.

Some barriers to client participation

Actively encouraging participation in assessment can be difficult. Vernon *et al.* (2000) suggested that the views of older people are rarely sought in the assessment process, which means that their perspective on declining health and functional ability is not formally gathered. The influence on assessment outcome is therefore at best *ad hoc*. Some patients may be unable to represent themselves or have the requisite skills for full participation in assessment. The client can often be viewed as having limited reciprocity, with professionals consequently focusing on the management of the resource associated with care plans rather than challenging the adequacy or relevance of the resource for that patient. Patients need information in order to make informed choices about future care and increasingly, like their social service colleagues, nurses may face issues around unmet needs and need to know how and if these issues are made clear to clients. It is likely that unless patients and carers are supported to enable them to participate in the assessment process, their needs will continue to be marginalised (Cahill 1998).

Some patients, by virtue of their frailty or limited capability, may be unable to access the vital information required for positive participation. Therefore a further question that needs to be considered within the assessment process is whether patients have what the World Bank (2002: p28) refers to as the 'assets and capabilities' to access the benefits of any proposed health plan. Do the social fabric, social infrastructure and socialisation processes affecting the patient militate against this? Health plan assets can be physical in origin (material resources, infrastructures), financial (access to credit, capital, savings) or interpersonal (personal abilities, qualities such as assertiveness, etc.). Interpersonal assets relate to the patients' capabilities, which are equally as important. For example, do we appreciate their human resources (education, specialised skills, experience and organisational capability)?

On a community level, what organisational resources or social capital does the patient have access to? Relationships among peer groups within communities are an asset that can help to establish networks that yield health information or promote social health activity. If there is a paucity of resources available or accessible to the patient, this will have an impact upon future health behaviour. Capability therefore enables a person to function, exercising freedom to access useful health resources and entitlements.

The role of the nurse

From this perspective, social assessment is not simply a matter of considering the available health-related resources but of recognising and enhancing the capability of people to access the available resources. The role of the nurse in comprehensive social assessment is to determine which assets and capabilities are present and which are lacking. There is an additional need to include an analysis of whether these capabilities can be developed. For example, both Callista Roy and Dorothea Orem in their respective nursing assessment frameworks define capability as the person's abilities to adapt (Roy) or self-care (Orem). The assessor is charged with the responsibility to examine the person's capacity to positively adapt or self-care. Orem calls this self-care agency. They both emphasise the educational requirements inherent in the process of fostering social adaptation processes to engage in and capitalise on the existing assets available to the individual and community. Similarly the assessor needs to be mindful of the view that social barriers exist that can obstruct people from accessing the health resources they require. Barriers may exist in an institutionally embedded form. These barriers are often applied along social lines and reinforced by certain stakeholders. Stimson *et al.* (2003) refer to this within their structural perspective, arguing that factors such as the local social, economic and legal environments are influential in the construction of institutions. Consequently any social assessment would have to explore the social assets, capabilities of the client and the social barriers that might be at work within the patient's community.

All communities have systems through which people express interests. All such systems have some degree of inclusion and exclusion. Understanding local and traditional forms of participation is crucial to designing an effective health participation system. Professionals working with community groups will require a local awareness of how social participation is organised and who are the key stakeholders that control these processes. Each situation or community encountered will include customary forms of participation that are proper subjects for recognition within a social assessment.

Equality in participation is challenging for the assessor. It is, however, a concept that is real and even compelling, particularly in terms of marginal, vulnerable and poor people. In short, any health plan emerging from an assessment of patient need should not attempt to impose a rigid template, based solely on a professional view, over an existing system but rather should relate the health plan to the existing structural context.

Institutional rules/behaviours

A comprehensive assessment of health would need to encompass an analysis of the relationship between organisations and institutions within the community; that is, the formal and informal rules of the important relationships played out in societies that influence the health of a community. This is critical because many health development interventions, including community projects and policy reforms, depend for their implementation on institutional change. For example, the strategies within the White Paper *Saving Lives: our healthier nation*

(DoH, 2000b), which may be vital for our patients, may require policy changes such as those envisaged within the *NHS Plan* (DoH, 2000c) and the subsequent Modernisation Agenda. Institutions such as those involved in the broad social and health agenda within the UK work within codes or rules of practice that govern their behaviour.

Institutions can be thought of as a form of social capital. Social capital reflects how relationships between people enhance those people's ability to get things done. The World Bank (2002: p19) stated that:

> 'Social capital can have vertical and horizontal dimensions. Vertical social capital describes connections between people that operate through institutions where one person has power over another. Horizontal social capital inheres among peer groups.'

When the nurse undertakes an assessment through the social dimension, they need to be aware of the various institutions, their rules and behaviour in order to capture the character and nature of vertical social capital. The relative influence or social impact of each of these institutions can vary from community to community. Figure 8.3 outlines a number of established supportive institutions involved in the healthcare arena that the assessor will have to consider.

An appreciation of all the agencies and institutions involved in the provision of health- and social care is essential for the nurse considering the assessment of patients. It not only provides a context within which the nurse can identify the appropriate agencies that are involved or need to be involved in the future care of the patient but it helps them to understand relationships and influence within the sector. Figure 8.3 clearly indicates the flow of influence embedded in policy from central government through the sectoral levels down to agencies and eventually the professional interacting with patients.

Social risk

All health assessments and consequent actions have inherent risks attached for all the stakeholders. The key question in this dimension of assessment is 'What can go wrong?'. The World Bank (2002) proposed five risk categories, which would be equally valid for the health assessor. By taking these categories as a basis for discussion here, a new set of five categories has been adopted:

- vulnerability
- community risk
- institutional risk
- iatrogenic risk
- political-economic risk.

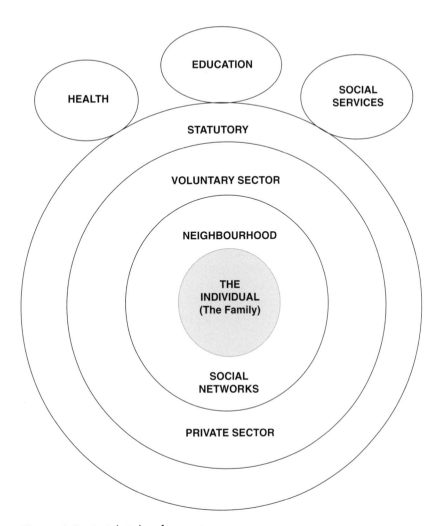

Figure 8.3 Social circles of support

Vulnerability

Healthcare professionals may already be dealing with individuals and groups who could be classed as vulnerable or at risk. A planned assessment of health need should throw into sharp focus the dimensions of vulnerability and the risks associated with the identified need, care intervention or non-intervention. Furthermore, the assessment process itself can be viewed as interventionist and has the potential to stir up all sorts of reactions within the patient; for example, the assessment of patients with psychosocial difficulties associated with forms of abuse/incest within the family or community. Wilson (1998) illustrates how a frequent finding in inquiries into failures of mental health services both here and overseas is a lack of robust risk assessment and management.

Community risk

The potential risk factors associated with people who have severe and enduring mental illnesses in the community and their 'lack of social skills' mean they are in danger of social exclusion. This can lead to further disengagement and non-compliance in these clients. It is against this backdrop that Ford & McClelland (2002) argue that risk is and will always be the most important consideration when addressing care in the community for people with severe and enduring mental illness. The assessor would need to be mindful of this and other potential risks associated with such an exploration.

It is important to examine how these risks can be managed within the total health assessment. Risks may be associated with specific environmental factors such as high density or poor housing. Earlier in this chapter it was outlined how these factors can lead to higher rates of childhood accidents, for example. Risks associated with social disengagement or dysfunctional engagement and exclusion (forced or self-imposed) would also have to be identified. Some community assertive outreach teams employ risk assessment with the use of risk profiling and individual relapse signatures for patients. If these are linked to appropriate contingency planning then risk can potentially be managed effectively. There is an argument that contingency planning could be widened to incorporate other patients where the social risks are at a level that would cause concern. There can also be risks associated with the advice generated from the assessment that may affect the existing social infrastructures such as family and family relationships or dynamics, employment and social/leisure engagement.

Institutional risk

As services develop within the modernisation initiatives associated with the new NHS, there are significant risks linked to these institutional changes. There is a need for all assessors to have clear understanding about the services that may be required for the patient. If there is a lack of understanding then risks can be created through inappropriate referral or inaccurate interpretations of existing support. For example, as 'intermediate care teams' (ICT) emerged to support patients within the community, there was a need for their working practices and protocols to be fully understood by assessors who may need information from them as part of the assessment or information about the remit of the service so they can refer appropriately. The dilemma facing practitioners here is that, by their own admission, the members of the ICT were also coming to terms with what was in reality an evolving service. One consequence of this evolution was that protocols were constantly being amended and in some cases written from scratch because of the uniqueness of the service environment. Furthermore, all the tensions highlighted earlier in the section discussing institutional rules and behaviours about interagency working can equally apply here.

Iatrogenic risk

This type of risk is related to those problems generated by the professional intervention itself. We have already mentioned the fact that the actual intervention of assessment can stir up a whole range of reactions in the patient. Risk analysis is not a risk-free process. For example, the assessment may be performed poorly with a lack of insight into key personal or community stress triggers. This can have a detrimental effect on the patient. This is always a possibility when you are dealing with an unknown; indeed, the whole assessment process is based upon a starting position which is one of a relatively unknown quantity.

Political-economic risk

These are risks posed by the prevailing political and economic conditions affecting the patient's community, which can hamper the availability of health resources. Slevin (2003) suggests that globalisation in itself poses a significant social risk driven by predominantly economic factors. He uses the example of major disasters to illustrate his point, such as the Chernobyl atomic energy accident, which was manmade. The assessor should develop 'a greater sense of watchfulness in respect of potential or emerging risks and in particular the sudden threats of disaster or terrorist attack' (p822). The social environment within which patients live can also be influential here. For example, those living close to chemical or nuclear plants may be classed as more at risk. In addition, there is the risk of scapegoating particular ethnic groups in the wake of incidents or in times of terrorist threat. Other broad issues that should be considered include the social, economic and environmental costs of progress and the advances of science, for example:

- scientific advances that have a direct detrimental effect on the global environment, such as greenhouse gas emissions
- water fluoridisation
- the growth and then decline in the use of pesticides
- nuclear science
- the sometimes unscrupulous actions and impact of transnational corporations
- the threat of global disease transmissions, such as HIV and more recently avian influenza and severe acute respiratory syndrome (SARS).

Activity

• What are the current global/national and local political issues that are having an impact upon health and social care provision?

The levels of social assessment

So far within this chapter we have explored the entry points or dimensions of social enquiry. These factors and inter-related components within these dimensions can be explored from various levels. The levels outlined here are based on the work of Stimson *et al.* (2003) within *The Rapid Assessment and Response Technical Guide* (TGRAR). TGRAR suggests that the levels of assessment mentioned for each entry point discussed are significant. Factors discussed at each entry point could impact on the social state of the client. The questions posed below do not form an exhaustive list and it is suggested that they may be used as a starting point for a more detailed social assessment.

Outlined below are the types of information and questions to consider during social assessment of a client.

The individual level

• Age
• Gender
• Address and type of accommodation
• Type of work (social class)
• Ethnicity
• Culture
• Religion
• Marital status
• Next of kin/any children/family members
• What kind of lifestyle does the patient lead?
• Does the client drink alcohol? If so, how much and how often?
• Does the client smoke cigarettes? If so, how many daily?
• Is the client stigmatised or marginalised because of their health problem/s or behaviour or the group to which they belong?
• Does the client's health problem affect their social and economic role in society?
• Do those health problems lead to greater need for social, economic and other support?
• Is there discrimination in terms of access to resources such as healthcare, housing, welfare and job opportunities' often referred to as the 'postcode lottery'.

- Does the client engage in illegal activity and do they and others suffer as a consequence?
- Are there consequences for their interpersonal relations with family and friends?

The community level

- How do community norms affect or exacerbate the social consequences of health behaviour, health problems or particular groups?
- What is the influence of community settings and contexts (such as housing, neighbourhoods where people live)?
- How are communities affected by the health problem or behaviour?
- What are the social consequences for families (including children) and friends, e.g. economic and social resources needed?
- What are the social consequences for other people and the wider community?

The structural level

- What is the social impact of local and national policies on the client?
- Is the client subject to special legal or other interventions because of their health problem, behaviour or status?
- Is the client offered special additional support and welfare benefits?
- What is the impact of the social, economic and legal environment on the client?
- What is the significance of public attitudes on the health problem or the population group?

Summary

Within this chapter we have examined the social dimensions of the nursing and health assessment processes. A framework for social analysis has been proposed that can form the basis for a comprehensive examination of nursing need. The assessment can be explored on three levels: the level of the individual, the level of community and finally on a structural level related to societal institutions and organisation. The current health and social care policy agenda within the UK is aimed at providing a more integrated approach to the care of patients and making real progress in tackling the major health problems affecting the population. In addition, there is a significant attempt to address the problems associated with all the aspects of social exclusion that can be so damaging to the health of individuals and communities alike.

References

Busby, C & Scott Cato, M (1997) Death rates from leukaemia are higher than expected in areas around nuclear sites in Berkshire and Oxfordshire. *BMJ* 315: 309.

Cahill, J (1998) Patient participation: a review of the literature. *Journal of Clinical Nursing* 7: 119–28.

Department of Health (1989) *Working for Patients*. HMSO, London.

Department of Health (1990) *The NHS and Community Care Act*. HMSO, London.

Department of Health (1997) *The New NHS: modern, dependable*. HMSO, London.

Department of Health (2000a) *National Service Framework for Older People*. HMSO, London.

Department of Health (2000b) *Saving Lives: Our Healthier Nation*. HMSO, London.

Department of Health (2000c) *The NHS Plan*. HMSO, London.

Department of Health/Social Services Inspectorate (1991) *Care Management and Assessment. Practitioner's guide*. HMSO, London.

Edelmann, R (2000) *Psychosocial Aspects of the Healthcare Process*. Prentice Hall, Harlow.

Ford, K & McClelland, N (2002) Assertive outreach: development of a working model. *Nursing Standard* 16 (23): 41–4.

Ford, P & McCormack, B (1999) Determining older people's need for registered nursing in continuing healthcare: the contribution of the Royal College of Nursing's Older People Assessment Tool. *Journal of Clinical Nursing* 8 (6): 731–42.

Leathard, A (2000) *Health Care Provision: past, present and into the 21st century* 2nd edition. Stanley Thornes, Cheltenham.

Lewis, J & Glennerster, H (1996) *Implementing the New Community Care*. Open University Press, Buckingham.

Lockwood, A & Marshall, M (1999) Can a standardized needs assessment be used to improve the care of people with severe mental disorders? A pilot study of 'needs feedback'. *Journal of Advanced Nursing*. 30 (6): 1408–15.

Meredith, B (1993) *The Community Care Handbook*: the new system explained. Age Concern, London.

Miller, C, Freeman, M & Ross, N (2001) *Interprofessional Practice in Health and Social Care*. Arnold, London.

Naidoo, J & Wills, J (2000) *Health Promotion: foundations for practice*. Baillière Tindall, London.

National Statistics (2004) *Social Trends: United Kingdom*. Stationery Office, London.

Neuman, B (1995) *The Neuman Systems Model*, 3rd edition. Appleton and Lange, Norwalk, Connecticut.

Orem, D (2001) *Nursing: concepts of practice*, 6th edition. Mosby, St Louis.

Philippe, M & Whittaker, N (2004) Stroke. In: Whittaker, N (ed.) *Disorders and Interventions*. Palgrave, Macmillan, Basingstoke.

Rogers, M E (1989). Nursing: a science of unitary human beings. In: Riehl-Sisca, J P (ed.) *Conceptual Models for Nursing Practice*, 3rd edition. Appleton and Lange, Norwalk, Connecticut.

Roper, N, Logan, W W & Tierney, A J (2000) *The Roper, Logan, Tierney Model of Nursing*. Churchill Livingstone, Edinburgh.

Roy, C (2005) *The Roy Adaptation Model*, 3rd edition. Prentice Hall, New York.

Slevin, O (2003) Global dimensions: nursing in the risk society. In: Basford, L & Slevin, O (eds) *Theory and Practice of Nursing: an integrated approach to caring practice*, 2nd edition. Nelson Thornes, Cheltenham.

Stimson, G, Donoghoe, M, Fitch, C, Rhodes, T, Ball, A & Weiler, G (2003) *Rapid Assessment and Response Technical Guide Version 1.0*. Department of Child and Adolescent Health and Development, and Department of HIV/AIDS, World Health Organisation, Geneva.

Townsend, P, Davidson, N & Whitehead, M (1988) *Inequalities in Health. The Black Report and the health divide*. Penguin, Harmondsworth.

Vernon, S, Ross, F & Gould, M (2000) Assessment of older people: politics and practice in primary care. *Journal of Advanced Nursing* 31 (2): 282–7.

Waterworth, S & Luker, K (1996) Reluctant collaborators: do patients want to be involved in the decisions concerning care? *Journal of Advanced Nursing* 15 (8): 971–6.

Wilson, J (1998) *Guidelines for Clinical Risk Assessment and Management in Mental Health Services*. Ministry of Health for New Zealand, New Zealand.

World Bank Group (2002) *Social Analysis Electronic Sourcebook*. www.theworldbank.org.

Psychological assessment

J. H. Parkes

Learning objectives

- Define such concepts as the 'self', the 'self-concept', 'self-esteem' and 'personality'.
- Outline the range of possible explanations for conducting a psychological assessment.
- Discuss the possible causes of poor psychological functioning, including stress and anxiety.
- Describe the nurse's role in supporting the individual who may feel unable to cope with stress or a possible change in lifestyle.
- Explain how to practically and objectively conduct the psychological assessment.

Introduction

Humans are fully interconnected biopsychosocial, cultural and spiritual beings and a perceived threat to one dimension can have direct implications in the other areas of their life. This chapter will examine the importance of conducting an assessment of psychological functioning and the aspects that should be included in such an activity. The aims are to address these key aspects of the assessment process, with particular focus on the emotional, cognitive and behavioural dimensions of the individual.

What is psychological health?

The beliefs of holistic philosophy advocate that individuals have physical, emotional, intellectual, sociocultural and spiritual dimensions to their being, which constantly interact with each other and the environment surrounding them (Sivik, 2000; Spurgeon, 2002). These dimensions are separate, yet interconnected. People live in a social and cultural context, subject to their own cognitions, emotions and behaviour, and biology. In each of these aspects, individuals engage in a dynamic 'homeostatic' process to maintain 'equilibrium'. This status of balance and harmony is where the body is trying to maintain the stability of its internal world in the face of environmental changes and internal demands.

Arguments have been presented concerning the correlation between lifestyle, health and illness. Among other researchers, Vanitallie (2002) has strongly argued that stress can cause illness (or at least be a significant contributing factor) and that its alleviation is probably instrumental in recovery. It would appear from the results of some research that both physical and mental illness might, to an extent, have their causes in stressful life events (Cohen *et al.*, 1998; Marnocha, 1999; Mizoguchi *et al.*, 2000; Paykel, 2000). It has also been suggested that there is a correlation between psychiatric disorder and psychological distress and coronary heart disease (Stansfeld *et al.*, 2002).

Illness itself can exact a demanding toll from patients and their carers, from worrying about the symptoms they are experiencing, through to receiving a diagnosis and facing possible treatment. The potential ramifications of experiencing 'illness' range from temporary discomfort and disability through to significant lifestyle changes. People may experience fear, anger, pain, loss, disability, anxiety, frustration and even depression. They may experience difficulties in their personal relationships, financial pressures and changes in their roles and responsibilities and may suffer from loss of self-esteem. Different people will face such crises in different ways, depending on previous experience, current sources of social support and personal resources.

Activity

- Write down some situations that have caused you to become stressed.
- What coping strategies did you use to 'help' you in these situations? Were they effective?
- Ask a friend whether they have been in similar situations and what coping strategies they used.
- Were there any differences between the coping strategies that were used?

Having carried out the activities above, you will have noted differences in the way individuals react to crisis. Not all individuals will hide behind a personal defence mechanism or experience some traumatic psychological challenge as a result of being faced with such personal threat. Allport (1963, 1968) suggested that the vast majority of people will face most problems 'head on' and will only evoke personal defence mechanisms in exceptional circumstances.

All individuals are challenged with personal difficulties throughout life and generally learn to adapt and cope in the face of adversity. However, on occasions our personal support systems may prove inadequate and ineffective and psychological distress may be the result. Psychologic homeostasis has been altered and the satisfaction of psychological needs is being threatened. Emotional stress can cause people to feel anxious, fearful, overwhelmed and not in personal control. If such feelings become prolonged and/or intensify, the individual may suffer psychological crisis. While, in many cases, such experiences are self-limiting and most will progress through the stages of adaptation successfully, on occasion the individual may 'stall' in a particular phase of adaptation or may embark on a maladaptive path towards resolution. It has been suggested that nursing intervention is indicated when stress caused by biological, psychological, family or medical care stressors leads to ineffective coping (Gammon, 1998; Rustoen & Hanestad, 1998).

Why conduct a psychological assessment?

Nurses, and to some extent other healthcare professionals, are expected to monitor the psychological, social, cultural, physical and spiritual responses of the clients and their family to illness. Nursing preparation in particular includes a unique core of knowledge about biopsychosocial responses to illness. This theoretical and experiential base can then be used to assess clients' coping strategies and intervene therapeutically when ineffective coping is occurring due to the presence of actual or potential psychological risk factors (Davidhizar & Newman-Giger, 1998).

Additionally, nursing is about helping and caring for the client, whether it is in a hospital ward or in their own home. As a practice, its purpose and philosophy are fundamentally based on the therapeutic patient–nurse relationship (Freshwater, 2002). It is an interpersonal activity, which clearly relies on good communication and interpersonal skills.

If the activities of the nurse practitioner are explored more fully, a number of aspects can be identified as explicit to the role:

- talking with and listening to patients, assessing patients
- giving and receiving information during ward handovers

- educating patients about their health, helping individuals cope with their worries
- carrying out or assisting individuals with physical activities, such as personal hygiene and comfort (Whiting, 1999).

Further examination of these activities highlights the fact that there is a psychological dimension to patient care giving, alongside the physical aspects of care and treatment. This clearly illustrates the concern that nurses should be able to integrate and demonstrate both psychological and social as well as physical, spiritual and cultural knowledge in their assessment and care of the client.

By forming relationships with the patients in their care, the nurse will be best placed to identify not only that patient who can marshal personal coping strategies when faced with emotional stress but also those who are displaying ineffective methods of coping and/or abnormal neurological functioning. It has been suggested that with good interpersonal skills, empathy and support, the nurse may avoid or prevent emotional crisis and may even be able to reverse the pre-crisis types of maladaptive processes such as depression, anxiety and other signs of inadequate coping. With an astute and thorough psychological assessment as part of the admission and ongoing evaluation of the individual's care, the maladaptive process can be identified, recognised and properly treated. This forms the fundamental basis for the psychological assessment, to determine if the individual understands the nature of the healthcare process and the information that is being given to them, and can make decisions about their healthcare accordingly.

What to assess

The discussion which follows will briefly outline those aspects of all human beings which will need to be explored by the nurse practitioner, when conducting a psychological assessment. The emotional, cognitive and behavioural facets of human character will be explored, with the intention of extending the clinician's knowledge base concerning the psychological functioning and well-being of the clients in their care.

Personality

When people are asked what 'psychology' is actually about, they will frequently respond that it is the study of 'personality'. We use this term extensively in everyday interactions; we may refer to people as having a 'pleasant' or difficult' personality. Yet, when we try to explore this concept further, it seems very difficult to define. Most people agree that it is closely linked to the concept of 'self' and that, in the process of 'self-discovery', we try to uncover and understand the nature of our 'personality'. As with the 'self', a number of theories have been offered to explain and describe the characteristics of 'personality' but it remains a difficult concept to grasp. The study of personality has been the focus of several eminent and seminal theorists in the field of psychology (Allport, 1963; Eysenck, 1967; Freud, 1933). It is their work that forms the basis for this chapter.

It is generally accepted that the 'personality' is a unique pattern of thoughts, feelings and behaviours that characterise an individual and influence the way the person interacts with their environment. It is that set of characteristics which distinguishes us from each other. Less agreement seems to have been reached on whether it is a 'constant' and 'consistent' aspect of the individual, which remains fixed in any set of circumstances or over time. One group of theories have suggested that the 'personality' is genetically transmitted and remains fairly static throughout life (Eysenck, 1967; Cattell, 2002); however, others argue that we acquire our personalities as we interact with and learn from other people during our life (Allport, 1963). It is probably true that some aspects of 'personality' are acquired at birth, temperament and physical characteristics for example, but equally possible that other aspects of our 'personality' are acquired through the process of socialisation.

The concept of 'personality' is particularly relevant in the context of healthcare, as an individual's personality to an extent determines their reaction to and even the nature of their illness. In 1987, Friedman & Booth-Kewley found a clear link that personality may affect health. They suggested that people with high levels of anxiety, depression and anger/hostility seemed to be prone to developing a variety of illnesses, particularly heart disease. Kobasa *et al.* (1982) have also argued that individuals who exhibit specific personality traits, frequently referred to as 'hardiness', such as commitment, control and a willingness to respond to change, may be 'protected' by those characteristics from high rates of physical illness. This has been supported by research carried out by Taylor *et al.* (2000), who found that psychological beliefs such as 'optimism, personal control, and a sense of meaning' are protective of not only mental health' but also physical health. Their programme of research into 'the implications of cognitive adaptation theory and research on positive illusions for the relation of positive beliefs to disease progression among men infected with HIV' found that 'even unrealistic optimistic beliefs about the future may be health protective'. This reinforces the idea that the concept of 'control' does appear to be an important factor in understanding the relationship between stressful experience, behaviour and health, an issue we will return to later.

The self-concept

The idea of the 'self-concept' is closely related to the existence of our 'personality'. It develops over time and is 'shaped' by external influences, such as the feedback we receive from significant others and comparing ourselves to those around us. It is a set of ideas we discover about ourselves; what we are, who we are and what we are like. It incorporates the way we perceive ourselves to be physically (body image), how we value and measure our abilities and achievements (self-esteem) and the person we would like to be (ideal self). The major components of 'self-image' are our knowledge of our personality, our body image and our knowledge of what we do. Throughout life, we interact with our environment through a number of roles and relationships; we may be a father, teacher, son, manager or wife. In each of these roles, we may adopt an image, or 'persona', which we present to those we encounter. As the public/professional 'self' begins to dominate, the private true 'self' may shrink and hide from the gaze of others. As we embark on the process of self-discovery, it is often the desire to understand our 'true, real' self that becomes our focus (Burnard, 2004).

Model of the self: public and private worlds

Burnard's model of the 'self' (1990, 2004; Andersen et al., 1998) offers a very clear way of comprehending the interplay between the 'public' and 'private' worlds of people (see Figure 9.1).

The public self

Behaviour, being the 'public' world, is the method by which we convey our inner 'private' world, such as thoughts and feelings, to the people around us and we communicate these insights through both verbal and non-verbal means. Verbal means would include the way we speak and the words we choose to use, the speed and tone of our conversation and the manner in which we communicate. We learn to read another person's message through their words but also through their non-verbal communication such as eye contact, facial expressions, physical proximity, bodily posture, volume of speech and hand movements. While we must always be aware of cultural variation, we can still 'read' another's feelings through both their verbal and non-verbal expressions of feelings. As previously suggested, 'basic' emotions appear to be a universal form of human language. Even when the specific understanding of what is being said eludes us, due to it being expressed in a different language, we seem to be able to recognise when someone is happy or sad.

The private inner self

The 'private' world constitutes our cognitive and emotional being. Thoughts are frequently described as cognitive or mental processes and include problem solving, decision making and ideas, whereas feelings can be described as happiness, grief, love and anger. These basic emo-

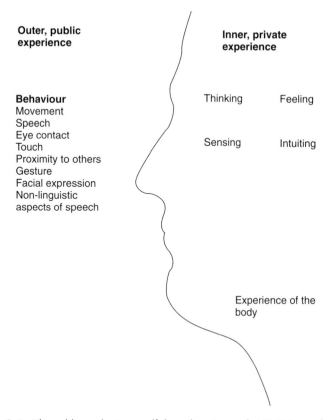

Figure 9.1 The public and private self (based on Burnard, 1990) (reproduced with permission from Heinemann Professional Publishing)

tions are apparently universal and can be found in all cultures to similar degrees. However, Burnard (1990) stresses that dimensions of thinking, feeling and behaving are intimately linked and clearly overlap and as such we should consider them in their totality.

Feelings would include the expressions of emotion, anger, grief, fear and embarrassment, and according to Burnard (2004), to express these feelings is entirely healthy. Suppressed emotions can influence normal psychological functioning, through the distortion of cognitive thought processing. Part of becoming 'self-aware' involves exploring our own emotional aspects, as well as reflecting on the way we think and behave. By recognising these elements of our own 'being', we can begin to recognise these processes in those around us. It is a skill that can be enhanced through training and forms the basis of all observational practices, particularly within nursing. Being able to accurately interpret the thoughts, feelings and actions of the people receiving care is clearly a core skill in the healthcare environment.

The 'experience of the body'

The Burnard (1990, 2004) model talks about 'the experience of the body', which is the inseparable link between mental activity and its effect on the body, and vice versa. Burnard suggests that information we glean from our body can enable us to appreciate something about our psychological status. Some have suggested that the 'self' is a separate entity from the physical body. However, the physical aspects of self very much influence our 'body image' and perception of 'self' and therefore cannot be seen as separate. How others see us and how we view ourselves are very much based on how we see ourselves to be physically. One only has to look at people who experience anorexia to see how much 'body image' is a part of psychological well-being.

Positive 'self-concept'

It has been suggested that the development of a positive 'self-concept' and 'self-esteem' can be instrumental in assisting the individual to cope with life's events and challenges. 'Self-esteem' can be described as a sense of personal worth and incorporates a number of significant factors, which converge to form the 'whole'. These are intelligence, competence, degree of emotional adjustment and popularity. If we consider ourselves to be able to successfully think, solve problems and offer appropriate answers and responses, then we may consider ourselves to be 'competent'. These achievements, together with demonstrating emotional stability in the face of stress and crisis, may result in admiration, affection and validation from those around us. Questions which focus on whether we like ourselves, consider ourselves to have a valuable role and purpose in society and how successful we are form the basis of our 'self-esteem'.

Activity

- List the types of disorders and medical interventions that can affect self-concept.
- Select one example from your own field of practice and suggest the type of data that you might collect to assess the impact of the disorder or intervention on the client.

Anxiety, stress and coping

As we have discovered, we all respond to life's events and experiences in different ways and to varying degrees. We all experience 'anxiety' because it is a normal reaction to perceived threats. We all adopt a range of different strategies to manage and handle the stressful situations we find ourselves in and sometimes we 'cope' and sometimes our personal resources seem to have been completely depleted. We all have different personalities, vary in our levels of social support and are shaped by our upbringing, education and relationships. So, as individuals, we differ in our reaction and response to stress. The question that arises is when does our 'normal' reaction to life's difficulties become 'abnormal' and 'out of character', and what effect does it have on our 'normal psychological functioning'?

Fear is an emotion which usually triggers a number of bodily changes, including rapid heartbeat and breathing, dryness of the throat and mouth, perspiration, trembling and a sinking feeling in the stomach. Most of these physiological changes occur during emotional arousal and result from the activation of the sympathetic nervous system as it prepares the body for emergency action (Atkinson *et al.*, 2003). Feeling 'frightened' can be the emotional response to anything that is a potential threat to either our own personal well-being or the well-being of those around us. The number of potential threats to a person's physical or psychological well-being is extensive, some of which may be encountered as 'actual' threats while others may remain as only perceived threats. A reaction to these triggers always seems to occur in three phases: perception of a threat, physiological response and awareness of the emotion.

The production of 'anxiety' is the natural and relatively common response when we consider ourselves to be under threat, whether perceived or actual harm. As a construct, it describes aspects of the individual's internal state, the experience of negative affect and physiological arousal and it manifests itself in the individual's behavioural response to the potentially frightening scenario (Cox, 2002; Davison & Neale, 2001). In 1990, Peplau provided the following comprehensive framework of the construct, which remains useful in succinctly presenting the complexity of this naturally occurring phenomenon:

- a subjective affective (emotional) experience – uneasiness, dread, apprehension, etc.
- is an energy that cannot be observed directly – what is noticed are its effects
- is triggered cognitively by an input of real or imagined, internal or external, personal or situational material, perceived as a threat
- is an immediate physiological reaction (as described earlier)
- is an awareness of apprehension, felt discomfort and physiological reactions, often in the absence of awareness of the precise nature of 'cause'
- is adaptive, in the sense that it warns of impending threat to survival, particularly the survival of the self system
- occurs in different degrees
- may reflect a predisposition in families.

Generalised anxiety is viewed as a response to the inability to cope with many everyday occurrences. People who experience generalised anxiety tend to be unrealistic in their appraisal of the situation, especially where the danger is remote. This constant feeling of 'threat' means that the autonomic nervous system is frequently in a state of heightened arousal and readiness. The person will experience unwanted and repetitive intrusive thoughts that are difficult to extinguish. This can lead to the individual engaging in ritualistic and obsessive behaviour, in an attempt to neutralise these destructive and sometimes abhorrent thoughts.

In phobic behaviour, the individual's anxiety is not precipitated by any particular set of circumstances, as in the case of 'free-floating', generalised anxiety, but is triggered by a specific object or situation, such as spiders or flying. In such cases, the person's 'phobia' endures because they engage in extreme and elaborate behaviours to avoid the stimulus of their anxiety; therefore, they are prevented from dispelling their fear.

Individuals employ a variety of approaches to cope with stressful situations: stress avoidance strategies such as 'defence mechanisms' (see Box 9.1), problem-focused strategies that are designed to actively change the situation and finally, emotion-focused approaches, which help them to manage the distress (Jungbauer & Angermeyer, 2003; Lazarus, 1998; Rosche et al., 2004).

It has been suggested that the use of internal and unconscious drives to repress unacceptable or 'threatening' impulses can be a contributory factor in the development of more stable anxiety disorders and also in depression. Such thoughts are perceived as potentially threatening to self-esteem, and possibly relationships with those around us, if verbally expressed. The individual does not easily explain these unconscious feelings of anxiety and apprehension, as they are usually in the process of employing techniques of psychological protection, such as the defence mechanism.

Box 9.1 presents the defence mechanisms initially isolated and described by Sigmund Freud (1933), which were subsequently elaborated and summarised by his daughter, Anna (Freud, 1993). A similar process occurs in the case of depression, which has been described as a pervasive lowered mood. This altering of affect (mood) tends to represent a reaction to loss. The original loss can be the withdrawal of parental affection towards a child, which is later triggered by a more recent loss, such as loss of role, employment or a relationship. People who are experiencing such loss may experience anger towards the object of loss, repress their feelings and consequently alienate those closest to them. Finally, it has been argued that low self-esteem and feelings of worthlessness associated with depression stem from a child-like need for approval and the later loss merely triggers the regressive behaviour of the individual to an earlier state.

Box 9.1 Defence mechanisms, based on Sigmund Freud's work (1933) and elaborated on by his daughter, Anna (Freud, 1993).

- Repression
  - 'An unconscious mechanism that keeps thoughts that might provoke anxiety out of our conscious mind' (Banyard, 1996: p33)
- Displacement
  - Choosing to take your feelings out on someone or something else, because you are unable to express them to the appropriate person, e.g. kicking the car
- Denial
  - When something is too frightening or upsetting, the person refuses to acknowledge that it exists
- Suppression
  - A deliberate effort to put a stressful memory out of one's mind
- Projection
  - This is an unconscious process where the individual describes how another is overtly displaying the feelings and behaviours that they are subconsciously feeling themselves
- Rationalisation
  - Offering apparently reasonable explanations for actions which arise from emotions in an attempt to limit painful feelings or disappointment
- Intellectualisation
  - Consists of dealing with or confronting a stressor on an abstract intellectual level
- Sublimation
  - Redirecting negative and potentially destructive personal energies into socially acceptable and constructive activities, e.g. sport and exercise
- Regression
  - Reverting back to behaviour associated with earlier stages of human development, i.e. childhood (Gross, 1996)

People also utilise a range of external resources in managing stress and anxiety, such as social support, financial and material resources, and intrapersonal resources, such as personal qualities and self-esteem. People who feel they can control the situation, can make choices, have robust support mechanisms and have 'hardiness' in terms of personality seem to cope with life's difficulties more successfully than those who feel that life controls them, who are isolated and have no choices.

'Healthy' psychological functioning not only concerns our ability to cope with stress but also includes our motivation, motor ability, intellectual development, perception, speech, personality, decision-making ability and many other aspects of 'self'. If a person is physically and mentally healthy, all psychological functions will work to promote a sense of well-being. The person will feel emotionally stable, aware of who they are, where they are and what time of day it is. They will be able to concentrate and focus on activities they are engaged in, such as working, driving or reading. They will be able to plan, make decisions, solve problems, have ideas, be creative and reflective. The individual will be able to remember previous experiences and recall earlier life events. Finally, the person will be able to maintain a social life, as observed through their ability to sustain a variety of roles, responsibilities and relationships. Unfortunately, however, normal psychological functioning does falter on occasions and the individual is faced with the need to cope and adapt. It is important for the nurse to recognise when an individual is experiencing increased mental stress, in the face of psychological trauma.

How to conduct the psychological assessment

At the outset of any patient's journey through the healthcare process, the holistic assessment should form the cornerstone of their diagnosis, care and treatment. The needs of the patient/client should be at the heart of any form of this process. Trying to identify those needs, and address them appropriately, is the whole essence of this aspect of the nursing process. In order to elicit this information as accurately, honestly, objectively and swiftly as possible, the practitioner must create a safe environment, where the individual can feel respected, worthwhile, valued and secure. The nurse must employ a range of communications and intrapersonal skills to build up as complete a picture as possible of the person before them. They must listen, question, empathise, support and document the information offered, in as unbiased, caring and accurate a way as possible.

Nurses' role in assessment

'Although assessment may involve a wide range of functions, in nursing the assessment may seek an answer to the question 'what does it mean to be this person?'. (Barker, 2004: p6)

Assessment is about seeing the client in front of you as a unique individual with a life and relationships outside the clinical setting. The assessment should seek to understand that particular individual and how they are coping with their needs and difficulties. Any holistic assessment should take account of strengths, weaknesses, threats and opportunities (SWOT analysis) and should include a robust personality and coping profile of the patient.

The practitioner needs to develop not only the skill of assessing the person presenting before them, with their own personality, behavioural traits, attitudes, emotions and past experiences, but also the awareness of their own feelings, thoughts and actions. The nurse needs to be able to form an objective estimation of the patient's personality and how they may react to a variety of different situations while remaining 'in tune' with their own attitudes, emotions and behaviour. The nurse–patient relationship is fundamentally an interpersonal process that takes place between two unique beings. The psychological assessment is about measuring the characteristics that different people have in common and plays an important role in telling us how one person differs from another. It tells us what makes each person unique.

The assessment process

The assessment of the client's holistic requirements is about much more than just addressing their physical needs. This process of information gathering will include the collection of data concerning their physical well-being but also a comprehensive investigation of their social, cultural, spiritual and psychological functioning. As we have constantly maintained throughout this text, the individual before us operates on multidimensional levels and these dimensions are fully integrated to form the 'whole' being. Therefore, the same credence should be given to assessing and supporting the person psychologically as caring for and treating them physically.

The psychological assessment is vitally important for several reasons. The first is to clearly exclude any physical factors which may be directly impacting on the individual's speech, memory, concentration, balance, perception, attitude and behaviour. This may include pain, medication, physical illness, mental illness, non-prescribed drugs and alcohol. The assessment process also informs us of the needs of potentially vulnerable groups and may help us to ascertain the individual's ability to cope with the impact of illness and the prospect of disability and lifestyle change. Finally, the ultimate goal of the psychological assessment is to determine whether the patient is capable of understanding and making decisions about their healthcare and whether caring relationships and a positive 'self-concept' are being preserved (Lyke, 1992).

Objectivity: validity and reliability

The assessment of psychological needs differs from the assessment of physical needs and these differences pose a number of associated problems. The first is that the nurse may experience difficulty in being objective. The successful appraisal of a patient's psychological needs is founded on the nurse's ability to attend to their thoughts and feelings and observe their appearance and behaviour without forming any judgements, making any inferences or drawing any premature conclusions. The documented information must be devoid of any bias. Milne (1993) defines bias as taking 'many forms, such as selectively attending to certain parts of a client's behaviour while ignoring others, because one expects to observe certain things'. The nurse may also encounter hurdles when forming impressions of clients' statements and behaviour. The client may have difficulty expressing their concerns and feelings. For a variety of reasons, clients may try to conceal their fear, pain or discomfort and may adopt a 'mask' of coping even though, internally, their emotions may be in turmoil. On such occasions, some clients may also appear to be very awkward, frustrating and even aggressive. There may be a variety of explanations why clients exhibit behaviour that at times may appear socially unacceptable, which may include physical illness, mental disorder, pain, fear and medication, and the nurse must strive to keep an open mind and investigate the possible causes of such behaviour.

As well as ensuring that the assessment of the client is objective, the nurse must also ensure that the information is reliable. It is difficult to do this solely using interview techniques but a number of other methods have been developed, largely by psychologists, for trying to measure the individual's thoughts, feelings and behaviour. The options available to the practitioner are psychometric tests (Beck *et al.*, 1961, 1988; Snaith *et al.*, 1982; Zigmund & Snaith, 1983), observation, self-reporting, interview schedules and history taking. During the course of an admission assessment, when both the physical and social needs of the patient will be explored, such complex tools as psychometric tests are unlikely to be used but the practitioner will need to obtain a personal history. In order to obtain a full psychological picture, they will need to interview the client, observing both the client's verbal and non-verbal behaviour. The practitioner must also be constantly reflecting on their own thoughts and feelings. They must constantly monitor both 'self' and 'other' simultaneously, in order to guard against personal opinions and beliefs which may distort their own thinking and so bias the results of the assessment. Equally, the nurse must respect the client's own view of their 'self', as they are in the best position to communicate how they are thinking and feeling. Being able to self-monitor and evaluate in all three psychological dimensions is a significant aspect of the assessment process for both parties engaged in the process – the clinical practitioner and the client.

The interview

The psychological assessment will primarily follow an interview format. This should take place in an environment where the practitioner and patient can feel comfortable and relaxed, free from interruption or distraction. The privacy, dignity and confidentiality of the individual should be protected at all times throughout this process. The person should be able to discuss and disclose their intimate thoughts in a 'psychologically safe' environment and feel that the interviewer can cope with their potentially troubling thoughts and fluctuating emotions.

The admission profile

The interviewer begins by taking some biographical details, using open-ended questions, in order to obtain a picture of the person in front of them. We cannot assess the individual without knowing something of who they are. These personal details, which may have been obtained earlier, will include name, age, sex, marital status, family, religion, domestic situation, occupation, financial status, medical history, personal history and social history. During the psychological phase, we will want to discover something about the person's relationships, work, likes/dislikes, routines and desires. Initially we are trying to create a trusting relationship where we get to know the person inside the 'patient'. Barker (2004) stresses that the history should never be a routine administrative chore: 'it should aim to search out something about the real person'.

Taking the personal history

The second phase of the psychological interview will aim to explore the psychological functioning of the individual: their emotional, cognitive and behavioural dimensions of 'self'. It should be stressed here that this assessment is not designed to be an extensive psychological examination. It is intended to inform the student clinical practitioner how to conduct an assessment of normal psychological functioning, in an attempt to identify any psychological maladaption. It is to be expected that the individual may experience chronic emotional stress as a result of their perceived personal health threat and therefore altered mood and some behavioural changes. But this assessment will not suffice where there is evidence of a severe functional psychiatric condition. If such a presentation is thought to be evident, the inexperienced practitioner should refer to a more senior professional.

In order to complete this phase of the interview, it may be helpful for the nurse to use a similar format to the Mini-Mental State Examination (Folstein et al., 1975; Green, 1996; Puri et al., 2002). The headings used in the Mini-Mental State Examination are shown in Box 9.2. The following discussion concerning the assessment of the individual's cognitive, emotional and behavioural functioning will be based on this structure.

The aim of this assessment is to elicit signs of psychological distress, which will allow us to distinguish organic brain syndromes, physical conditions which may impact on psychological functioning, intoxication and mental disorders, and provide us with evidence of abnormal psychological functioning.

Appearance

Begin with a description of the individual's physical presentation: height, weight, build, hair colour and how the person is dressed. It may

---

> **Box 9.2** Components of the Mini-Mental State Examination (based on Folstein *et al.*, 1975).
>
> - Appearance
> - Behaviour
> - Manner
> - Speech
> - Mood
> - Thought
> - Cognition
> - Insight
> - Language
> - Level of consciousness

include attention to personal hygiene, condition of clothes and application of make-up. We must be very careful to keep our observations factual and avoid value-ladened terminology. Evidence of self-neglect may point towards dementia-type conditions or a depressive mood, while inappropriate levels of dress may indicate a more chaotic thought process. When taking note of appearance, the practitioner should also observe how the individual interacts during the assessment process. The appropriateness of eye contact, appearing distracted, general posture, appearing relaxed or tense, and ability and willingness to converse should also be recorded as objectively as possible.

Behaviour
The individual's behaviour may appear entirely appropriate to the situation or they may present as agitated, distressed, bizarre or confused. Some individuals may sit and quietly and concisely answer the questions asked, others may pace the room, some may be tearful, while others may seem to respond to a third person in the room when no one else is present. It is important to record the individual's behaviour factually, including their gestures, mannerisms, posture and ability to interact.

Manner
Many individuals are co-operative during the assessment process but some refuse or are unable to speak. Some individuals are suspicious, guarded or hostile to the questions being asked. Sometimes it may be extremely difficult to establish a rapport with the individual; this may be because they refuse to make eye contact with you or to answer your questions. On occasion, some individuals may appear overfriendly and familiar with you, or hostile, making the assessment quite a difficult process. It may be necessary to end the assessment at this point or summon assistance in order to continue.

Speech

Issues associated with communication have been addressed in some detail during the course of this text but it is important to stress here that the manner in which individuals communicate with each other can indicate a lot about their thoughts and feelings. It can provide tremendous insights into how psychologically stressed or disordered somebody is. In terms of speech, it is critical that the assessor takes note of the tone, pitch, speed and content of what is being expressed. Somebody who is depressed may appear slow to answer questions, withdrawn, negative, tearful, guilty and lacking hope. In some conditions, such as mania, speech may appear to be 'pressured' (speeded up), may rhyme and may appear crammed full of ideas, which may not always appear realistic. If speech seems chaotic, 'made up', not based in reality, lacking insight and in response to external stimuli (such as a third person who is not present), the person may be experiencing a psychotic episode or an organic disorder.

Mood

The term 'mood' has been defined as 'a pervasive and sustained emotion that, in the extreme, markedly colours the person's perception of the world' (Puri *et al.*, 2002: p65). All of us are subject to 'moods' all the time, because they are closely linked to our emotions, the way we are feeling. They constantly fluctuate, within a 'normal' range, in response to both internal and external factors which can have a direct impact on the way we are feeling. These factors may include illness, stress, pain, medication, hormones, light and the seasons.

The quality of an individual's mood can be objectively determined during the course of taking the history, by observing their appearance, behaviour, speech and posture. Somebody who is low in mood (anxious or depressed) may appear to be not self-caring, hunched up, avoiding eye contact, slow to respond to questions and talk about 'being unable to cope'. A subjective assessment can be obtained by getting the person to try to describe how they are feeling inside and by asking them about the ideas and thoughts they experience. It is a myth that talking to a suicidal individual will prompt them to act on their ideas of self-harm. In fact, by exploring somebody's ideas and plans of self-destruction, we may be able to identify those that are at risk and refer them to a more appropriate professional accordingly. Finally, the practitioner completing the psychological assessment must be aware of the possibility of incongruence between what the person is describing and their apparent behaviour. Frequently, people may describe themselves as feeling fine when they are clearly in pain or patients may seem awkward and challenging when they are actually frightened or experiencing discomfort, either physically or mentally. We must not make assumptions about appearance without a full assessment and possible physical investigations. As we have discussed previously, people are perfectly able to wear a mask to hide their true self.

Thought

When we talk about the concept of thought, as with speech, we are considering two aspects: form and content. The form of thought is often reflected by speech. If thoughts are chaotic, it is fair to assume that speech will also be difficult to follow or understand. Speech may appear 'pressured' (rapid), which could indicate that the individual's thoughts are racing and tumbling over each other, as in the case of mania. Equally, the person may experience sudden gaps in speech (thought blocking), which may occur due to the sudden intrusion of distressing thoughts, as in the case of schizophrenia, in which the individual may be responding to unseen voices (hallucinations). Individuals may appear preoccupied and withdrawn, concerned with feelings of worthlessness and guilt. It is important to record all thought processes as accurately as possible and without placing any value judgement on what is being verbally expressed. Each response should be written as stated, to avoid misinterpretation or incorrect inferences being drawn.

Cognition

An individual's cognitive assessment is quite a complex aspect to consider and includes their orientation, attention, concentration and memory. Cognitive tests are designed to elicit signs that may point to organic mental illnesses or physical illnesses, which may have a direct influence on the individual's psychological functioning. An example might be the clouding of consciousness due to hallucinations, which may indicate a delirious state (organic brain syndrome) arising from infection or hypoxia (Green, 1996). When exploring an individual's orientation, it is usual to try to ascertain if they are orientated to time, place and person. In organic brain syndromes, this ability is gradually eroded and eventually lost altogether. It is possible to be temporarily disorientated to time, day, place or all three for a number of reasons, including lack of sleep, intoxication or acute illnesses, but generally this function returns on full recovery.

Attention and concentration describe the individual's inability to focus on the task in hand. The person may appear to be easily distracted and unable to maintain their attention on the activity for any length of time. This could be due to a variety of reasons such as anxiety, depression, a psychotic episode or organic brain syndromes and a thorough investigation by trained practitioners is frequently required to ascertain the cause more accurately.

A number of factors can directly influence the way we perceive the world and the people around us. Perception, according to Coon (2004), is 'the process of assembling sensations into a useable mental representation of the world'. This process involves collecting information from our senses (eyes, ears, nose, mouth and touch) so that our brain can interpret and use it. Some of the information is acted on almost instantly but much is stored for future reference in a storage facility known as memory. Memory is clearly associated with the process of learning, where information is gathered, organised and stored for future use. Some information is retained for a very brief period of time, usually seconds (short-term memory); other information may be remembered for years (long-term memory).

Information can also be lost (forgotten) for a variety of reasons but one of the more significant causes is deterioration of the memory itself. Memory loss can occur for a variety of reasons but is quite apparent in dementia, where the function gradually deteriorates over time. In these cases, during the earlier stages, it is usually short-term memory which is lost initially; however, the disease is progressive and eventually most memory functions will fade away.

The final piece of the information-processing puzzle is the concept of intelligence. This aspect of psychological functioning describes the individual's ability to learn. Some people are more likely to learn things, and learn them more quickly, in the same environmental context than others. As a concept, intelligence has been studied extensively by psychologists over the years but it is still difficult to define and measure. What we can say is that it seems to describe the ability to learn and benefit from previous experience, abstract thinking, reasoning and the ability to solve problems, and includes the repertoire of skills that enable the individual to adapt to their environment. In relation to assessment, it is unlikely that we would formally test levels of intelligence, though IQ tests are available, but we would wish to understand someone's ability to solve problems, make decisions, think abstractly and recognise the nature of their problems or difficulties.

Insight

The term 'insight' describes the way the person sees their problem, difficulty or illness. Some may not be able to recognise that the problem actually exists. This is frequently referred to as 'lacking personal insight' and has major implications for the professionals involved. The person does not feel they are in need of treatment as there is nothing wrong with them; therefore, compliance with treatment regimes is not always consistent.

Language

Patients suspected of experiencing the effects of dementia may be unable to find the word to describe everyday objects. They may find it problematic to construct a simple sentence or read a short paragraph in a book. Where there is parietal or frontal lobe (brain) damage, as in the case of dementia, the individual may demonstrate an inability to think in abstract terms. The content of their conversations may appear very 'singular', more commonly referred to as 'concrete thinking'.

Level of consciousness

The final aspect of psychological functioning to consider when engaged in assessing an individual is 'consciousness', a term that describes the ability to be aware. Human beings possess a sense of who they are and the impression they make on others. Level of consciousness describes the extent of our awareness concerning our surroundings. In neurological terms, levels of consciousness may range from fully awake and alert (conscious), through to no response to deep pain or evidence of any spontaneous movement (unconscious: see Chapter 6). Many disorders can cause impaired levels of consciousness: delirium, fugue, clouding of consciousness, damage to the brain and acute physical conditions.

Accurate reporting and documentation

As has been stressed throughout this process of taking the history, it is crucial that the practitioner remains as open and unbiased in their judgements as possible. Barker (2004) stresses the need to be 'scrupulously objective' and not to jump to any conclusions as to why a person might be behaving in a particular way. There may be many explanations as to what is happening to the individual, ranging from physical distress, cultural and spiritual beliefs (see Chapter 10), through to major mental disorders. The student practitioner is not engaged in a comprehensive mental health investigation but in trying to identify if there are any underlying concerns or anxieties that may be triggering a psychological reaction. If any aspect of the assessment causes the assessor to feel vulnerable, inexperienced or unsafe, they should refer to a more experienced practitioner, who may in turn need to refer to a more appropriately qualified professional or even to another service.

It is also vital that all answers to questions asked and all personal observations are recorded as fully and objectively as possible, devoid of personal judgements, values and beliefs. Any evidence of risk, such as suicidal thinking, must be recorded and reported immediately, so that action can be taken to ensure the person's safety. Finally, on completion of the assessment, the practitioner should communicate the essence of their findings to the practitioner in charge and care should be planned which takes account of the individual's psychological needs. All information gathered during the assessment should be documented accurately and in line with NMC (2004) guidelines for record keeping (see also Chapter 5).

Summary

The purpose and philosophy of nursing is to help and care for the person who is in need of support and understanding – the patient. This individual is a complex being, who functions on multiple dimensional levels, biologically, socially and psychologically. A disturbance in any aspect of these dimensions is certain to have a direct impact on the psychological or physical well-being of that individual. As practitioners concerned to care for the whole being, we cannot avoid engaging with each of these dimensions as we seek to support the person through the healthcare process. Therefore, we must strive to understand all of their healthcare needs, their fears, hopes, anxieties and ability to cope. We need to understand how they are feeling, what they are thinking and why they are behaving the way they do. A psychological assessment, together with the physical, social, cultural and spiritual assessments, is the process we use to understand holistically the person behind the label of 'patient'.

Activity

(1) Consider the following terms that have been used throughout this chapter and define their meanings:
- the 'self'
- the self-concept
- self-esteem
- self-image
- personality.

(2) Outline the possible physiological reactions to stress.

(3) What are the different approaches that may be adopted by individuals to cope with stress or anxiety?

(4) What must the practitioner guard against when conducting a psychological assessment?

References

Allport, G W (1963) *Pattern and Growth in Personality*. Holt, Rinehart and Winston, New York.

Allport, G W (1968) *The Person in Psychology: selected essays*. Beacon Press, Boston.

Andersen, S M, Glassman, N S & Gold, D A (1998) Mental representations of the self, significant others, and non-significant others: structure and processing of private and public aspects. *Journal of Personality and Social Psychology* 75: 845–61.

Atkinson, R L, Atkinson, R C, Smith, E E, Bem, D J & Nolen-Hoeksema, S (2003) *Hilgard's Introduction to Psychology*, 14th edition. Thomson Learning, Belmont, California.

Banyard, P (1996) *Applying Psychology to Health*. Hodder and Stoughton, London.

Barker, P J (2004) *Assessment in Psychiatric and Mental Health Nursing*. Nelson Thornes, Cheltenham.

Beck, A T, Ward, C H, Mendelson, M *et al.* (1961) An inventory for measuring depression. *Archives of General Psychiatry* 4: 561–71.

Beck, A T, Steer, R A & Garbin, M G (1988) Psychometric properties of the Beck Depression Inventory: twenty-five years of evaluation. *Clinical Psychology Review* 8: 77–100.

Burnard, P (1990) *Learning Human Skills. An experiential guide for nurses*, 2nd edition. Heinemann Nursing, Oxford.

Burnard, P (2004) *Acquiring Interpersonal Skills. A handbook of learning for health professionals.* Nelson Thornes, Cheltenham.

Cattell, R B (2002) Enriched behavioural prediction equation and its impact on structured learning and the dynamic calculus. *Psychological Review* 109 (1): 202–5. http://gateway.ut.ovid.com/gw2/ovidweb.cgi/

Cohen, S, Frank, E, Doyle, W J, Skoner, D P, Rabin, B S & Gwaltney, J M (1998) Types of stressors that increase susceptibility to the common cold in healthy adults. *Health Psychology* 17: 211–13.

Coon, D (2004) *Introduction to Psychology: gateways to mind and behaviour*, 10th edition. Wadsworth Publishing Co/Thomson Learning, Belmont, California.

Cox, S M (2002) *What are Anxiety Disorders? How can I tell which one I have?* National Anxiety Foundation, Lexington, Kentucky.

Davidhizar, R & Newman-Giger, J (1998) Patient's use of denial: coping with the unacceptable. *Nursing Standard* 12: 44–6.

Davison, G C & Neale, J M (2001) *Abnormal Psychology*, 8th edition. John Wiley, New York.

Eysenck, H J (1967) *The Biological Basis of Personality*. Charles C Thomas, Springfield, Illinois.

Folstein, M F, Folstein, S E & McHugh, P R (1975) Mini-Mental State: a practical method for grading the state of patients for the clinician. *Journal of Psychiatric Research* 12: 189–98.

Freshwater, D (2002) *Therapeutic Nursing: improving care through self-awareness and reflection.* Sage Publications, London.

Freud, A (1993) *The Ego and the Mechanisms of Defence*. Chatto and Windus, London.

Freud, S (1933) *New Introductory Lectures on Psycho-Analysis*. Hogarth, London.

Friedman, H S & Booth-Kewley, S (1987) The 'disease-prone' personality. *American Psychologist* 42: 539–55.

Gammon, J (1998) Analysis of the stressful effects of hospitalisation and source isolation on coping and psychological constructs. *International Journal of Nursing Practice* 4: 84–96.

Green, B (1996) *Problem-based Psychiatry*. Churchill Livingstone, London.

Gross, R (1996) *Psychology: the science of mind and behaviour*, 3rd edition. Hodder and Stoughton, London.

Jungbauer, J & Angermeyer, M C (2003) Coping strategies in spouses of schizophrenic patients. *Psychotherapy and Psychosomatics* 53: 295–301.

Kobasa, S C, Maddi, S R & Puccetti, M C (1982) Personality and exercise as buffers in the stress-illness relationship. *Journal of Behavioural Medicine* 5: 391–404.

Lazarus, R S (1998) *Stress and Emotion*. Springer, New York.

Lyke, E M (1992) *Assessing for Nursing Diagnosis: a human needs approach*. Lippincott, Philadelphia.

Marnocha, S (1999) Chronic stressors increased susceptibility to colds. *Evidence Based Nursing* 2: 54.

Milne, D (1993) *Psychology and Mental Health Nursing*. Macmillan/The British Psychological Society, London/Leicester.

Mizoguchi, K, Yuzurihara, M, Ishige, A, Sasaki, H, Chui, D H & Tabira T (2000) Chronic stress induces impairment of spatial working memory because of prefrontal dopaminergic dysfunction. *Journal of Neuroscience* 20: 1568–74.

Nursing and Midwifery Council (2004) *Guidelines for Records and Record Keeping*. NMC, London.

Paykel, E S (2000) Forward. In: Murray, L & Cooper, P (eds) *Post-partum Depression and Child Development*. Guilford Press, New York.

Peplau, H E (1990) Interpersonal relations model: principles and general applications. In: Reynolds, W & Cormack, D (eds) *Psychiatric and Mental Health Nursing: theory and practice*. Chapman and Hall, London.

Puri, B K, Laking, P J & Treasaden, I H (2002) *Textbook of Psychiatry*. Churchill Livingstone, London.

Rosche, J, Uhlmann, C & Weber, R (2004) Changes of coping strategies in patients with therapy refractory epilepsy in the course of a ward based treatment with a holistic therapeutic approach. *Psychotherapy and Psychosomatics* 54: 4–8.

Rustoen, T & Hanestad, B R (1998) Nursing intervention to increase hope in cancer patients. *Journal of Clinical Nursing* 7: 19–27.

Sivik, T (2000) *Psychosomatic Medicine: why fix it if it ain't broken? Psychotherapy and Psychosomatics* 69: 178–80.

Snaith, R P, Baugh, S J, Clayden, A D *et al.* (1982) The Clinical Anxiety Scale: an instrument derived from the Hamilton Anxiety Scale. *British Journal of Psychiatry* 141: 518–23.

Spurgeon, A (2002) Models of unexplained symptoms associated with occupational and environmental exposures. *Environmental Health Perspectives* 110: 601–5.

Stansfeld, S A, Fuhrer, R, Shipley, M J & Marmot, M G (2002) Psychological distress as a risk factor for coronary heart disease in the Whitehall II Study. *International Journal of Epidemiology* 31: 248–55.

Taylor, S E, Kemeny, M E, Reed, G M, Bower, J E & Gruenewald, T L (2000) Psychological resources, positive illusions, and health. *American Psychologist* 55: 99–109.

Vanitallie, T B (2002) Stress: a risk factor for serious illness. *Metabolism* 51: 40–5.

Whiting, L S (1999) Maintaining patients' personal hygiene. *Professional Nurse* 14: 338–40.

Zigmund, A S & Snaith, R P (1983) The Hospital Anxiety and Depression Scale. *Acta Psychiatrica Scandinavica* 67: 361–70.

Cultural and spiritual health assessment

S. Allen and A. Crouch

Learning objectives

- Define the term 'culture'.
- Discuss how cultural beliefs may influence a person's behaviour during an illness and describe how such behaviours may impact on the assessment process.
- Identify and discuss some of the reasons why the incidence of certain medical and mental health conditions is higher in some cultural groups than in others.
- Describe how the cultural needs of patients may be assessed.
- Define the terms 'spiritual' and 'spirituality'.
- Discuss some of the possible influences of spirituality on health and illness.
- Give an outline of how the spiritual needs of a patient could be assessed.

Cultural health assessment

Before we can explore appropriate mechanisms to assess the cultural needs of patients and clients, we need to think about why culture is important as part of the nursing process. Archer (1998: p1) suggests that culture is very difficult to describe and remains vague despite little dispute that it is a core concept. Shanahan & Bradshaw (1995: p457) would agree that: 'the culturally diverse person's health beliefs and practices are often not well understood and explored'. Archer

(1998: p1) suggests that culture is 'grasped' so what is this grasp that the nurse must have in the array of assessment skills they need to acquire?

Activity

Before we go on to explore this further, take a few minutes to reflect on what is in your mind just now. What picture do you hold in your mind when you think of culture? What are the factors that you initially think are important?

This picture will probably lead to the questions you think you need to ask patients and clients to ensure you have considered cultural needs and will also help to identify any knowledge gaps you may have. Within your sociology curriculum you will have debated such concepts of culture and have some understanding of how the predominant cultural environment of which an individual is part shapes beliefs and values. Leninger (1985: p450) describes the word 'culture' as the: 'learned, shared and transmitted values and beliefs, norms and lifestyle practices of a particular group that guide thinking, decisions and actions in patterned fashions'.

For the nurse, the challenge is to have sufficient understanding of an individual's uniqueness to be able to provide culturally sensitive care. The Nursing and Midwifery Council (2004) requires a registered nurse or midwife to be personally accountable for ensuring the promotion and protection of: 'the interests and dignity of patients and clients, irrespective of gender, age, race, ability . . . lifestyle, culture and religious or political beliefs'.

Within this statement from the NMC, culture and religious beliefs are linked together but this relationship, although sometimes very strong, should not be assumed. *The Code of Ethics for Nurses* (ICN, 2000) and the introduction of the Patient's Charter (DoH, 2001) placed a responsibility on healthcare professionals to show respect for the religious, spiritual and cultural needs of all who use the health service. Prior to that, the importance of improving access to services for all users had been emphasised in a number of government publications (DoH, 1998a,b, 1999). Therefore part of the aim of this chapter is to explore some of the cultural beliefs, values and practices that may influence the assessment process and the provision of care. Later on in the chapter, we will discuss some issues in relation to the assessment of patients' spiritual needs, which includes the assessment of religious needs.

Cultural frame

Culture is often referred to as 'the way we do things around here' and this may have an impact on health behaviours of different groups. For example, in some parts of England Friday night is 'fish and chip' night, associated with social interaction and the signalling of a rest from the week of work. This kind of subculture may have implications for health promotion activity and ensuring patients comply with treatment regimes to maintain a healthy lifestyle. Indeed, Archer (1998: pxvii) suggests that the: '. . . cultural system and sociocultural life do not exist or operate independently of one another; they overlap, intertwine and are mutually influential'.

According to Mazanec & Tyler (2003), values, beliefs and rules of conduct within cultural groups continually evolve; hence achieving cultural competence is a continual process. Everybody lives within a 'cultural' frame and for some it may be easier to fit in with the predominant culture where care is taking place but for others the potential for care to be compromised due to lack of thought or understanding on the part of healthcare individuals can be more problematic. So for nurses to be able to provide culturally and spiritually sensitive care, they need to be aware of how culture and spirituality are part of the fabric of both their own and their colleagues' lives and how their patients and clients view illness, health, the health system and the different cultural and religious practices.

Influence of culture on health, illness and assessment

Cultural background tends to inform many people's understanding of illness. Thus cultural beliefs could influence a person's behaviour following an illness. In Vietnamese culture, for example, it is disrespectful to ask a doctor a question (Shanahan & Bradshaw, 1995). Within that culture, it is also believed that individuals who do not complain of pain or discomfort are strong in character (Shanahan & Bradshaw, 1995; Wills & Wooton, 1999).

Activity

With reference to the above information on some Vietnamese individuals:

- What effect do you think such a belief might have on an individual's behaviour during illness?
- What impact is such behaviour likely to have on the health assessment process?

Activity		
Country/ group	**Examples of cultural belief/s**	**Possible behaviour when ill/impact on assessment and care planning**
• Some West Africans	• May believe that illness has come about as a result of juju; beliefs usually acceptable in such cultural groups	
• Asians	• Most Asians believe that the sick, postnatal women and those who have had surgery should stay in bed. The sick patient is expected to express suffering and anxiety openly. S/he is not expected to be active or cheerful	
• Muslims	• A central tenet of Islam is the concept of *hiya* (modesty). Nudity/nakedness is extremely offensive. Traditionally, except for their faces during the day, women are clothed from head to toe. Men are obliged to cover from the waist to knee (Maternity Alliance, 2004)	
• Filipino-Americans	• Belief in *bahalana*, i.e. one must endure great suffering because it is God's will (Villanueva & Lipat, 2000)	
• Japanese	• Eye contact is confrontational and adversarial (Lester, 1998)	
• Some tribes in Zimbabwe	• Making direct eye contact is considered disrespectful	

The above activities indicate that cultural beliefs could influence how one reacts to an illness. Such reactions could in turn determine the outcome of the illness. In a comparative study of patients in India and the US who experience chronic malignant pain, for example, Kodiath & Kodiath (1995) found that soon after noticing any physical changes in their bodies, the Americans sought medical advice and help. They therefore experienced very little or no pain in connection with the condition. The Indians, on the other hand, experienced high levels of pain and only sought help when it had become intolerable, because pain is viewed as part of a normal life.

Health status in different cultural groups

Certain conditions appear to be more prevalent in certain cultural groups. Dyson & Smaje (2001), for example, reported higher incidence of hypertension within Caribbean, Pakistani and Bangladeshi groups as compared to the white population. The incidence is, however, lower in the Chinese and Indian populations (Dyson & Smaje, 2001). African-Americans also have a higher incidence of stroke and stroke mortality than their white counterparts (Horner *et al.*, 2003).

Incidence of diabetes mellitus and the rate of death due to diabetes are also said to be high for all countries compared to England and Wales (Dyson & Smaje, 2001).

Inherited blood diseases such as sickle cell disorders tend to affect mainly, but not exclusively, people from Africa, the Caribbean, India, Mediterranean origin and Middle East (DoH, 2004; Dyson, 2001; Streetly, 2005). Beta-thalassaemia is another genetically inherited blood disorder which affects mainly, but not exclusively, people of Mediterranean origin, with particular reference to Cypriots, plus those from the Middle East, India, Pakistan and China (DoH, 2004; Dyson, 2001; Streetly, 2005).

The National Statistics (ONS, 2004) also reported that children from Bangladesh, India, Pakistan and China were less likely than other ethnic groups, or the general population, to report any form of acute illness. Afro-Caribbean and Pakistani young females were also more likely to be obese than those in the general population (Saxena *et al.*, 2004).

Whilst this information is significant, it is also of interest that these areas are receiving high-profile interest through the National Service Frameworks, as both the incidence and mortality and morbidity are on the increase in the UK. This is a phenomenon which relates to a number of factors, which can be attributed to both cultural and subcultural lifestyle influences.

The Reed Report (1994) and Iley & Nazroo (2001) suggest that the admission rate to mental health hospitals for Afro-Caribbean people is higher, with the likelihood of being diagnosed as suffering from psychotic illness, particularly cannabis psychosis and schizophrenia, 3–6 times higher than the white population. However, the incidence of depression seems significantly lower than the white population (Iley & Nazroo, 2001).

Socio-economic factors are said to contribute to disproportionately high levels of mental health symptoms nationally and internationally. For example, it has been shown that the likelihood of having a neurotic disorder or depression increases as household income falls (ONS,

2003). Also, in Lima-Costa *et al.*'s study (2003: p7), the poorer elderly in Bambui (a town in south eastern Brazil) were found to have reported more psychiatric symptoms compared to the 'better off'.

Different views about illness challenge professionals to provide treatment and care in a way that is meaningful (McGee, 2000: p33) and an awareness of different concepts of health is fundamental to providing this care. Current Western notions of health (McGee, 2000) encompass a range of states in which the individual responds and adapts to a number of factors such as age, social circumstances and the environment. This range of states can include the presence of disease or disability, meaning that individuals can describe themselves as 'healthy' even though they have an illness (Seedhouse, 1991). Helman (2000) refers to the Indian Ayurvedic system of medicine that is based on the concept of harmony and balance between various parts of the body; illness is a state of disharmony, meaning that health and illness cannot co-exist.

Assessment of cultural needs

Effective communication with all patients, clients and their families is an essential element of nursing practice and is essential in the assessment of cultural needs. Consequently, the fundamental questions of 'what?', 'when?' and 'how?' are of equal importance in the assessment of cultural needs.

Culturally competent care means being sensitive to the context in which questions are asked. For example, physical closeness and eye contact may be interpreted differently. How will you know what is the right stance to take? In many situations in the hospital environment, resources may be available to give you guidance but don't be afraid to ask patients, relatives or indeed an interpreter if custom related to body language is different from the context with which you are familiar. Cultural competence is also about respecting clients' wishes in how they are addressed and the appropriateness of using first names, etc. This will differ between age as well as cultural groups and should be considered as part of the process of gaining consent from the patient and carers.

Nurses also come from diverse cultural backgrounds themselves and this will influence their perception of the world around them. It may be helpful to reflect on a recent situation where you have made assumptions about people based on your own experience.

Within the healthcare system, diversity is strength within nursing and other healthcare professional teams. This means that role modelling is important behaviour and so care needs to be taken with the use of language which may be potentially disrespectful. For example, in the author's part of the country it is quite common for the terms 'me duck' and 'me love' to be heard in all environments where interaction takes place. For nurses from overseas, copying the language but using it out of context can be a big problem. Any misunderstandings can have embarrassing and frustrating consequences. So being culturally sensitive applies just as much to work colleagues as it does to patients and clients.

Millon-Underwood (2000) highlighted some of the questions nurses in Britain need to ask to ensure they come to informed decisions about the appropriate care for patients. The example relates to breast cancer but could be supplemented in respect of any other condition. These questions are just the beginning to enable the nurse to achieve knowledge and skill in providing culturally competent care (Campinha-Bacote, 2002):

- What is the incidence of (breast cancer) among members of black or other ethnic minority groups?
- What do members of these different groups think (cancer) is?
- What beliefs about and attitudes towards (cancer) do members of these groups hold?
- How would you explain (cancer) and the importance of screening and early detection to a member of a black or other ethnic minority group? (Millon-Underwood, 2000)

McGee (2000) suggests that to provide care in a meaningful way means moving away from the 'recipe' approach of providing the right food, finding an interpreter and knowing what to do when someone dies, although these important factors need to be included.

For people to thrive spiritually, even in the context of life-threatening illness, requires skilled interpersonal effectiveness from nurses and carers, adding to the sense of meaning in the communication rather than detracting from it by failing to recognise the cultural needs of patients and their families. Asking questions is easier than listening to the responses; ask yourself if you actively listen to the clients with whom you interact. Watch body language; listen to what they are *not* saying as much as what they are saying; think through some of the emotional consequences which may be running alongside admitting they have an illness.

Assessing the needs of clients in a multicultural society is a partnership between the nurse and the patient. Often the assumption is made that the lived experience within the predominant culture is a positive one. We know very often this is not the case which is as significant for the person who has always been part of British society as for those from outside it.

Evidence suggests higher levels of self-reported ill health amongst immigrants, which might be linked to poorly paid jobs in deprived environments (Dyson & Smaje, 2001). One group that may have significant psychological needs are refugees or asylum seekers. McGee (2002) reports on a Foundation of Nursing Studies seminar which focused on 'meeting the needs of refugees in hospital'. It was noted that many refugees suffer poor health as a result of their experiences both before and after arrival in the UK. At least 134 countries are known to routinely use torture and abuse as a means of punishment, repression and maintaining control. This is most likely to be sexual and psychological. In assessing such patients, four key issues need to be addressed:

- *Communication.* Careful and clear explanations of interventions are essential. Interpreters should be selected with care to avoid the revelation of distressing information linked with repressive regimes.
- *Consent.* Consent must never be assumed, even for minor interventions.
- *Compliance.* Recognise that compliance with healthcare regimes may not always be a priority for those struggling with the complexity of new social situations.
- *Procedures.* Recognise that some interventions, e.g. catheterisation, may be very similar to past experiences of torture. Be sensitive to patients' past experiences and believe what they tell you.

The above seminar was held under the auspices of the Transcultural Nursing and Healthcare Association, set up in the UK in 1998 to promote knowledge and understanding of cultural issues to help healthcare professionals provide the best care to all their patients.

Spirituality and spiritual needs

Spirituality as a subject and the need to address patients' spiritual needs are issues which are sometimes not addressed by nurses. Research findings do, however, suggest that where spiritual needs are identified and care interventions take place, there is a sense of well-being amongst nurses and patients feel 'comfortable and supported' and 'appear peaceful, relaxed, calm and grateful' (Narayanasamy & Owens, 2001: p453).

Literature suggests (Mickley & Cowles, 2001; Sherwood, 2000; Thompson, 2002) that humans have four spiritual necessities in sickness and in health. These are the need:

- for meaning and purpose in life
- to give hope and receive love
- for creativity
- for forgiveness.

Other needs that have been identified by other authors include faith, connectedness and the need for the right relationship with self, others and 'God'/deity (Narayanasamy *et al.*, 2004; Sherwood, 2000; Tanyi, 2002).

Providing meaningful care includes care that meets the spiritual needs of patients. It is not possible for nurses and midwives to meet such health needs unless they are spiritually aware and have some knowledge of how their clients view illness, health, the health system and the different spiritual and religious practices. To provide good spiritual care, healthcare professionals need to be able to carry out a thorough assessment of the patient's spiritual/religious needs. Before they can do so, however, they also need to have some idea of what is meant by the terms 'spiritual' and 'spirituality' and to be self-aware of their own beliefs and values. So prior to reading the rest of this chapter, it would be useful to spend a few minutes reflecting on the terms 'spiritual' and 'spirituality'.

Activity

- Now jot down on a piece of paper what the terms mean to you.
- Do you feel that you have any spiritual needs? If so, what are they?
- If you do not have any spiritual needs, why do you think that is?
- Now compare your answers with that of your colleagues.

You will probably notice that you had some difficulty in arriving at any answers. If you did manage to get any answers, they are probably quite different from those of your colleagues. You may also find that unlike the term 'culture', the terms 'spiritual' and 'spirituality' are elusive concepts (McSherry, 2004; Narayanasamy & Owens, 2001; Tanyi, 2002).

Definitions of spirituality

Search for meaning and purpose

Some authors view the spiritual dimension as a search for meaning (Frankl, 2004; Watkinson, 2002). Narayanasamy (2000) suggests that clients with mental health illness often struggle to find meaning and purpose in their lives. It has also been suggested that the spiritual dimension strives for answers about the infinite and comes into focus during health crises, with particular reference to death (Narayanasamy *et al.*, 2004; Russell, 2002).

Spiritual distress could occur due to a total inability to invest life with meaning (Burnard, 1987). It may be characterised by spiritual pain, guilt, anger, anxiety, loss and despair (Thompson, 2002). Apart from emotional, mental and physical pain, for instance, spiritual wrestling is often triggered when a life-threatening diagnosis such as cancer is given (Sumner, 1998). Cancer patients and their families also tend to give more thought than before to spiritual questions; they could, for example, become preoccupied with issues about death, the purpose of life, life after death and the existence of God (Kuupelomaki, 2000, 2002). Mazanec & Tyler (2003) advocate that patients could be helped to recognise meaning and purpose in their lives if encouraged to tell their life stories.

Relationship with self, others and/or things of world

It is worth noting that not everyone has faith in God. An atheist, for instance, denies the existence of God and an agnostic is unsure of God's existence; hence their spirituality might be focused on 'strong beliefs in significant relationships, self-chosen values and goals instead of a belief in God' (Burnard, 1988; Stoll, 1989; Tanyi, 2002: p503). This means that some people explore spirituality through connection with others; Buddhists, for example, explore their spirituality through connection with Siddhartha Gautama (the Awakened One, the Buddha) through lighting candles, burning incense and meditating in the presence of his statue (BBC, 2004). For the Buddhists, their main goal in life is to reach enlightenment, a state that goes beyond suffering by enabling the mind to be at peace through meditation (BBC, 2004). So the Buddhist who practises such beliefs is perhaps more likely to be hopeful for an escape from suffering than those who do not.

Also, in a study of women with breast cancer, Moch (1998) found that meaning and purpose in their lives were identified through connectedness with the environment, self and others. The sample studied by Moch was small but the findings suggest that for some people, spirituality may not be related to a connection with or belief in deity but in people or things around them and they may consider the search for meaning as a spiritual journey. Hence, their needs will probably be more related to the search for the right relationship with the self and with others (Narayanasamy et al., 2004), as well as for the meaning and purpose in life. Coyle (2002: p4) refers to such dimensions of spirituality as the 'value guidance approach'.

Relationship/connectedness with God/deity

The word 'spirituality' has also been defined as 'one's relationship with God/Deity, Supreme Being' (Mattis, 2000). This implies a sense of connectedness with God and may be expressed through prayers, meditation (Black, 2003; Dossey, 2002), presence, physical touch (Kendrick & Robinson, 2000) or an appreciation of spiritual music. It is important to note that people's perceptions of who or what God is differ. Muslims, for example, believe in one God (Maternity Alliance, 2004), referred to as Allah (Rasool, 2000). Many Christians also believe in one God, referred to as the Lord God (Jesus Christ). Mattis' study (2000) highlighted the need for participants to feel connectedness with God or a higher power, which contributed to their health. This suggests that the sense of connectedness appears to be beneficial to health, which will be discussed later on.

Stoll (1989) also referred to spirituality as her being, the inner person, expressed through her thought, body, judgement and what she does. It is through spirituality that she appreciates God and the things around her. She is also motivated to worship and communicate with God. This means her relationship with God is expressed through her beliefs, nature and interactions with herself and with others. It also means it is the spirituality within her that gives her God-consciousness and increased self-awareness. People who express spirituality in this way are probably more likely to search for the right relationship with God/deity and for forgiveness in time of health crisis or death (Mickley & Cowles, 2001; Narayanasmy *et al.*, 2004).

Vital principle of man or breath of life

Schofield (1986) explained that it is the spirit part of a person which allies them to the spiritual creation and gives them God-consciousness. This implies that the spirit links human beings to and helps them to interact with the spiritual realm. Since the word 'spirit' means 'air in motion', 'wind or breath' or 'breath of a man or woman', Stoter (1995: p3) sees spirituality as 'the vital principle of man or breath of life, which gives life to the physical organism'. This also means that spirituality is an integral component of humans (Narayanasamy, 2000; Wright, 2000) and that the body without the spirit is dead. This in turn implies that 'spirituality' is the presence of the divine (God) in human lives, as Black (2003) suggests. Coyle (2002: p4) refers to definitions of spirituality which appear to highlight God/deity as an essential feature as the 'transcendence approach'.

In a study of patient's religiosity and spirituality Woods & Ironson (1999) found that the patient's beliefs and connectedness to a higher power, self or others promoted a sense of hope. This means that a patient's sense of hope is likely to be promoted especially at point of death, irrespective of who they perceive deity to be and has implications for practice in the assessment of one's spirituality.

Spirituality and religion

Some authors draw distinctions between spirituality and religion (McSherry, 2004; McSherry & Ross, 2002) but others seem to have difficulty in separating the two. Barnes *et al.* (2000), for example, suggest that in connection to children, the two concepts are best understood as highly related, with blurred boundaries in everyday life. Likewise, for many Christians spirituality is directly related to religion (Kuupelomaki, 2002).

The word 'religion' has been defined as 'an organised system of worship' by Kozier *et al.* (2003), examples of which include Buddhism,

Hinduism, Islam, Judaism, Jehovah's Witnesses (Arianism), Mormons, Rastafarianism, Sikhism and the Christian religion, examples of which are Baptist, Church of England, Roman Catholicism, Methodism, Pentecostalism, Presbyterianism and Seventh Day Adventists.

Benefits of spirituality/religiosity

Being spiritual and/or having faith in some form of belief system have been associated with certain benefits and the concepts of connectedness, self-transcendence and inner strength components all appear to add to the meaning of spirituality. Having faith or some form of belief system, for example, appears to generate inner strength and peace. Religiosity has also been linked to better cognitive function, greater social support, fewer depressive symptoms and greater co-operativeness (Koenig et al., 2004) and to health-related physiological processes including cardiovascular, neuroendocrine and immune function (Seeman et al., 2003). Barnes et al. (2000) also reported lower levels of drug misuse in religious children, as well as better decision making and well-being, with less violence and fewer behavioural problems in adolescents. Barnes et al. also suggested that a child's sense of spirituality or involvement in religious activities in a community may provide a structure for positive coping strategies. Low religiosity, on the other hand, has been associated with higher rates of drug misuse, smoking, teenage pregnancy and drinking (Borowski et al., 1997). Such findings suggest that one's spirituality could influence how one behaves in society and one's health-related behaviours and have implications for practice.

Possible influence of spirituality on behaviour during an illness

One's spirituality may also influence how one responds to an illness. Asser & Swan's study (1998), for example, revealed that some parents in America decided not to resort to medical treatment since doing so may have been seen as a lack of faith. The parents believed that prayer could substitute for conventional treatment of children with medical conditions. Some parents may also not have their children immunised and this could lead to increased morbidity and mortality in their children (Rodgers et al., 1998).

Research findings also suggest that spiritual beliefs could influence how people perceive the cause of an illness. Some Chinese patients, for example, believe that suffering before death is a way of reparation for any sins committed so if they do not suffer whilst alive, they will do so later (Mazanec & Tyler, 2003). There may also be some cultural aspects to such beliefs. This does, however, mean that the patient might not express pain to the health professional during health assessment. Such patients may also refuse pain-relieving agents. This suggests that behaviour during an illness could affect the assessment process as well as impact on the care planning for and with the patient.

The points listed in the activity below are not comprehensive but are examples to provoke some thought. It is important to be aware that members of particular cultural groups will react differently to difficult situations or to an illness. Lack of acceptance and understanding of such individuals could lead to stereotyping. Stockwell (1984), for example, described how a patient was labelled as 'unpopular' and antagonistic because she detached herself from other people and used very limited forms of communication after experiencing a major loss. Such labelling and the consequent stereotyping should be avoided.

Activity		
Religious or cultural group	**Examples of spiritual/religious beliefs**	**How are they likely to behave during an illness or on admission to hospital?**
• Apostolic (oneness Pentecostals)	• Belief in repentance and baptism by complete immersion in water in Jesus' name for the remission of sin, the receiving of the Holy Spirit and living in accordance with scripture teaching (*Acts* 2:38; 10:43–8)	
• Buddhist	• Need to practise *lamrim* (a set of 21 meditations) daily (BBC, 2004)	
• Church of England	• Sacraments (these include baptism and Holy Communion) are important (Green, 1992a)	
• Hindus	• Women wear nuptial thread around neck. Men wear sacred thread around arm, which indicates adult religious status attainment. Religious customs must be adhered to ensure good quality of one's next life	
• Jehovah's Witnesses	• Blood represents life itself; based on Bible teaching that refers to blood as the soul of the flesh (*Gen* 9: 3–4, *Acts* 15: 20, 28–9, 21: 25)	
• Jewish (orthodox)	• Need to observe the Sabbath as per Bible teaching to keep it holy and treat it as a day of rest (Exodus 16: 22–9, 20: 8–11)	

Continued

Religious or cultural group	Examples of spiritual/religious beliefs	How are they likely to behave during an illness or on admission to hospital?
• Lakota people	• Believe in spiritual healers; herbs, songs and prayers can cure illness or disease (Pickrell, 2001)	
• Muslims	• Need to pray 5 times daily facing Mecca. Fasting during daylight hours is important during Ramadan. Forbids ingestion of pork and meat that is not halal (Rasool, 2000)	
• Rastafarians	• Fear of contamination of the body (Green, 1992b)	
• Roman Catholics	• A sacrament for the sick is a symbol of Christ's healing. Belief in the last rite, i.e. need to confess sins (Green, 1992a: p28)	
• Sikh	• Have 5 traditional symbolic marks for men: long hair, comb to keep hair in place, a steel bangle on the right wrist, a sword, and a pair of shorts to symbolise spiritual freedom. Sikhs also use in holy water from the Gurdwara	

Activity

Work individually or in groups.

- Can you think of other individuals, cultural or religious groups of people who have spiritual beliefs and practices that are different from the examples given in the activity above?
- How could their needs be met?

Spiritual assessment: questions to consider

A thorough spiritual assessment will help you identify the spiritual needs of a patient as well as helping you to plan and implement good spiritual care. The use of appropriate and relevant questions could facilitate spiritual assessment and allow the patients to explore their feelings, fears and beliefs. Such exploration requires time, skills and sensitivity (McSherry & Ross, 2002) and has implications for nursing practice. In their research, Narayanasamy *et al.* (2004) found that listening plays a very important part in the identification and assessment of the spiritual needs of patients. Mickley & Cowles (2002) and Narayanasamy *et al.* (2004), also found that following a diagnosis of cancer, some patients use forgiveness to clarify personal values and help eliminate negative feelings from inflicted hurt. When assessing spiritual needs, the patient should therefore not only be observed but also be listened to very carefully.

The following are questions/points to consider when assessing spirituality:

- What is your source of hope and strength?
- What gives your life meaning? (Dossey, 1998: p46)
- Do you have a sense of purpose in life? (Dossey, 1998: p46)
- What is your concept of God/deity?
- Do you participate in any religious activities? (Dossey, 1998: p46)
- Who are the significant people in your life?
- How does spirituality impact on your state of health?
- To whom do you turn when you are ill or distressed?
- What has bothered you most about being ill (or what is happening to you)? (McSherry, 2000: p78)

Observation
Observe the patient closely for clues including possession and/or use of:

- Holy Bible, Torah, Koran or other religious/spiritual books
- necklace with a cross on the chain
- prayer beads/rosary/mat
- star of David
- musical equipment for meditation
- bracelets/rings
- special tattoos.

Also, note what TV programmes your patient prefers to watch and whether they observe the Sabbath, e.g. Jewish religion.

Listening
- Listen carefully to expressed concerns about the patient's relationship with God, deity or higher power.
- Listen carefully for expressions such as 'speaking in tongues', especially when the patient is distressed or in pain or when praying (Pentecostal faith).
- Listen carefully to patients expressing the need to forgive or be forgiven.

- Listen carefully to the patient expressing the need to see certain people or relatives.

Summary

From the above discussion, we note that everyone lives within a 'cultural' frame; this may be the predominant culture within the region or country where care is taking place. Spirituality is also a concept that is difficult to define and is unique to each individual irrespective of belief or religious orientation. Care could be compromised due to lack of thought or understanding on the part of healthcare individuals. Nurses need to be aware of how culture and spirituality are part of the fabric of individuals and how their clients view illness, health, the health system and the different cultural and religious practices, to help provide culturally and spiritually sensitive care.

Please complete the following activity after reading this chapter.

Activity

Spend a few minutes alone. Think about an incident or an event that involved cultural/spiritual issues and then try and address the following questions.

- What happened, how did you act and why?
- How did you feel about it at the time? How do you feel about it now?
- Could your reaction/actions have been different and if so, how?
- What have you learnt about yourself from this situation?

References

Archer, M S W (1998) *Culture and Agency. The place of culture in social theory.* Cambridge University Press, Cambridge.

Asser, S M & Swan, R (1998) Child fatalities from religion-motivated medical neglect. *Pediatrics* 101 (4): 625–9.

Barnes, L, Plotnikoff, G, Fox, K & Pendleton, S (2000) Spirituality, religion, and pediatrics: intersecting worlds of healing. *Pediatrics* 106 (4) (suppl): 1–19.

BBC (2004) www.bbc.co.uk/religion/buddhism/worship/index.shtml/.

Black, D Y (2003) *Racial identity, spirituality and health attitudes among African Americans.* MA thesis. Central Connecticut State University. New Britain, Connecticut. http://fred.ccsu.edu:8000/archive/00000110/02/etd-2004-1.pdf.

Borowski, I W, Hogan, M & Ireland, M (1997) Adolescent sexual aggression: risk and protective factors. *Pediatrics* 100 (6): 7–17. http://pediatrics. application.org/cgi/content/full/100/6/e7.

Burnard, P (1987) Spiritual distress and the nursing response. Theoretical considerations and counselling skills. *Journal of Advanced Nursing* 12 (3): 377–82.

Burnard, P (1988) The spiritual needs of atheist and agnostics. *Professional Nurse* 4: 130–2.

Campinha-Bacote, J (2002) Cultural competence in psychiatric nursing: have you asked the right questions? *Journal of the American Psychiatric Nursing Association* 8 (6): 183–7. www.ingentaconnect.com/search/expand.

Coyle, J (2002) Spirituality and health: towards a framework for exploring the relationship between spirituality and health. *Journal of Advanced Nursing* 37 (6): 589–97.

Department of Health (1998a) *Our Healthier Nation.* Stationery Office, London.

Department of Health (1998b) *The New NHS: modern, dependable.* Stationery Office, London.

Department of Health (1999) *Clinical Governance. Quality in the new NHS.* DoH, London.

Department of Health (2001) *Your Guide to the NHS.* DoH, London.

Department of Health Sciences (2004) *A Survey of Haemoglobinopathy Screening Policy and Practice in England, October 2001.* DoH, London. www.kcl-phr.org.uk/haemscreening/.

Dossey, B M (1998) Holistic modalities and healing moments. *American Journal of Nursing* 98 (6): 44–7.

Dossey, L (2002) How healing happens. Exploring the NonlocalGap. *Alternative Therapies in Health and Medicine* 8 (2): 12–16, 103–10.

Dyson, S (2001) Midwives and screening for haemoglobin disorders. In: Culley, L & Dyson, S (eds) *Ethnicity and nursing Practice. Sociology in nursing practices. Part II.* Palgrave, Basingstoke.

Dyson, S & Smaje, C (2001) The health status of minority ethnic groups. In: Culley, L & Dyson, S (eds) *Ethnicity and Nursing Practice. Sociology in Nursing practices. Part I.* Palgrave, Basingstoke.

Frankl, V E (2004) *Man's Search for Meaning.* Rider, London.

Green, J (1992a) Christianity. *Nursing Times* 88 (3): 26–9.

Green, J (1992b) Death with dignity. Rastafarianism. *Nursing Times* 88 (9): 56–7.

Helman, C (2000) *Culture, Health and Illness: an introduction for health professionals.* Hodder Arnold, London.

Horner, R, Swanson, J, Bosworth, H & Matchar, D (2003) Effects of race and poverty on the process and outcome of inpatient rehabilitation services among stroke patients. *Stroke* 34: 1027–31.

Iley, K & Nazroo, J (2001) Ethnic inequalities in mental health. In: Culley, L & Dyson, S (eds) *Ethnicity and Nursing Practice. Sociology in nursing practices. Part I.* Palgrave, Basingstoke.

International Council of Nurses (2000) *Code of Ethics for Nurses.* ICN, Geneva.

Kendrick, K & Robinson, S (2000) Spirituality: its relevance and purpose for clinical nursing in a new millennium. *Journal of Clinical Nursing* 9 (5): 701–5.

Kodiath, M F & Kodiath, A (1995) A comparative study of patients who experience chronic malignant pain in India and the United States. *Cancer Nursing* 18: 189–96. http://gateway.uk.ovid.com/athens.

Koenig, H G, George, L K & Titus, P (2004) Religion, spirituality, and health in medically ill hospitalised older patients. *Journal of the American Geriatrics Society* 52 (4): 554–62. http://gateway.ut.ovid.com/gw2/ovidweb.cgi.

Kozier, B, Erb, G & Berman, A J (eds) (2003) *Fundamentals of Nursing. Concepts, process and practice*, 6th edition. Prentice Hall, New York.

Kuupelomaki, M (2000) Cancer patients', family members' and professional helpers' conceptions and beliefs concerning death. *European Journal of Oncology Nursing* 4 (1): 39–47.

Kuupelomaki, M (2002) Spiritual support for families of patients with cancer: a pilot study of nursing staff assessment. *Cancer Nursing* 25 (3): 209–18.

Leninger, M (1985) Transcultural care diversity and universality: a theory of nursing. *Health Care* 6 (4): 208–12.

Lester, N (1998) Cultural competence. A nursing dialogue. *American Journal of Nursing* 98 (8): 26–34.

Lima-Costa, M F, Barreto, S M, Firmo, J O A & Uchoa, E (2003) Socioeconomic position and health in a population of Brazilian elderly: the Bambui Health and Aging Study (BHAS). *Revista Panamericana de Salud Publica* 13 (6): 7. www.scielosp.org/scielo.php.

Maternity Alliance (2004) *Experiences of Maternity Services. Muslim women's perspectives.* www.maternityalliance.org.uk/documents/muslim womenreport/.

Mattis, J S (2000) African American women's definitions of spirituality and religiosity. *Journal of Black Psychology* 26 (1): 101–22.

Mazanec, P & Tyler, M K (2003) Cultural considerations in end-of-life care: how ethnicity, age and spirituality affect decisions when death is eminent. *American Journal of Nursing* 103 (3): 50–8. http://gateway1.uk.ovid.com/ovidweb.cgi.

McGee, P (2000) Health, illness and culture. *Nursing Standard* 14 (45): 33.

McGee P (2002) *Meeting the needs of refugees in hospital.* Winter newsletter. Transcultural Nursing and Healthcare Association, London.

McSherry, W (2000) *Making Sense of Spirituality in Nursing Practice. An interactive approach.* Churchill Livingstone, Edinburgh.

McSherry, W (2004) Meaning of spirituality. *Journal of Clinical Nursing* 13 (8): 934.

MCSherry, W & Ross, L (2002) Dilemmas of spiritual assessment: considerations for nursing practice. *Journal of Advanced Nursing* 38 (5): 479–88. http://gateway.uk.ovid.com/gw2/ovidweb.cgi.

Mickley, J R & Cowles, K (2001) Ameliorating the tension; use of forgiveness for healing. *Oncology Nursing Forum* 28 (1): 31–7. http://gateway.uk.ovid.com/gw2/ovidweb.cgi.

Millon-Underwood, S (2000) Reducing the cancer burden among African Americans. *Cancer* 83 (S8): 1877–84. www.interscience.wiley.com/cgi-bin/abstract.

Moch, S D (1998) Health-within-illness. Concept development through research and practice. *Journal of Advanced Nursing* 28: 305–10.

Narayanasamy, A (2000) Spiritual care and mental health competence. In: Lyttle, J, Thompson, T & Mathias, P (eds) *Lyttle's Mental Health and Disorder*, 3rd edition. Bailliere Tindall, London.

Narayanasamy, A & Owens, J (2001) A critical incident study of nurses' responses to the spiritual needs of their patients. *Journal of Advanced Nursing* 33 (4): 446–55.

Narayanasamy, A, Clissett, P, Parumal, L, Thompson, D, Annasamy, S & Edge, R (2004) Responses to the spiritual needs of older people. *Journal of Advanced Nursing* 48 (1): 6–16.

Nursing and Midwifery Council (2004) *Code of Professional Conduct: standards for conduct, performance and ethics*. NMC, London.

Office of National Statistics (2003) *Prevalence of Neurotic Disorders among Older People: by sex and gross household income. Social trends*. National Statistics online. www.statistics.gov.uk/STATBASE/Product.asp.

Office of National Statistics (2004) National Statistics online. www.statistics.gov.uk/cci/nugget.asp.

Pickrell, K D (2001) A crosscultural nursing experience on the Rosebud reservation. *Nurse Education* 26 (3): 128–31.

Rasool, G H (2000) The crescent and Islam healing, nursing and the spiritual dimension. Some considerations towards an understanding of the Islamic perspective on caring. *Journal of Advanced Nursing* 32 (6): 1476–84.

Reed, J (Chairman) (1994) *Report of the Working Group on High Security and Related Psychiatric Provision*. Department of Health, London.

Rodgers, D V, Glinder, J S, Atkinson, W L & Markowitz, L E (1998) High attack rates and case fatality during a measles outbreak in groups with religious exemption to vaccination. *Pediatric Infectious Disease Journal* 12: 288–92.

Russell, P (2002) Dying, death and spirituality. In: Hogston, R & Simpson, M (eds) *Foundations of Nursing Practice. Making the difference*, 2nd edition. Palgrave, Basingstoke.

Saxena, S, Ambler, G, Cole, T J & Majeed, A (2004) Ethnic group differences in overweight and obese children and young people in England: cross-sectional survey. *Archives of Disease in Childhood* 89: 30–6.

Schofield, C I (1986) *Holy Bible. The first Schofield Study Bible. King James version.* Barbour and Company in co-operation with Oxford University Press, Oxford.

Seedhouse, D (1991) *Liberating Medicine*. John Wiley, Chichester.

Seeman, T E, Dublin, L F & Seeman, M (2003) Religiosity/spirituality and health: a critical review of the evidence for biological pathways. *American Psychologist* 58 (1): 53–63. http://gateway.uk.ovid.com/gw2/ovid/ovidweb.cgi.

Shanahan, M & Bradshaw, D L (1995) Are nurses aware of the differing health care needs of Vietnamese patients? *Journal of Advanced Nursing* 22: 456–64.

Sherwood, G (2000) The power of nurse–client encounters. *Journal of Holistic Nursing* 18 (2): 159–75.

Stockwell, F (1984) *The Unpopular Patient*. Croom Helm, London.

Stoll, R (1989) The essence of spirituality. In: Carson, V (ed.) *Spiritual Dimensions of Nursing Practice.* WB Saunders, Philadelphia.

Stoter, D (1995) *Spiritual Aspects of Healthcare.* Mosby, St Louis.

Streetly, A (2005) Screening for major haemoglobinopathies. *Midwives* 8 (2): 62–3.

Sumner, C H (1998) The right to receive care that respects individual spiritual values was recently added to the Joint Commission standards. Here are some points to consider as you strive for maximum effectiveness in this aspect of patient care. Recognising and responding. *American Journal of Nursing* 98 (1): 26–30.

Tanyi, R A (2002) Towards clarification of the meaning of spirituality. *Journal of Advanced Nursing* 39: 500–9.

Thompson, I (2002) Mental health and spiritual care. *Nursing Standard* 17 (9): 33–8.

Villanueva, V & Lipat, A (2000) The Filipino American culture: the need for transcultural knowledge. In: Kelley, M & Fitzsimons, V (eds) *Understanding Cultural Diversity.* Jones Bartlett, Sudbury, MA.

Watkinson, G (2002) Promoting health. In: Hodgston, R & Simpson, M (eds) *Foundations of Nursing Practice. Making the difference,* 2nd edition. Palgrave, Basingstoke.

Wills, B S H & Wooton, Y S Y (1999) Concerns and misconceptions about pain among Hong Kong Chinese patients with cancer. *Cancer Nursing* 22 (6): 408–13. http://gateway1.uk.ovid.com/ovidweb.cgi/.

Woods, T E & Ironson, G H (1999) Religion and spirituality in the face of illness. *Journal of Health Psychology* 4: 393–412.

Wright, S (2000) Life, the universe and you. *Nursing Standard* 14 (52): 23.

Glossary

Abdomen: The area of the body between the diaphragm and the pelvis. Anatomists have divided the abdomen into nine regions to identify the location of organs.

Abdominal cavity: Superior aspect of the abdomino-pelvic cavity containing the stomach, pancreas, spleen, liver, gall bladder, the small intestine and part of the large intestine.

Abdomino-pelvic cavity: Inferior portion of the abdomino-pelvic cavity.

Abduction: Movement away from the midline.

Acute: Rapid onset and severe symptoms.

Adduction: Movement towards the midline.

Adrenal glands (suprarenal): Two endocrine glands located superior to each kidney.

Aetiology: The study of causes of disease.

Agnosia: Inability to recognise the form and nature of objects or persons.

Agraphia: Inability to write.

Alert: Able to respond to commands, orientated to time, place and person, and comprehends verbal and written language.

Alopecia: Partial or complete lack of hair resulting from ageing, cytotoxic medication, skin disease or endocrine disorder.

Alveoli (lungs): Air sacs in the lungs where gaseous exchange takes place.

Alzheimer's disease: A type of dementia characterised by dysfunction and loss of specific cerebral neurons, causing intellectual impairment, disorientation and personality changes.

Amnesia: A loss or lack of memory.

Anatomical position: A position used for anatomical descriptions. In this position, the body is erect, the eyes face forward, the upper limbs are at the sides, the palms face forward and the feet are flat on the floor.

Anatomy: The study of the structure of the body.

Aneroid BP manometer: Blood pressure machine with a calibrated dial and an indicator that points to numbers representing the blood pressure.

Angina: Cardiac pain due to myocardial ischaemia, frequently occurs on exertion. The pain is typically felt in the centre of the chest and may radiate to the left arm and lower jaw.

Anorexia: Loss of appetite accompanied by a lack of interest in food.

Anoxia (hypoxia): Lack of oxygen in the body.

Antenatal: Before birth.

Anterior: Nearer to the front of the body.

Anterior chamber: Space superior to the pupil and iris.

Anthropometry: Study of the physical measurement of the human body.

Apex of the heart: The lower portion of the heart.

Aphasia: Impairment or absence of speech.

Arrhythmia (dysrhythmia): A disturbance in the rate, rhythm or conduction of the heart.

Articulation: Joint or connection between two or more bones.

Ascites: Abnormal accumulation of fluid in the peritoneal cavity.

Assessment: The collection and analysis of subjective and objective data on the patient's health status. The first stage of the nursing process.

Ataxia: Unco-ordinated voluntary muscle movements.

Atherosclerosis: Narrowing and hardening of the arteries caused by fatty plaques in the arterial walls.

Auscultation: Listening to sounds within the body.

Axilla (armpit): Small hollow beneath the arm where it joins the body at the shoulders.

Babinski sign: Extension of the big toe (with or without fanning of the other toes) in response to stimulation of the outer aspect of the sole. Indicative of damage to descending motor pathways (after the age of 18 months).

Balanced diet (healthy diet): Food or drink considered with regard to its nutritional qualities, composition and effects on health.

Bartholin's glands: Glands located between the labia minora of the vagina and the hymen. Produces a clear, viscid and odourless fluid, important for viability and motility of sperm along the female reproductive tract.

Base of the heart: Upper part of the heart.

Blood pressure: A measure of the force exerted by the flow of blood against the arteries. It is a function of cardiac output and peripheral resistance.

Body mass index (BMI): Indicator of the body composition; weight in kilograms divided by the square of height in metres.

Borborgymi: Audible abdominal sounds (rumbling, gurgling) produced by hyperactive intestinal peristalsis.

Bradycardia: Pulse rate less than 60 beats per minute.

Cachexia: Wasting caused by extreme malnutrition.

Carpal tunnel syndrome: Pressure on the median nerve as it passes through the carpal tunnel in the wrist due to oedema. This leads to tingling and numbness in the hand.

Cataract: Opacity of the lens of the eye.

Cell: The basic structural and functional unit of all organisms.

Cephalic: Pertaining to the head.

Cervix: The narrow, lower part of the uterus that opens into the vagina.

Chronic obstructive pulmonary disease: A chronic progressive condition of the lungs characterised by diminished inspiratory and expiratory capacity. It includes chronic bronchitis, emphysema and asthma.

Cognition: The word originated from the Latin *cognition* which means to know, think, pay attention. Cognition is the act of knowing, thinking, remembering and also involves information processing.

Cognitive ability: Ability to know, think, remember, process information.

Coma: Unconscious state. Unable to be roused and does not respond to body and environmental stimuli.

Cryptorchidism: Failure of one or both testes to descend into the scrotum.

Cushing's disease: A metabolic disorder characterised by increased secretion of adrenocortical steroids caused by increased amounts of adrenocorticotrophic hormone (ACTH). It is characterised by 'moon face', 'buffalo hump' and pendulous abdomen. Cushing's syndrome includes all causes of excessive cortisol secretion.

Cyanosis: Slightly bluish or dark purple discolouration of the skin due to deficient oxygen in the circulating blood.

Cystitis: Inflammation of the urinary bladder.

Dementia: Any mental condition that is characterised by loss of memory, intelligence and orientation.

Diabetes mellitus: A condition in which there is either absolute (type I) or relative (type II) lack of insulin in the body. This leads to a rise of glucose levels in the blood, some of which is excreted in the urine.

Diastole: Relaxation of the heart.

Disease: A change from a state of health.

Dyspnoea: Shortness of breath.

Electrolytes: Any compound which when dissolved in water separates into ions and has the ability to conduct electricity.

Empathy: The skill of entering and feeling another person's world; being able to communicate such understanding to the person through reflection of facts and feelings (Egan, 2002).

Enzymes: Various complex substances that originate from living cells. Enzymes drive and regulate metabolic reactions in the body.

Erythema: Skin redness.

Ethics: Ethics is concerned with the study of moral knowledge and behaviour and what is considered to be right, just and good.

Evaluation: The assessment of the client's progress in achieving stated outcomes.

Exophthalmos: Abnormal protrusion of the eyeball seen in thyrotoxicosis.

Fibroids: Benign tumour of the uterus.

Foetus: The unborn human offspring. Human embryo from the sixth week of pregnancy.

Food: An edible substance; a complex mixture of different nutrients that can be used by the body to sustain growth.

Fremitus: Palpable vibration, resulting from air passing through the bronchopulmonary system.

Gene: A sequence of DNA that codes for a specific protein.

Glasgow Coma Scale: A 15-point scale for assessing conscious level by evaluating three behavioural responses: best verbal response, motor response and eye opening.

Glaucoma: Condition characterised by raised intraocular pressure that can damage the optic nerve as it leaves the eye and disrupt the visual field.

Glycosuria: Abnormal presence of sugar, especially glucose, in the urine.

Goitre: Enlarged thyroid gland.

Haematemesis: Vomiting of blood.

Health assessment: The systematic gathering of information about a person's health history and status.

Health beliefs: A set of attitudes towards health, which may influence behaviour.

Hemiparesis: Unilateral weakness.

Hemiplegia: Unilateral paralysis.

Hirsutism: Excessive body hair.

Holism: The belief that the 'whole' is more than the sum of its parts.

Holistic assessment: Assessment of the person as a whole, taking into account the physical, psychological, social, cultural and spiritual aspects of the person.

Homeostasis: The body's ability to maintain internal stability.

Hyperglycaemia: High blood glucose levels.

Hyper-resonance: Increased resonance caused by percussion.

Hypertension: Blood pressure which is constantly above 140 mmHg systolic and 90 mmHg diastolic.

Hypoglycaemia: Low blood glucose levels.

Hypotension: Low blood pressure, which is insufficient to maintain adequate perfusion.

Hypothermia: A fall in the body temperature to below 35°C.

Infarction: The development and formation of an infarct (localised area of necrosis in a tissue resulting from tissue anoxia caused by interruption in blood supply).

Inferior: Towards the lower part of a structure or away from the head.

Inspection: Systematic observation of the client during physical examination using the senses of vision, hearing and smell.

Institutional rules and behaviours: The relationship between organisations and institutions within any community; that is, the formal and informal rules of the important relationships played out in societies that influence the health of a community.

Integumentary system: Skin and its appendages (hair, nails, sweat glands, sebaceous glands).

Intercostal space: Space between ribs.

Intervention: Nursing action designed to achieve client's outcomes.

Jaundice: Yellowish discolouration of the skin, sclera and mucous membranes caused by an increase in bile pigments in the blood.

Kyphosis: Excessive convexity of the thoracic spine.

Learning disability: Impaired cognitive function. People with learning disability require support from parents, carers and professionals in order to be able to achieve their potential, access their community, use services and lead a fulfilling life.

Lethargy: Sluggish responses. Slowed mental and motor processes.

Light palpation: Superficial palpation, depressing the skin 1 cm.

Lordosis: An exaggeration of the lumbar curve.

Macronutrients: Bulk of the food we eat, including protein, carbohydrate and fat.

Makaton: A communication system that involves manual signing for use with people who have severe learning disability.

Mediastinum: Area between the lungs where the heart is located.

Megaloblastic anaemia: A reduction of red blood cells due to lack of folate or vitamin B12 for DNA synthesis.

Melaena: Black, tarry stool caused by bleeding in the upper digestive tract.

Memory: The ability to recall thoughts.

Meninges: Membranes covering the brain: from internal to external – pia, arachnoid and dura mater.

Micronutrients: A range of minerals and vitamins.

Midline: An imaginary vertical line that divides the body into equal left and right sides.

Midsternal line: Vertical line drawn from the midpoint of the sternum.

Morbidity: Relating to disease or abnormal condition.

Mortality: Death.

Murmur: Abnormal sound heard on auscultation of the heart, due to valvular disorders.

Myopia: A visual defect in which the person can see objects clearly at close range but not at a distance.

Myxoedema: An endocrine disorder due to excessive production of thyroxine, characterised by low metabolic rate.

Neural tube defect: Defect in the formation of the neural tube as occurs in spina bifida, where the arches of the back of the spine are incomplete. On occasion, there is only a bony gap (spina bifida occulta). Other conditions classified as neural tube defects include anencephaly, a gross malformation in which the cranial vault and the brain fail to develop. Such defects are linked to folic acid deficiency.

Nursing process: Systematic approach in nursing consisting of five stages: assessment, nursing diagnosis, planning, implementation and evaluation.

Nutrients: The components of food, namely carbohydrates, proteins, fats, vitamins, water and minerals.

Nutrition: The process of obtaining food for energy, growth and repair.

Nystagmus: Involuntary oscillation of the eye.

Objective data: Data obtained through observation and measurements; sign.

Oedema: Accumulation of fluid in the interstitial spaces.

Os: Means *opening*; so internal and external cervical os mean internal and external opening of the cervix.

Osteomalacia (adult rickets): A condition in which there is very painful softening of the bones due to vitamin D deficiency.

Palpation: One of the techniques of physical examination in which the clinician uses the sense of touch to feel pulsations and vibrations and to locate body structures.

Paraphrase: A restatement of what someone has said in your own words, without changing the meaning.

Participation in social assessment: The extent to which individuals or social groups can and do engage in the development of potential health plans constructed in collaboration with healthcare professionals.

Pathogen: A disease-producing micro-organism.

Percussion: A physical examination technique in which the clinician taps on the skin surface to assess size, border and consistency of internal organs as well as evaluating fluid in a body cavity.

Peristalsis: Successive muscular contractions along the wall of a hollow muscular structure (e.g. digestive tract), enabling its contents to move forwards.

Phenylketonuria: In this condition, there is a lack of the enzyme phenylalanine hydroxylase, which is necessary for the conversion of phenylalanine into tyrosine (an amino acid). The level of phenylalanine in the blood therefore rises, some of which is excreted in the urine as phenylpyruvic acid. The build-up of phenylalanine in the body leads to brain damage, blue eyes, fair hair and dry skin if undetected and treated early. All newborn babies in the UK are screened for this condition. Early treatment with a low-phenylalanine diet can result in good recovery.

Phimosis: Tightness of the prepuce of the penis that prevents retraction of the foreskin over the glans.

Posterior: Nearer to or at the back.

Precordium: Area of the chest over the heart.

Prolapse: A dropping or falling down of an organ (e.g. prolapse of the uterus or rectum).

Proximal: Near to the point of origin or attachment.

Pulse: The alternate expansion and recoil of an artery with each systole.

Retroflexed: Bent backwards.

Retroverted: Turned backwards.

Rickets: A condition in which the calcification of bone is deficient due to lack of vitamin D.

Sickle cell anaemia: A severe, chronic haemoglobinopathic, anaemic condition that occurs in people homozygous for haemoglobin S (Hb S).

Snellen chart: Chart used for testing distance vision.

Social diversity: The range of groupings that may be identified on the basis of gender, social class, ethnicity, religion, age, culture and social role as well as 'spatial' (geographical) and economic characteristics within a society.

Social risk: The extent to which individuals and groups within society are classed as vulnerable.

Sociogram: A diagrammatic representation of the social relationships in a group.

Stakeholders: Stakeholders are essentially the individual or groups of individuals within society who are subject to the process of health assessment.

Stenosis: An abnormal narrowing of a duct or opening.

Subjective data: Information provided by the client and/or relatives; symptom.

Synapse: The junction between two neurons or between a neuron and an effector organ.

Synovial joint: Freely movable joint that is lined by synovial membrane and has synovial fluid for lubrication.

Systole: The phase of contraction of the heart.

Tachycardia: Pulse rate greater than 100 beats per minute in an adult.

Thoracic cavity: Superior portion of the ventral cavity. Located above the diaphragm and contains the lungs, the heart and major blood vessels.

Thyrotoxicosis: An endocrine disorder due to excessive production of thyroxine, characterised by high metabolic rate.

Tinnitus: Ringing sounds in the ear.

Turgor: Elasticity of the skin.

Vasoconstriction: A decrease in the size of the lumen of the blood vessel, particularly the arterioles and the veins in the blood reservoirs of the skin, which contributes to the control of blood pressure and distribution of blood throughout the body. Vasoconstriction depends on stimulation of sympathetic nerves to the smooth muscle of blood vessels.

Vasodilation: An increase in the size of the blood vessel caused by inhibition of its constrictor nerves or stimulation of dilator nerves.

Vegan: One who does not eat any form of animal product at all. The diet is mainly composed of vegetables, oils and cereals.

Warts: Abnormal but benign growth of epithelial skin cells caused by a virus.

Xiphoid process: The inferior portion of the sternum.

References

Egan, G (2002) *The Skilled Helper: a systematic approach to effective helping.* Brooks Cole, California.

Index